THE AGING BRAIN
AND SENILE DEMENTIA

ADVANCES IN BEHAVIORAL BIOLOGY

Recent Volumes in this Series

A Continuation Order Plan is available for this series. A continuation order will bring delivery of each new volume immediately upon publication. Volumes are billed only upon actual shipment. For further information please contact the publisher.

THE AGING BRAIN AND SENILE DEMENTIA

Edited by
Kalidas Nandy

Geriatric Research, Educational, and Clinical Center
Veterans Administration Hospital
Bedford, Massachusetts
and Boston University School of Medicine
Boston, Massachusetts

and
Ira Sherwin

Research and Development
Veterans Administration Hospital
Bedford, Massachusetts
and Harvard Medical School
Boston, Massachusetts

PLENUM PRESS · NEW YORK AND LONDON

Library of Congress Cataloging in Publication Data

Symposium on the Aging Brain and Senile Dementia, Boston, 1976.
    The aging brain and senile dementia.

    (Advances in behavioral biology; v. 23)

    Includes index.
    1. Senile psychosis—Congresses. 2. Aging—Congresses. 3. Brain—Congresses. I.
Nandy, Kalidas. II. Sherwin, Ira. III. United States. Veterans Administration. IV.
Title.
RC524.S94 1976   616.8'983   77-8190
ISBN 0-306-37923-6

Proceedings of the Symposium on The Aging Brain and
Senile Dementia sponsored by the Veterans Administration
held in Boston, Massachusetts, June 2-4, 1976

© 1977 Plenum Press, New York
A Division of Plenum Publishing Corporation
227 West 17th Street, New York, N.Y. 10011

Printed in the United States of America

Preface

There are currently about 21 million people over 65 years in the United States and over a million of them suffer from a severe degree of mental impairment. This number will undoubtedly increase as more and more people attain their full lifespan. The Veterans Administration is acutely aware of this problem in the population it serves. Currently, there are about 31 million veterans in the United States. About 13 percent of these veterans are over 65 years of age and the number is expected to increase to 40 percent by the turn of the century. In recognition of the pressing need to address this problem, eight Geriatric Research, Educational and Clinical Centers (GRECC) have been established under the auspices of the Veterans Administration and the guiding spirit of Dr. Paul Haber, Assistant Chief Medical Director for Professional Services, Veterans Administration. The purpose of these centers is to develop a better understanding of the complex biomedical and socio-economic problems of the aged in general and to enhance the quality of life of the older veterans in particular.

Gerontologists working towards a better understanding of the aging process and better care of the aged have made major progress in the biomedical field in the last decade. Among the efforts made by the Veterans Administration, the department of Extended Care and Academic Affairs have sponsored a number of symposia in the field of Gerontology. Leaders in the field of the Neurobiology of Aging gathered in Boston to present and discuss State-of-the-Art and recent scientific advancements relating to the aging process of the brain and senile dementia. This book covers the proceedings of this symposium in two sections. The first section of the book deals primarily with the neuroanatomical, neurochemical and physiological changes which occur in the mammalian brain during aging. The second section of the book is devoted to the neuropathological, immunological and clinical aspects of brain aging and senile dementia. An additional chapter correlating the clinical aspects of senile dementia with neuropathological, anatomical, and immunological changes has been added for the benefit of clinicians. Similarly, an introductory chapter has been added to review fundamental concepts of aging in general for the benefit of scientists working in other disciplines. It is our hope that this book will be useful to basic scientists, clinicians, graduate students, and others interested in the field of gerontology.

ACKNOWLEDGEMENTS

The editors express their appreciation to the publisher for continued cooperation and understanding in dealing with the numerous problems arising during the preparations of the manuscripts. We also express sincere thanks to John D. Chase, M. D., Chief Medical Director, Veterans Administration, for the permission to publish the proceedings of the symposium. We are especially thankful for the encouragement and assistance given to us by Dr. Richard Filer, Acting Assistant Chief Medical Director for Extended Care, and Mr. Phillip Haines, Coordinator of GRECC, V. A. Central Office. We also appreciate the cooperation of the members of the Planning Committee of the symposium, Director, Bedford GRECC, and the Management Staffs of the Bedford V. A. Hospital and the Boston Outpatient Clinic. The editors are also grateful to Mrs. Terry Laffey for her excellent typing and hard work in the preparation of the manuscripts. The help and support of Mead Johnson and Ciba-Geigy Pharmaceutical Companies is gratefully acknowledged.

Kalidas Nandy, M.D., Ph.D.
Ira Sherwin, M.D.

Contents

BIOMEDICAL ASPECTS OF AGING RESEARCH

Paul A. L. Haber

Asst. Chief Medical Director for Professional Services,
Department of Medicine and Surgery, Veterans Administration,
Washington, D. C. and Asst. Clinical Professor of Medicine,
George Washington University School of Medicine

Few subjects available to intellectual scrutiny at the present
time offer the author of an introductory chapter as much challenge
and breadth of scope as does this - THE BIOMEDICAL ASPECTS OF AGING
RESEARCH which opens this text of AGING BRAIN AND SENILE DEMENTIA.
The array of subject material is vast; the evidence leading to any
one set of conclusions is confusing and contradictory; the interest
is intense.   Theories of aging develop rapidly only to fall into
discard within a few short years or even months and lines of
investigation that seemed to hold promise a short while ago are
found to be "blind alleys".

To those of us who have worked in the field of aging for most of
our professional lives it is difficult to understand the rapidly
crescendoing interest in aging and aging research which has been
taking place in the past half decade since the second White House
Conference on Aging; difficult because no new factors have entered
the basic equation.   That there are growing numbers of aging Americans
(and indeed growing number of humans worldwide who are reaching old
age) comes as no surprise.   Demographers have been telling us for
years that there would be more older people around.   But the fact
that interest in Aging is on the increase is undeniable.   To attest
to such public interest one need only be reminded of the recent
creation of the new National Institute of Aging in the National
Institutes of Health, of the enlargement of the Administration on
Aging, of the proliferation of various consumer groups representing
the aging population, of the passage of a flood of legislation
affecting the elderly such as the Older American Acts and the
resurgence of attention paid by a large number of governmental
agencies such as the Department of Health, Education, and Welfare,

the Department of Housing and Urban Development, the Department of
Transportations and The Veterans Administration to the problems of
the aged and aging.

The phenomenon that may help explain the interest in aging is
the recent juxtaposition of two previously extant factors: one is
the admitted increase in the physical presence of augmented numbers
of older Americans - now totalling some 10.5% of the 220 million
and there are expected to be almost 24 million by 1980; the other
factor is the growing concern of Americans about health care in
general (Source Book of Health Insurance Data, 1975-76). A great
deal of popular attention is manifest in public forums, in the
press, in the news media centers about health care these days and
since older people are greater consumers of health services than the
general population (accounting for more hospital admissions, days
of hospital and long-term care, and visits to physicians' offices)
it follows that more attention is paid to the aging segment of the
population than any other. As one example, the number of visits to
physicians' offices in 1974 by populations of all ages was 4.9 visits
per year, while the number of visits for both sexes over the age of
65 was 6.8 visits per year. In sum, the reasoning goes something
like this: health care is rapidly growing more expensive amounting
to 104.2 billion dollars in 1974 (representing 7.7% of the GNP) and
the elderly are the most significant group of health care consumers
in proportion to their numbers, and the numbers of elderly are
daily increasing; therefore, anything that can reduce the morbidity
and mortality of the elderly becomes exceedingly important. Not only
does the general population feel that way but the elderly themselves,
increasingly aware of their growing political and economic strength
and importance, are beginning to have a larger voice in the decision
making processes that determine the national policy.

It has been brought to our attention by Hayflick and many others
that although the phenomenon of aging is not new, it has not until
recent times been of any particular significance. The parsimony of
biology dictates that the individual has little value for the
survival of the race once the child bearing function has been con-
summated. Since the vigorous young animal in the post pubertal state
is designed for optimal function in producing progeny and in raising
offspring, his survival past young middle age is a biological luxury.
It remained for the species Homo Sapiens in the latter half of the
twentieth century to accumulate the material wealth and the sagacity
to be able to indulge that luxury. Never before in the history of
living things have so many individuals survived beyond the period
during which they were needed for the continuation of the race.

But while the relative and absolute numbers of aging and aged
individuals has reached an all time high, the life span of older
individuals seems to have remained relatively constant. For awhile

the chances of an individual at birth to live to the full extent of
the life span seem measurably greater than ever before, the number
of years of life allotted to any individual entering old age has
not increased since biblical times. True there are probably more
centenarians alive today than ever before, but the ultimate limit of
longevity even for the hardiest of them is about 125 to 130 years.
What we are seeing is the squaring of the Gompertz curve of population
survival. The gradual decline of the curve showing the force of
mortality as aging progresses has given way to a straight line
running through the early and middle age years and then showing a
rapid drop-off in old age. Mathematical formulations of the Gompertz
equations reveal two sets of phenomena, neither of which is unexpected; first, that although the average force of mortality for
populations seems to be decreasing until old age has been achieved,
the average life span of the aged individual has remained relatively
constant; second, that as we age, fewer survivors remain in any given
time frame.

It would be useful at this point to present a brief review of
the various theories of aging. But first a few general considerations
should be elaborated. In the first place, there is general acceptance
that at present no single theory of aging seems to explain satisfactorily all the problems one would wish to consider. Second,
although there seem to be as many theories as there are theorists,
many theories really interconnect with one another and, if one digs
deeper, turn out to be only different manifestations of the same
basic explanation. Thirdly, no theory which serves at any level
more complex than the molecular is uniformly applicable across
all species of all living things.

Probably foremost among the still reputable theories of aging
is the Free Radical Theory. Free radicals are produced in the course
of oxygenation of a great multiplicity and variety of organic substances through the chemical and physical means of the exchange of
electrons. Free radicals thus produced are highly reactive and may
result in degradation mechanisms. Examples of free radical inter-
ference occurring in ordinary processes are the aging and cracking
of rubber, the rancidity of butter, the failing of plastics. At a
cellular level, free radicals have been unfavorably implicated in
the degradation of membranes, of mucopolysaccharides, of collagen,
elastin and other connective tissue elements, of the accumulation
of inert waste products within the cell itself. Probably more
important than these effects, however, is the likely effect of free
radicals on DNA. The interaction between free radicals and DNA
causes the formation of intermediate substances which are notoriously
unstable and which work to alter the DNA so that deleterious information is transmitted to the RNA which may in turn cause mutant proteins
to form imperfect enzymes which may result with harmful effects to
the cell.

The Free Radical Theory, though not new, seems to have acquired the distinction of being periodically rediscovered and given new emphasis among theorists of aging. One particularly vexing problem has been the association of free radicals with the problem of un-saturated fatty acids in diet (Herman, 1960). There has been a great deal of information recently about the harmful effects of diets rich in saturated fatty acids with the associated low iodine number. But proponents of the Free Radical Theory of aging point out that the disruptive effect of free radicals is maximized in their interaction with unsaturated fatty acids, these effects tending to result in damage to arterial wall structure.

In an attempt to neutralize or combat the putative ill effects of free radicals on the aging process, a number of agents known to be anti-oxidants in the chemical sense have been used with some encouraging but by no means universally accepted results. Thus BHT (butylated-hydroxytoluene) and antoher antioxidant related to the mercaptans 2-mercaptoethylamine have been used. In lower mammals they have been found to have a life prolonging effect. More recently Vitamin E has been proposed as the agent with most promise to antagonize the oxidation effect of free radicals. Vitamin E has been found to be effective in preventing spoilage of certain foods. Vitamin E was therefore proposed to prevent the accumulation of fat degradation products particularly ceroid which tends to build up in cells which contained fat (Tappel, 1970). Nor is the anti-oxidant capability of certain chemicals related only to the prevention of ceroid accumulation. It has been pointed out that lipofuscin buildup is also slowed by the action of anti-oxidant materials.

Closely related to the Free Radical Theory of aging is the in-crimination of radiation as a basic cause of aging. In the aftermath of the Hiroshima cataclysm a great deal of interest was focused on the effects of ionizing radiation as a cause of aging. Many reputable scientists felt that the effects of the atom-blast provided a usable model of "instant aging" and for awhile in the mid nineteen-fifties it was fashionable to attempt to equate the damage wrought by radiation as synonomous with the effects of the aging process. We now know that though there are similarities between the processes of aging and radiation induced damage, there are more profound differences between them. The mere fact that there is a correlation between increased death rates and force of mortality on the one hand and the quantity of radiation exposure and the force of mortality on the other does not necessarily speak for a relationship between the two observations. Radiation probably produces its lethal effects in a variety of mechanisms, but the one that most closely resembles aging is through the production of free radicals such as those which are liberated within the cell after cellular water has been radiated to form electrons, hydrogen ions, and hydroxyl radicals. So powerful are the effects of free radicals that only one per 1.0×10^6 molecules,

which are produced by a given dose of radiation, is accompanied by
lethal outcome in half the exposed population. Further, there is
an estimate that if one molecule within a cell out of a million is
destroyed by radiation the cell may not survive. Considering that
the background radiation we are all exposed to is the equivalent
of 0.1 rad per year, there are some persuasive factors which
implicate radiation as one contributing factor in the process of
aging, and studies are being conducted in New York State and other
places which seek to determine the effects of shielding animal
populations from background radiation exposure and to correlate
those effects with possible increases in life span.

The free radical theory cannot be discussed without some
reference to the role of oxygen. Oxygen, necessary for the performance of metabolic activities within the cell, also gives rise through
some unclear mechanism to the production of peroxides which in
turn increase the amount of free radicals present in the cell.
Free radicals may exert their deleterious effects upon a number of
sites within the cell. One site thus affected is the nuclear membrane which is composed in part of lipid substances. It is the
oxidative effect on these lipids (particularly those which are made
up of polyunsaturated fatty acids) which tends to degrade membranes
and impede the smooth flow of membrane mechanics and perfusion dynamics. In the mitochondria where cellular oxidation takes place,
the effect of free radicals is felt despite the protective effect
of Vitamin E, a powerful antioxidant. Vitamin E and coenzyme Q (a
quinone substance) tend to be similar in function in mitigating the
oxidative effect of the free radicals so that oxidation can go on
without at the same time consuming the mitochondria themselves
(Pryor, 1971). Finally, free radicals exert an influence on DNA
causing unfavorable changes which perturb the production of messenger
RNA. This alteration inevitably lead to some form of protein
malsynthesis, incompatible with prolonged life.

Another important theory of aging has to do with the basic
concept of rate of energy expenditure. It is tempting to conjecture
that for any given species of animal (probably more so for mammals
than other vertebrates) the total endowment of energy production is
relatively constant and is peculiar to that species. Thus, despite
differences in the rate of energy consumption in different species
of animals the total lifelong energy consumption may be thought of
as relatively constant. The most convenient way of measuring
consumption of energy (rate of living) is the measurement of basal
metabolism. It has long been known that animals with high metabolic
rates tend on the whole to be smaller and have shorter life spans.
Part of this phenomenon is related to mass versus surface area. In
smaller mammals a greater proportion of total body mass is consumed
by the surface envelope providing for more rapid heat loss and
therefore requiring greater heat production and a higher metabolic

rate. In larger mammals the surface area is relatively less
proportional to the total body mass and heat dissipation is slower
requiring less heat production and lower specific metabolic rate.
But it is interesting to note that the lifespan also increases
proportional to the lower metabolic rate as the size of the mammal
increases.

Some illustrative data help confirm the above thesis. Thus,
the mouse has an average weight of 0.021 kg. Its basal metabolic
rate is 3.6 kcal/day or 171.5 kcal/kg/day, its lifespan (depending
on species) is between two and three years. By contrast, the pig
has a weight of 128 kg. Its basal metabolic rate is 2443 kcal/day
or 19.1 kcal/kg/day and its lifespan is 16 years. The domestic
horse, largest of these three mammals we are considering, weighs
441 kg. with a basal metabolic rate of 4990 kcal/day or 11.3 kcal/
kg/day and its lifespan is 30 years (Kleiber, 1961).

In humans the BMR tends to increase during the first few days
of life as the infant struggles to adapt to its new environment,
then there is a decrease during the first decade which gradually
decelerates in its rate of change. Human data have been studied
extensively and various relationships have been proposed, but for
the present, none of them seems to lead to theses which can be
manipulated with the thought of prolonging life. It has been shown,
however, that in lower animals dietary deprivation and exposure to
lower than normal ambient temperatures is correlated with a longer
life span. Such data have not been definitely confirmed in higher
mammalian forms.

Finally, some theorists have postulated a link between rate of
living as measured by the basal metabolic rate and entropy production
and some go so far as to state that the prolongation of life requires
a decrease in entropy production. This decrease may be related to
observations about life prolongation in decreased ambient temperature
situations since it is recognized that there is an optimum life
temperature at which temperature entropy production is minimal
(Hershey, 1974).

We must turn now to the consideration of yet a third story of
aging that is concerned with the effects of cross-linking. The effects
of cross-linking are found in many types of tissues and indeed within
the cell itself, but probably is of most importance in its role in
aging collagen. Collagen is formed as soluble tropocollagen and as
it ages there is an increase in the number of cross links which bind
the parallel polymer strands. The increasing degree of cross-linking
can be measured in many ways - the inhibition of the tendency to
undergo shortening with thermal stress on the part of aging tendon
tissue or the inhibition of the tendency to undergo swelling in
certain kinds of solution. But whatever measure is used, it is clear

that as the animal ages the amount of cross-linking increases. The
inevitable result of this cross-linking is the loss of elasticity,
increased brittleness and rigidity of tissues and a certain loss of
vitality of the supporting tissues of the organism. The whole
process has been found similar to the tanning of leather and indeed
the similarity of aged (as opposed to young) skin to tanned leather
has been commented on for ages. Comment should also be made of the
fact that there is a relationship between the degree of cross-linking,
the presence of free radicals and the effects of oxidation and peroxidation. Another interesting correlation has been found with respect
to the rate of living and the degree of cross linking of collagen.
For example, it is known that rat tail tendon collagen is much more
densely cross-linked in old age (two and a half years) than a
comparably chronological matched human baby of two and a half years of
age. But when compared with a human of seventy years age, the
degree of cross linking was found to be similar. This gives rise
to the speculation that the metabolic rate is also somehow implicated
in the process of cross-linking of collagen (Kohn, 1971).

Cross-linking is also at work in the aging of elastin, but its
effects are either more subtle or less well understood. Two amino
acids, desmosine and isodesmosine, have been shown to be involved
in the cross-linking of elastin and they are known to increase
during maturation, but are presumed to hold fairly constant during
aging.

There is reason to believe that cross-linking also affects the
functioning of larger molecules such as DNA. This probably occurs
through the influence of the cross-linking process upon the usual
steric conformation of DNA. The specific effect on DNA is the
cross linking of two helices making it difficult for the template
function of the impaired helix to be served in a normal fashion. The
net result is, of course, formation of malsynthesized proteins. It
should be noted in passing that there are an abundance of naturally
occurring cross-linking agents such as a variety of aldehydes, metals
such as copper, aluminum and manganese, and several organic acids
like fumaric and succinic acid.

Yet another theory of aging has to do with the immunologic
phenomena of the intact organism. Immunologic events are of two
sorts with respect to the process of aging. On the one hand, the
immunocompetence of any organism is a vital factor in its defense
against invasion by other microorganisms. As this function declines
with age, it renders the aging animal more and more susceptible to
infections which in the younger animal do not hold the same portent
of lethality that they do in the older individual. On the other hand,
the mechanics of immunocompetence when perturbed by the process of
aging give rise to the process of autoimmunity. This in turn is
frequently accompanied by an attack on the organism's tissue as though

they were foreign and there may also be elaboration of abnormal proteins as an ancillary finding. The phenomena of immune reactions are based upon the fact that the body must be able to recognize self from alien tissue. It is tempting to philosophize that the organism does not recognize its aging tissues in the light of its early immunologic experience. According to Makinodan (1972) there are three postulates which govern the consideration of immunocompetence and aging. First, mortality increases due to infectious disease with advancing age; second, it is difficult, if not impossible, to establish immunization in older animals; third, there is an increase of age-related malignancies with a relationship to antigenically aberrant cells. There is an interesting apparent exception to this rule in that aged animals may have a profound anamnestic response to challenges by antigens experienced first in youth.

     Closely related to the immunologic theory of aging is the implication of somatic mutation. This variant of the immunologic theory holds that in the course of time mutations develop which in turn are immunologically foreign to the organism and set in motion the destructive processes of immunologic scavenging. This process is, of course, enhanced by radiation exposure and is influenced to some degree by the number of chromosomes; i.e. whether the animal is haploid or diploid.

     One theory which has been entertained for a long time is the accumulation of waste products theory. This sets forth the entirely reasonable notion that as the cell metabolizes, the end products of metabolism which cannot be dissipated or consumed, begin to pile up within the cell and disrupt the normal cellular activity. This theory called the "clinker" theory compares cellular activity to the functioning of a coal furnace in which the accumulation of ash (clinkers) ultimately reduces the effectiveness of the firing operation. One particular variant of this theory implicates lipofuscin as the most important culprit. Lipofuscin is a pigment substance whose origins are not fully known but they have been shown to be composed of complex fatty acid derivatives. Analysis has shown that they contain cholesterol ester, sphyngomyelin, lecithin and cephalin. It has been suggested that lipofuscin is the remnant of degenerated mitochondria, that it is the result of membrane degradation, or that is represents an organelle structure in itself, but none of these hypotheses has been definitely proved at this time. In any event, it is a matter of repeated demonstration that lipofuscin does increase with aging. The pigment is laid down in cells of many types but it is particularly demonstrable in cells with long lives such as neurone, myocardium, and skeletal tissue. In myocardium especially, the cellular mass is increasingly imposed upon by deposition of lipofuscin, both in terms of the number of cells which show lipofuscin accumulation and in the amount of pigment deposition per cell. The same observations have been made in neuronal tissues and there is a clear relationship between aging and the amount of pigment deposition observed, but there have been no correlations with loss of cellular function.

It should be noted in passing that a case has been made for the relationship between the accumulation of minerals and aging. Calcium in particular has been the subject of some investigations, but the finding of increased cellular binding of calcium with age has been inconsistent. Magnesium, too, has been thought to be related to age in terms of its intracellular deposition, but again no definitive conclusions have been reached. In general, the same inconsistencies have been noted in all particulars of the "clinker" theory.

Some mention should be made of the altered endocrine activity in aging. A great deal of work has been done by researchers in the field of endocrine metabolism which goes towards relating altered endocrine function with age. This alteration takes place in virtually all the endocrine organs, testis and ovary, pituitary, thyroid, adrenal, and pancreas to name the principal ones. Decline of gonadal function with age is well known and amply documented. Indeed, the obverse is true, in that preservation of sexual activity into late chronological age is viewed as proof of youthful vigor. Some have attributed many of the commonly seen features of old age - thickened dry skin, decrease in appetite, slow dysarthric speech, gastro-intestinal hypomotility - as but a reflection of the symptomatology of classic hypothyroidism. Finally, the reduced functioning of the pancreas specifically in the Islets of Langerhans cells has been though to be related to the onset of adult diabetes.

Of course, the central problem with the endocrine theory of aging is the same which confounds other prominent theories. That is, the dilemma over which is cause and which is effect. Does decreased endocrine function cause aging or is it the result? No certain answers are as yet forthcoming.

There are a number of other theories which seek to account for the process of aging and it may be useful to consider them very briefly. For example, there is a theory that aging is due to the accumulated stresses of living, the "wear and tear" philosophy. An interesting comparison has been made with the life expectancy of drinking glass tumblers in common cafeteria use and the process of aging in organic systems. Thus, the older the tumbler is, the greater likelihood of breakage on the basis of exposure alone. Curves drawn charting this likelihood bear some resemblances to curves for life expectancy of animals. Other theories seek to account for the phenomena of aging with disordered function of a particular organ system. Thus, the central nervous system, the cardiovascular system, the skeletal and supporting structures system have all been cited

as the central cause of aging on the thesis that their failure
predicts the failure of other organ systems which herald the advance
of aging.

In summary, we have looked at a number of theories which seek
to explain the process of aging. However, there is no theory of
aging which can satisfactorily explain all the manifestations of
aging. In many instances, the presentation of data which relates
changes in one or another parameter to aging may represent allied
phenomena and does not help determine which is cause and which effect.

Consideration of the theories of aging leads directly into an
assessment of areas which are ripe for further future investigation.
Biomedical research on aging needs to be done at several levels -
cellular, organ tissue, organismal, and population - and there must
be some interfacing among all the levels if we are to understand
the process of aging. The most basic biological levels will deal
with the changes in genetic composition and the alteration of DNA
and RNA. Damage done to DNA caused intrinsically or extrinsically
must be repaired if the organism is to survive into old age. There
is reason to believe that species endowed with efficient repair
mechanisms are inherently longer-lived than those which lack the
appropriate repair systems. The era of cellular biology has barely
begun. We are not even certain of all the functions of the intracellular contents whether organelle or cytoplasmic, let alone the
metabolic pathways and eventual fate of all the involved elements.

One classic observation, known as the Hayflick phenomenon, sets
limits on cellular life. In his now-famous series of experiments,
Hayflick showed that the number of cellular divisions was finite
and constant for any species. In the lung fibroblasts with which
he dealt, fifty cell divisions constituted that limit and even if
the division process was interrupted by freezing and rethawing the
number of divisions could not be altered.

Even the cell membrane, once thought to be a relatively inert
structure which served only to envelope the cell's contents is now
known to be exceedingly complex and must be understood in terms of
its own dynamics. But other cell structures-the mitochondria, the
ribosomes, the lysosomes must also be examined in greater detail if
we want to know about production of proteins, and the generation of
energy at a cellular level.

Studies should also proceed at an organ system level. Many of
the diseases commonly associated with aging can only be defined or
understood in terms of organ system dysfunction. Thus atherosclerosis
may be viewed as one example of aging of the cardiovascular apparatus;
similarly emphysema may be considered an instance of pulmonary aging,
and cataract formation as an example of lens aging. To understand

these diseases is to understand some of the basic alterations that
occur in aging. Aging of the supporting and connective tissue organ
systems is particularly demanding of the researcher's efforts, since
many of the degenerative diseases' processes of these tissues result
in the common complications of osteoporosis, osteomalacia, and the
dermatoses of aging. Central nervous system disorders associated
with aging have been particularly resistant to the probing of
research. While the affective psychoses have yielded (at least in
terms of clinical management) to the discovery of psychotropic drugs,
the more irreversible psychiatric disorders associated with aging
have not been as well influenced. Although a great deal of anatomical
and pathological research has been done on the central nervous
system, direct correlations between loss of structure and loss of
particular intellectual or mental function has yet to be precisely
defined.

A few words have to be said with respect to the problems of
aging research in general. It has not been widely appreciated that
effective research in aging demands the availability of colonies of
aging animals. To do well controlled studies in aging, one cannot
rely on the usual source of animals for experimentation. But the
carefully controlled environment which must be provided over
relatively long periods of time is extremely costly. Also a
variety of animal types must be provided. While lower forms of
animal life may be useful (or indeed preferable to higher species) for
certain kinds of studies, researches on integrated functioning almost
has to be performed in higher mammalian species. And, of course,
these animals are the most difficult and expensive of all to produce
in large numbers for aging research. It would be extremely useful
to pursue the idea of developing through some sort of consortial
arrangement a common source of aging animals raised under appropriate
conditions.

This introductory review has dealt with the common current
theories of aging in an effort to set the stage for the papers
which follow. Dealing with the central nervous system exclusively
they will offer a valuable insight into the movement at the frontiers
of research in aging of the brain. If there is one area where human
suffering and misery can be singled out which calls for solution
and intervention on behalf of afflicted patients, it surely must be
that of the impairment of brain function with age. Because of the
great numbers of patients so affected both in the United States and
Worldwide, even a modest gain in understanding the physiological,
psychological, and social deficits encountered in the so-called
"senile psychoses" will pay tremendous dividends.

REFERENCES

Harman, D. The free radical theory of Aging: the effect of age on
    serum mercaptan levels. J. of Gerontology 15:38, 1960.

Hershey, D. Lifespan and Factors Affecting it, Chas. C. Thomas,
    p. 137, 1974.

Kleiber, M. The Fire of Life, New York, pp. 181-205, 1961.

Kohn, R.R. Principles of Mammalian Aging, Prentice Hall, Englewood
    Cliffs, N. J., p. 38, 1971.

Makinodan, T. Epidemiology of Aging, US Dept. Health, Education and
    Welfare, DHEW Publication no. (NIH) 75-711, p. 161, 1972.

Pryor, W.A.   Free radical pathology, Chemical and Engineering News,
    p. 34, June 7, 1971.

Source Book of Health Insurance Data 1975-1976, Health Insurance
    Institute, New York, N.Y., p. 14, 1975-1976.

Tappel, A.J. Lipid peroxidation Damage to cell components. Presented
    to Federation of American Societies for Experimental Biology,
    Fifth Annual Meeting, April 16, 1970.

I.
Neuroanatomical, Biochemical and Physiological Aspects

CELL LOSS WITH AGING

Harold Brody and N. Vijayashankar

Department of Anatomical Sciences
School of Medicine
State University of New York at Buffalo
Buffalo, New York

There have been several techniques developed to determine the number of cells in the central nervous system. Probably the simplest and the most common technique has been the ocular micrometric method. This was originally used by Hammerberg in 1895 and while other techniques may be mentioned, it is at the present time the most consistent and dependable. It involves examination of tissue with the aid of a micrometer disc inserted into the ocular of a compound microscope. Cells which fall within the squares of the disc may then be counted and total counts made as well as graphs showing relative populations within any portion of the section. This is most useful in determining cell numbers within a brain stem nuclear structure since it is possible in serial section counting to obtain an impression of the cell population at any specific point. By examination in several planes, one may obtain a 3-dimensional impression of the nucleus, and to compare specific sites within the nucleus in a number of brain specimens when the nucleus is of similar size. Direct optical examination of tissue by the investigator also makes possible a differentiation of neurons from glial cells and discriminates fairly easily when there is an overlapping of cells.

Other methods which have been developed include: (1) projection of a section upon a screen with visual counting of cells (Dornfield, 1942); (2) cell counting from a photograph (von Economo and Koskinas, 1925); (3) semiautomatic counting with a spectrophotometer in which cell number is determined from the optical density of the cells (Ryzen, 1956); (4) homogenation and total counts of brain (Nurnberger, 1958); (5) chemical methods (Hyden, 1960) based on the idea that DNA content in a nucleus of a single cell is constant. Therefore, determining the DNA content in a specific volume of tissue and

dividing this number by the DNA content of a single cell will
provide the number of nuclei (cells) within that tissue. Of recent
development is the automatic method of quantification first developed
as the flying spot scanner of Causley and Young (1955) and more
recently as the Quantimet, an image analyzer which transfers an image
of the section onto a television screen and automatically counts
particles such as nucleoli depending upon that particle's size,
shape and intensity of staining as determined by the investigator.

These methods each present advantages and disadvantages.
Certainly, the automatic devices show promise for future studies
although at this time no publications have been forthcoming from
the few laboratories which have been working with the Quantimet.

Possibly because of the difficulty in managing the techniques
of quantification, there have been few studies of nerve cell number
either in the normal or as a consequence of pathology. Where
calculations have been done, they have usually been performed on few
specimens and little attention has been given to the possible effects
of aging or to changes which might occur in pathological states.
To cite one example, while neuropathology textbooks state that the
number of nerve cells in the substantia nigra decreases in
Parkinsonism, no specific counts have been performed and no studies
of this nucleus have been performed to determine whether there may
be an age-related change in cell number. Therefore, one should
question the original premise regarding the effect of disease on
this group of cells.

Will cell number present the entire story for an understanding
of changes in nervous system function? We do not believe it will.
However, we contend that since the cell is the essential unit of the
nervous system, we need more information on cell populations in both
brain maturation and aging to relate to morphological changes which
may be occurring such as are described elsewhere in this volume
(Feldman, 1977; Scheibel and Scheibel, 1977), as well as chemical
and functional aspects presented in other chapters of the book.

The originator of the concept that increasing age might be
related to neuronal loss was Hodge. In 1894 he examined the brains
of young bees caught in the act of crawling out of the brood cells
and old bees with worn and frayed wings. When a beehive was opened,
he observed a bee quietly humped up taking neither part nor interest
in the general commotion. Hodge found that the young bees contained
2.9 times more cells than the old bees.

In 1919 and 1920, Ellis reported a 35-50% decrease in Purkinje
cells with age. Inukai, in a 1928 study which was technically
excellent, showed that the Purkinje cell packing density of the white

rat cerebellum is reduced with advancing age by approximately 20%. There have been other studies in which no significant change is reported for Purkinje cell numbers (DeLorenzi, 1931). The most recent study by Hall, Miller and Corsellis (1975) upon 90 normal human brains very carefully sampled, indicates that in spite of a wide variation from person to person at any given age, the Purkinje population decreases during adult life at an average of 25% over the age span of 100 years. These authors emphasize that such a generalization may be oversimplifying the problem since they did not identify an appreciable fall in the proportion of the total population in either sex until the 6th decade. These findings indicate that at least one category of neuron, the Purkinje cell, is prone to die off during the latter half of adult life. Whether the same is true of other neuronal populations in the human brains, or at least of those above the level of the hindbrain remains an open question.

Further quantitative studies are proceeding in several laboratories. Let us continue in this review by examining other portions of the neural axis.

Inferior Olive

Monagle and Brody (1974) have examined the main nucleus of the inferior olive and found no significant change in the number of cells from birth to 89 years of age despite more than a doubling in the size of the nucleus.

Facial Nucleus

Maleci (1936) examined the facial nerve nucleus after staining it with a modification of the Weigert method and found a curvilinear decline of cells with age approximating a loss of about 0.25% or 16 cells each year of adult life. These findings were not supported by van Buskirk in his 1945 study of this nucleus although the study was not strictly speaking, age related.

Ventral Cochlear Nucleus

Konigsmark and Murphy (1970) have examined this nucleus in 23 specimens ranging from the newborn to 92 years of age and found no significant change in cell number.

Abducens and Trochlear Nuclei

We have now completed cell counts in these two structures and find in each that there is a doubling in the length of the nucleus between birth and adulthood but no significant change in cell number during the remaining life span. Although individual variation was

evident in some specimens, the average number of cells was 6,454
in the abducens nucleus (Vijayashankar and Brody, 1971 and 1977a)
and 2,115 in the trochlear nucleus (Vijayashankar and Brody, 1977b).

Locus Coeruleus

Our recent studies of this structure indicate that this is the
only brain stem nucleus examined so far which shows a significant
decrease in cell number. Twenty-four specimens 14 years to 87 years
have been studied in sections 10μ in thickness. Except for one
specimen (12,070) in the group below the age of 63 years the cell
number within the locus coeruleus of one side is in the range of
15,360-18,790 cells. After that age, again with the exception of
one specimen of 68 years with a cell count of 18,950 cells, the
range is between 9,310 and 13,670 with no counts above 11,590 after
71. This would account for an approximately 40% decrease in cell
number in a structure which has assumed much importance and interest
recently because of its widespread connections within the central
nervous system, its relations to the catecholamine system, and its
possible relationship to sleep physiology.

Cerebral Cortex

Studies of the cerebral cortex are difficult becasue of a sampling
problem and variations from one specimen to another makes comparison
risky. From early studies performed on the cerebral cortex (Brody,
1955, '70), it was found that a significant decrease in cell number
occurs in the superior frontal gyrus, superior temporal gyrus,
precentral gyrus and area striata but no significant change was
found in the postcentral gyrus or inferior temporal gyrus. In
addition, while there was a decrease in neuron number in all areas,
the most marked loss occurred in the second and fourth layers, the
external and internal granule layers where the Golgi type II short
axoned cells are characteristic of the associational cells of the
human cerebral cortex. These findings have since been verified in
several laboratories, by Colon in 1972, Shefer in 1973 (by direct
optical study) and by Tomlinson (1976) using the Quantimet.

In summing up the present status of cell loss in aging brain,
we believe that we have a long way to go. Few areas of the nervous
system have been examined quantitatively in relation to function.
Incidentally, a most recent study by Landfield et al. (1977)
demonstrates a marked decrease in neuronal elements of the hippocampus
in aged Fisher rats. Interestingly, earlier behavioral studies have
shown memory deficiency in those rats. More correlative work such
as this needs to be done.

It is obvious from an examination of the literature that the
whole brain cannot be dealt with as a single organ. Cell decrease
does not occur generally but in relation to specific areas. These

marked differences must be taken into account in explaining variations in structure, function, response to stress, and relationship to aging.

Why are there these differences? Are they related to morphological differences between cell groups or chemical structure? What is the role of the microcirculation and the blood-brain barrier in aging of the nervous system? Can function play a role in determining longevity of cells or is there a "pacemaker" or "time clock" within the central nervous system or within cells, which controls the life of the cell?

In this regard, isn't it curious that brain stem structures which develop early show little change while cerebellar and cerebral cortex, developing later, show rather marked cell decrease? Even within neuronal types, in the cerebral cortex, the type II neurons remain less differentiated for a long time period. The tangential connections within cerebral cortex are also formed late being provided by type II cells (Morest, 1969). These same type II late developing cells decrease to the largest degree in human cerebral cortex and also show marked decrease in the neocortex of the aging Fisher rat.

The possible relationship between the early development of the central nervous system and the later effects of aging is intriguing and deserving of consideration. Finally, the question of "neuronal plasticity" and what happens to synaptic sites which are left vacant by the death of the cell whose processes originally occupied those sites, is at present unanswered. Does the old cell lose its ability to grow collateral branchings and to regenerate? There is mixed information on this point but studies here may provide the answer to whether changes in function after cell death are a response to the absence of neurons or to disorganized regrowth of remaining neurons.

REFERENCES

Brody, H. Organization of cerebral cortex. III. A study of aging in the human cerebral cortex. J. Comp. Neurol. 102:511-556, 1955.

Brody, H. Structural changes in the aging nervous system. In: Interdisciplinary Topics in Gerontology. (Ed. Blumenthal, H.), Karger, Basel/Munchen, 1970.

Buskirk, van, E.C. The seventh nerve complex. J. Comp. Neurol. 82: 303-335, 1945.

Causley, D. and Young, J.Z. Counting and sizing of particles with flying spot microscope. Nature 4479:453-454, 1955.

Colon, E. J. The elderly brain. A quantitative analysis of cerebral cortex in two cases. Psychiat. Neurol. Neurochir. 75:261-270, 1972.

DeLorenzi, E.   Constenza numerica delle cellule del Purkinje in individui di varia eta. Bull. Soc. ital. biol. sper. 6:80-82, 1931.

Dornfield, E. J., Slater, D.W. and Scheffe, H.   A method for accurate determination of volume and cell numbers in small organs. Anat. Rec. 82:255-259, 1942.

Economo, C. and Koskinas, G.   Die Cytoarchitektonik der Hirnrinde des erwachsenen Menschen. Leipsig, 1925.

Ellis, R. S.   A preliminary quantitative study of Purkinje cells in normal, subnormal and senescent human cerebella. J. Comp. Neurol. 30:229-252, 1919.

Ellis, R. S.   Norms for some structural changes in the human cerebellum from birth to old age. J. Comp. Neurol. 32:1-33, 1920.

Feldman, M.   Dendritic changes in aging rat brain. In: Aging Brain and Senile Dementia. (Eds. K. Nandy and I. Sherwin), Plenum Press, New York, 1977.

Hall, T. C., Miller, A.K.H. and Corsellis, J.A.N.   Variations in the human Purkinje cell population according to age and sex. Neuropath. Appl. Neurobiol. 1:267-292, 1975.

Hodge, C. F.   Changes in ganglion cells from birth to senile death. Observations on man and honey bee. J. Physiol. 17:129-134, 1894.

Hyden, H.   The Neuron. In: The Cell. (Eds. J. Brachet and A.E. Mirsky), Academic Press, New York, 1960.

Inukai, T.   On the loss of Purkinje cells with advancing age from cerebellar cortex of Albino rat. J. Comp. Neurol. 45:1-31, 1928.

Konigsmark, B. W. and Murphy, E. A.   Neuronal populations in the human brain. Nature 228:1335, 1970.

Landfield, P. W., Rose, G., Sandles, L., Wohlstadter, T. C. and Lynch, G.   Patterns of astroglial hypertrophy and neural degeneration in the hippocampus of aged, memory deficient rats. J. Geront. 32:3-12, 1977.

Maleci, O.   Sul rapporto numerico tra le cellule dei nuclei di origine e le fibre di nervi motor encefalici dell'uomo, con osservazioni sulle differenze qualitative delle dette fibre. Arch. Ital. Annt. Embriol. 35:559-583, 1936.

Monagle, R. D. and Brody, H. The effects of age upon the main
     nucleus of the inferior olive in the human. J. Comp. Neurol.
     155:61-66, 1974.

Morest, D. K. The differentiation of cerebral dendrites. A study
     of the post-migratory neuroblast in the medial nucleus of the
     trapezoid body. Z. Anat. Entwicklungsgeschichte 128:271-289,
     1969.

Nurnberger, I. I. Direct enumeration of cells of the brain. In:
     Biology of Neuroglia. (Ed. Windle, W.F.), Charles C. Thomas,
     Springfield, 1958.

Ryzen, M. A microphotometric method of cell examination within the
     cerebral cortex of man. J. Comp. Neurol. 104:233-245, 1956.

Scheibel, M. E. and Scheibel, A.B. Differential changes with aging
     in old and new cortices. In: Aging Brain and Senile Dementia.
     (Eds. K. Nandy and I. Sherwin), Plenum Press, New York, 1977.

Shefer, V. G. Absolute number of neurons and thickness of cerebral
     cortex during aging, senile and vascular dementia and Pick's
     and Alzheimer Disease. Neurosci. Beh. Physiol. 6:319-324, 1973.

Tomlinson, B. E. Some quantitative cerebral findings in normal and
     demented old people. In: Neurobiology of Aging. (Eds. R. O.
     Terry and S. Gershon), Raven Press, New York, 1976.

Vijayashankar, N. and Brody, H. Neuronal population of human
     abducens nucleus. Anat. Record 169(2):447, 1971.

Vijayashankar, N. and Brody, H. A study of aging in the human
     abducens nucleus. J. of Comp. Neurol., 1977a, in press.

Vijayashankar, N. and Brody, H. Aging in the human brainstem: A
     study of the nucleus of the trochlear nerve. Acta Anatomica,
     1977b, in press.

DENDRITIC CHANGES IN AGING RAT BRAIN: PYRAMIDAL CELL DENDRITE

LENGTH AND ULTRASTRUCTURE

Martin L. Feldman

Department of Anatomy and Gerontology Center
Boston University School of Medicine
Boston, Massachusetts 02118

INTRODUCTION

For the past several years, studies have been underway to in-
vestigate age-related cytomorphological changes that occur in a
highly specified cell population. This population consists of the
pyramidal neurons of layers III and V in rat visual cortex (area
17, Krieg, 1946a, b; Schober and Winkelmann, 1975). The restriction of cell population is based upon the abundance of evidence
that the processes of aging may vary among cell groups in mode,
severity, and tempo. In view of this fact, it seems clear that
one avenue towards meaningful progress in understanding the effects
of aging in the brain is thorough study of the totality of aging
changes affecting particular cell types.

The various dendritic branches of the pyramidal neuron are
typically studded with dendritic spines, small protrusions that
form the principal postsynaptic structures of this cell type (Colonnier, 1968; Feldman, 1975; Gray, 1959). It is also known that
the pyramidal apical dendrites are preferentially bundled into
dendritic clusters during their ascent toward the pial surface
(Feldman and Peters, 1974; Fleischhauer, Petsche and Wittkowski,
1972; Peters and Walsh, 1972). This bundling, together with dendritic thickness and verticality, considerably facilitates the un-
equivocal recognition of apical dendrites in both the light and
electron microscopes.

The present series of studies began with the observation of
a gradual loss of layer V pyramidal dendrite spines with advancing age (Feldman and Dowd, 1974, 1975). It was also possible to

demonstrate a relationship between spine density and dendritic thickness, and evidence for an age-related decrease in apical dendrite diameter was presented (Feldman and Dowd, 1975). Later, it was shown that the layer V pyramidal perikarya also decreased in size with advancing age (Feldman, 1976). Ultrastructural examination of the neuropil within the dendritic clusters at the level of layer IV revealed a decrease in the number of synapses present, particularly axospinous synapses. Electron microscopic examination of the pyramidal apical dendrites showed that aging dendrites commonly contained various types of lamellar inclusions. The speculation was advanced that the dendritic inclusions were related to lost spines (Feldman, 1976).

The above findings raised a number of questions. Two such questions are: (1) If pyramidal neurons, as they undergo the progressive deafferentation represented by a spine loss, exhibit a decrease in apical dendrite diameter and a shrinkage of the cell body, is there also a reduction in the length of the dendritic branches? (2) Could the hypothesized relationship between the dendritic inclusions and lost spines be confirmed by demonstrating the absence of such inclusions in old dendrites which retained their normal spine complement? Anatomical methods exist for answering each of these questions. The first question may be investigated through study of Golgi preparations, and the second question by means of serial E.M. sections. These methods are presently being employed. This report summarizes the progress made to date.

METHODS

The animals used in this study are male albino Sprague-Dawley rats (Charles River Breeding Laboratories), free of grossly detectable pathology. For the study of dendritic lengths, rats aged 1 month (1 animal) and 34-36 months (4 animals) have been examined thus far. The E.M. serial sections were prepared from a single 36 month old animal. All animals were fixed by perfusion with aldehyde solutions. The tissue blocks used in the dendritic length study were impregnated by the Golgi rapid method (for further details, see Feldman and Dowd, 1975). Computer-assisted analysis of dendritic length was performed on the following dendrite systems: basal dendrites of layer III and V pyramidal cells, oblique branches emanating from layer V pyramidal apical dendrites in layer V, and oblique branches emanating from layer V pyramidal apical dendrites in layer IV. In all, 145 dendrites have been measured. The data obtained has been evaluated for statistical significance by means of the randomization test (Siegel, 1956). The computer-assisted measurements are being carried out in the Department of Anatomy, Washington University, St. Louis, using a PDP-12 computer coupled to a Zeiss Universal microscope. Total dendrite lengths, representing the sum of the lengths of the individual dendritic branch segments, were

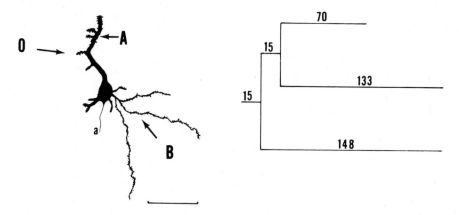

Figure 1. Left, a portion of the dendritic tree of a young adult layer V pyramidal neuron. The excrescences studding the dendrites are the dendritic spines. One basal dendrite is shown in its entirety (B). A, apical dendrite. O, oblique branches. a, axon. Computer measurement of the branch lengths of this dendrite generated the scaled-length Sholl (1956) diagram on the right. Branch lengths are in μm. Branch lengths are true 3-dimensional lengths and differ from those which would be measured on a 2-dimensional silhouette such as that shown on the left. This dendrite has three free endpoints and a total length of 381 μm. Calibration line, 50 μm.

measured in three dimensions (Zeiss Planapochromat x40, Optovar x1.25). Data was stored on magnetic tape and available for video display or permanent recording by means of DECwriter printout or Calcomp 565 X-Y plotter record (similar to Figure 1, right). The detailed operation of this system has been presented elsewhere (Wann et al., 1973; for one example of its application, see Woolsey, Dierker and Wann, 1975). Because of the technical problems involved in tracing long dendrites from section to section, only dendrites entirely contained within a single 125 μm section were analyzed for length. This excluded a considerable number of dendrites from the analysis and permitted the measurement of only some, never all, of the dendrites of any individual neuron. The second technique used in this study, the analysis of serial thin sections, was carried out on an uninterrupted 82-section series, oriented in the tangential plane through layer IV. Thus, the apical dendrite clusters were visualized cut in cross-section. Every section was examined and photographed at a minimum magnification of x4,000.

RESULTS

Dendritic Lengths

Qualitative observation of the Golgi material reveals a number of pyramidal dendrites in the old brains which appear to be
relatively short. But it is by no means certain from simple visual
inspection that dendritic lengths are reduced by comparison with the
young material. The reason for this uncertainty is the wide range
of dendritic lengths present in both the young and old material.
One subjective impression that is quite strong, however, is that an
old dendrite which is very short is often a dendrite which also is
relatively thin and which has a reduced complement of dendritic
spines.

Quantitatively, the computer-assisted measurements of 3-dimen-
sional length show a clearcut overall reduction in two of the four
dendrite systems examined. The data for basal dendrites of layer
III and V pyramidal neurons is presented in Figure 2. The mean
total dendritic length of the layer III basal dendrites decreases
29% with age. This drop, however, is only marginally statistically
significant. Caution would seem to be indicated in concluding that
these dendrites decrease in total length with age. Examination of
dendritic branching patterns in layer III basal dendrites does not
suggest any definite age-related change in this feature. One measure
of the extent of branching of a dendrite is the number of free
dendritic endpoints (see Figure 1). This measure correlates with
the number of branch points present along the dendritic tree. As
seen in Figure 2, the decrease in number of free endpoints for layer
III basal dendrites is not statistically significant. In contrast
to the layer III neurons, the basal dendrites emanating from layer
V pyramidal neurons appear to undergo a clear reduction in total
length with age. The reduction in mean dendritic length amounts to
approximately 50%. In addition, simplification of branching pattern
is indicated by a 43% decrease in number of free endpoints. With
respect to the oblique branches arising from the apical dendrites
of layer V pyramids, it turns out to be important to specify the
cortical layer in which the branch originates. If all oblique
branches, in layer IV as well as in layer V, are considered together,
highly statistically significant decreases of 36% in total dendrite
length and 21% in number of free endpoints are obtained. Separate
evaluation of the oblique branches arising in layer IV and those
arising in layer V, however, shows that the decreases are attributable
largely to the layer IV oblique branches, as shown in Figure 3.

The finding that the complexity of branching is reduced with age
for layer V basal dendrites and layer V oblique branches in layer IV
does not rest solely on the use of the free endpoint method of
measuring branching complexity. Analysis, for example, of the number

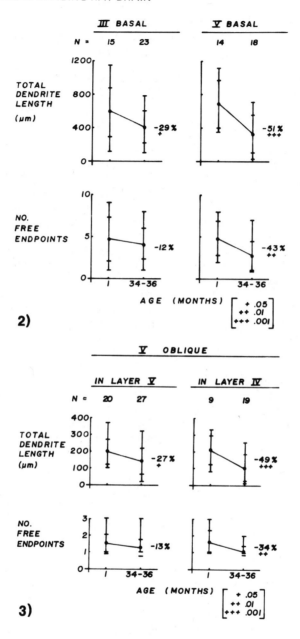

Figure 2. Age differences in total dendrite lengths and number of free endpoints. N's are numbers of individual dendrites measured. Mean, ± 1 standard deviation, and range is indicated for each condition. Statistical significance indicated by + signs.

Figure 3. As Figure 2, for oblique branches.

of branch orders for individual dendrites, where a branch order is
defined as one plus the number of branch points between a branch
and the cell body, leads to the same conclusion.

   The above data do not encourage the speculation that, with age,
dendrites shrink uniformly over their whole extent. If this were
the case, the number of free endpoints would remain unchanged, even
though total dendrite length would be reduced. Exactly how total
dendrite length decreases with age cannot be directly ascertained
by the present techniques. Nevertheless, the data do suggest a
possible mechanism. In considering ways in which dendrite length
might decrease, two models may be proposed, as illustrated in Figure
4. In the first model, whole dendritic branches are lost, at various
locations along the dendritic tree. In the second model, the distoproximal degeneration model, there occurs a dying back, a degenerative
process that begins preferentially at the dendritic tips. The
occurrence of a loss of whole branches initially affecting the distal
branches may be considered a variant of the distoproximal mechanism.
Note that these two models do not exhaust the possibilities. They
merely suggest themselves as plausible. There are several ways to
evaluate the liklihoods associated with the two models. One straight-
forward method, although not absolutely conclusive, is to measure
the furthest extent from the cell body of the distalmost dendritic
tip in the tree. A decrease with age in this value argues in favor
of the distoproximal hypothesis. Such a decrease is, in fact, found.
When measured in three dimensions, along the course of the dendrites,
the 14 young layer V basal dendrites have an average maximum extension
away from the cell body of 225 μm (range 144-310, S.D. 47.5); this
value for the 18 old dendrites is 164 μm (range 38-266, S.D. 57.6).
This difference is statistically significant (.01).

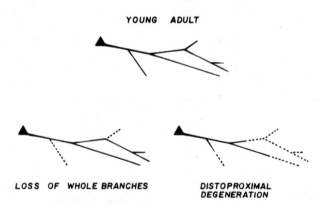

Figure 4.   Above, a schematic representation of a young adult pyramidal cell body and one basal dendrite. Below, two possible modes
of decrease in total dendritic extent with age.

Ultrastructural Observations

The aging apical dendrites reconstructed from serial sections were all of medium diameter and bore from approximately 2.5 to 3.5 spines per μm of dendritic length, a value consistent with that seen in normal young adults (Feldman, 1975). Virtually all of the spines which could be traced to their spine tips were postsynaptic to axon terminals. As judged by the shape of the dendritic profiles, the intermicrotubular spacing, and the mitochondrial density, none of the dendrites were shrunken. These were, then, dendrites which had survived the aging process relatively unscathed. They did, however, contain inclusions similar to those noted in the previous study (Feldman, 1976). The most frequently encountered inclusion was lamellar in form, roughly spherical or ovoid, and usually under 0.5 μm in diameter. The major axis of elongated inclusions was parallel to the axis of the apical dendrites. The typical lamellar periodicity was 50-60 Å, center-to-center. Some of the inclusions were of a vacuolar type (Figures 6a, 7c, 8), while others were relatively solid, with their interior filled with densely or loosely packed lamellae (Figure 10a). The number of lamellar inclusions within the dendrites examined varied from about 1.5 to 3.5 inclusions per μm of dendritic length, and did not appear to be closely related to number or position of dendritic spines. It must be concluded from these observations that the earlier hypothesis relating these inclusions to lost dendritic spines (Feldman, 1976) is not tenable.

A number of reconstructed lamellar inclusions are situated entirely within the confines of the apical dendrite. An unexpected finding, however, was that many of them appeared to communicate with the exterior of the dendrite (Figures 5-10). This probably explains the previously noted tendency (Feldman, 1976) for inclusions to be situated at the dendritic periphery. The communication with the exterior may be via a small finger-like channel (Figures 7, 8) or may consist of a perforation of the dendritic plasma membrane by the entire body of the inclusion (Figure 10b). In several cases, blind-ending finger-like channels, unconnected with larger intradendritic inclusions, were encountered (Figure 9). The most frequent site at which an inclusion or channel communicates with the dendritic exterior is where an axon terminal abuts but does not synapse with the dendritic shaft (Figures 5-10). Lamellar inclusions may also appear in smaller dendrites of uncertain identity (Figure 10), in axon terminals (Figure 5b), and in spine tips (s3 in Figure 5b).

DISCUSSION

Age-related reduction in the length of dendrites has been previously reported in human material. Mehraein, Yamada and Tarnowska-Dziduszko (1975) noted a clear shortening of vermal Purkinje cell dendrites in Alzheimer and senile dementia patients. They suggested

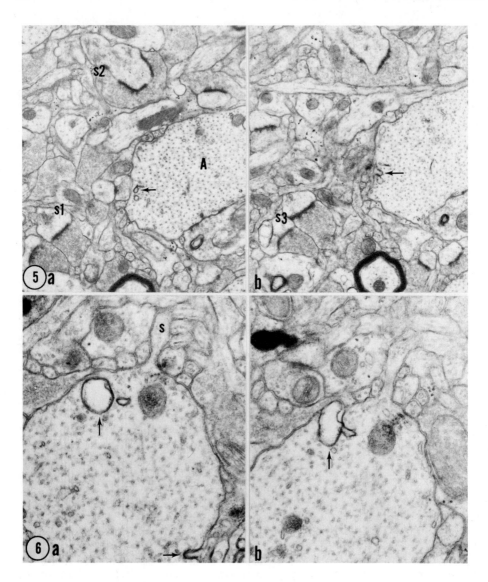

Figure 5. In <u>a</u>, a small lamellar inclusion (arrow) is seen in a
pyramidal apical dendrite (A). The inclusion appears to be open
to the dendritic exterior two sections away, in <u>b</u>. A similar inclusion is seen in the axon terminal at lower right. sl, dendritic
spine with normal spine apparatus. s2, spine with fragmented spine
apparatus. s3, spine with lamellar inclusion. x17,800.
Figure 6. Lamellar inclusion (<u>a</u>, upper arrow) within an apical dendrite and open to the dendritic exterior two sections away, in <u>b</u>.
s, stalk of a dendritic spine. Lower arrow in <u>a</u> indicates an invagination similar to that in Figure 5b. x38,000.

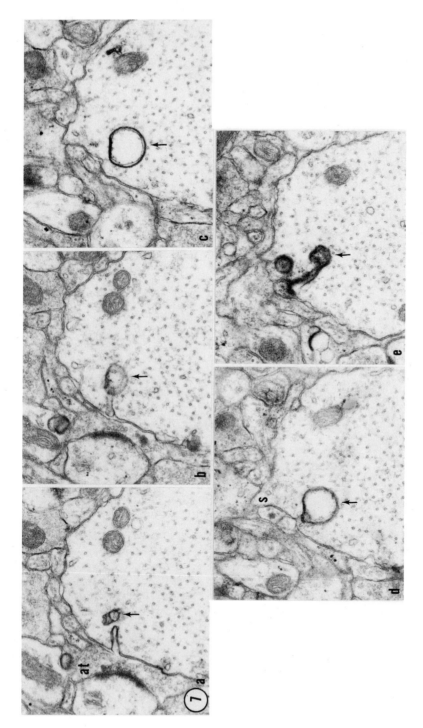

Figure 7. In a, a lamellar invagination protrudes into an apical dendrite near a lamellar inclusion (arrow). The inclusion appears to be continuous with the invagination in b, is sectioned equatorially in c, and appears to communicate with the exterior in d and e. s, stalk of a dendritic spine. x34,600.

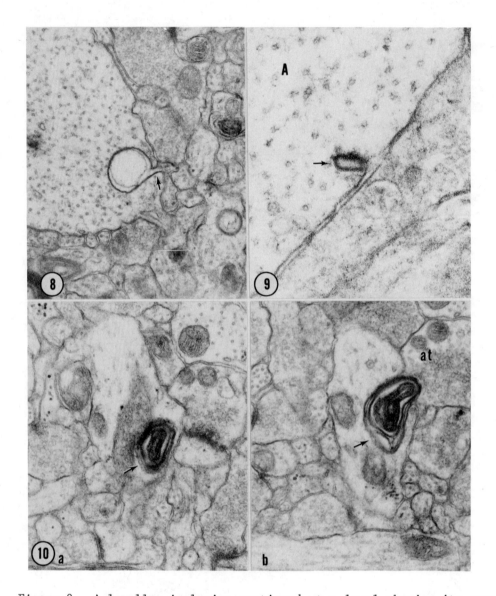

Figure 8. A lamellar inclusion sectioned at a level showing its communication with the exterior of an apical dendrite. x34,600.
Figure 9. An invagination (arrow) into an apical dendrite (A), showing the lamellar character of the wall. x86,000.
Figure 10. A lamellar inclusion (arrow, a) in a non-apical spiny
dendrite. Three sections away (b), the inclusion is seen to be open
to the dendritic exterior and contiguous with an axon terminal (at).
x38,300.

that disturbance of intradendritic transport (Schubert, Kreutzberg and Lux, 1972; Kreutzberg et al., 1973) was important in this phenomenon. Scheibel and Scheibel (1975), in a more extensive study, examined aged patients with and without evidences of senility. They described, particularly in layer III pyramids, in prefrontal and temporal cortex, a reduction and eventual loss of dendrites affecting principally basal and oblique branches. These changes were accompanied and perhaps precipitated by massive intraneuronal accumulations of tubular material (Terry and Wisniewski, 1970), and led to the death of the cell. The Scheibels' observations differ from those of the present study largely with respect to the terminal severity of the process and relative involvement of the layer III and V pyramids.

It seems reasonable to speculate that certain aging changes may not be wholly ascribable to factors intrinsic to the cell. Unfortunately, the identity of any extrinsic elements involved is not yet known. However, because of the dependence of normal dendritic structure upon an intact afferent input (Gelfan, Kao and Ling, 1972; Ghetti, Horoupian and Wisniewski, 1975; Globus and Scheibel, 1967b; Liu and Liu, 1971; Sadlack, 1972; Valverde, 1968), the suspicion arises that age-related changes in the axons synapsing with pyramidal cells may be involved in reduction of post-synaptic dendrites. Examples of possibly significant axonal changes include decrease in number of synapses (Feldman, 1976; Geinisman and Bondareff, 1976), impairment of axonal transport (Bondareff, Geinisman and Telser, 1976), and changes in neurotransmitter balance (Shelanski, 1976). In the specific case of the differential reduction of layer IV and V obliques, it may be noted that these two layers in rat visual cortex differ sharply in the extent to which they receive thalamic axon terminals (Peters and Feldman, 1976). Just how oblique branches in these layers may also differ with respect to intracortical input (Globus and Scheibel, 1967a) is more poorly understood.

Whatever extrinsic factors are involved, they probably interact with aging processes intrinsic to the cell. One intrinsic factor that may be of significance is the possible dependence of dendritic atrophy on distance from the soma. This hypothesis relates in an obvious way to the phenomenon of dendritic transport, mentioned above, and is consistent with the present observations concerning relative shortening of layer IV and layer V oblique branches and with evidence supporting the distoproximal hypothesis (Figure 4).

Intradendritic lamellar inclusions appear not to be direct consequences of the loss of dendritic spines with age. Whether or not the inclusions are at all related to spine loss or to dendritic shrinkage or retraction is not known. Although many inclusions communicate with the dendritic exterior, their multilamellar character suggests that they are not simple infoldings of the plasma membrane; similarly, they are not merely dilatations of the smooth E.R., with which some inclusions are in continuity (Feldman, 1976). The fact

that some serially reconstructed inclusions reside wholly within the
dendrite while others are open to the exterior raises the question
of the relationship between these two forms. It is not known whether
they are of similar origin or whether they are different stages of a
unitary process. Also unclear is their direction of movement, if any,
into or out from the dendrite. That either of these directions of
movement is plausible is suggested by reports of the ability of postsynaptic structures to surround and sequester degenerating presynaptic elements (Gentschev and Sotelo, 1973; Ghetti, Horoupian and
Wisniewski, 1975; Walberg, 1963), and by reports of "dendritic secretion", in which macromolecules are expelled from the dendrite
to the extracellular space (Kreutzberg, Toth and Kaiya, 1975). The
first of these two sets of observations is of particular interest
in view of the proximity of inclusion channels to axon terminals
(e.g., Figure 7a).

    Acknowledgements: This research was supported by N.I.H. grants
AG00001 and NS07016. The computer facility was made available through
N.I.H. grant EY01255 to Washington University; special thanks are due
to Dr. T. A. Woolsey and Dr. W. M. Cowan for their helpfulness with
this phase of the work.

REFERENCES

Bondareff, W., Geinisman, Y. and Telser, A. Age-related changes in
    axonal transport of glycoprotein in the rat septodentate pathway.
    J. Cell Biol., 70:332, 1976.

Colonnier, M. Synaptic patterns on different cell types in the
    different laminae of the cat visual cortex. An electron micro-
    scope study. Brain Res., 9:268-287, 1968.

Feldman, M. L. Serial thin sections of pyramidal apical dendrites
    in the cerebral cortex: spine topography and related observations.
    Anat. Rec., 181:354-355, 1975.

Feldman, M. L. Aging changes in the morphology of cortical dendrites.
    In: Neurobiology of Aging. (Eds. Terry, R. D. and Gershon, S.),
    Aging, vol. 3, Raven Press, New York, 1976.

Feldman, M. L. and Dowd, C. Loss of dendritic spines in aging cere-
    bral cortex. Anat. Embryol., 148:279-301, 1975.

Feldman, M. L. and Dowd, C. Aging in rat visual cortex: light micro-
    scopic observations in layer V pyramidal apical dendrites. Anat.
    Rec., 178:355, 1974.

Feldman, M. L. and Peters, A. A study of barrels and pyramidal den-
    dritic clusters in the cerebral cortex. Brain Res., 77:55-76,
    1974.

Fleischhauer, K., Petsche, H. and Wittkowski, W. Vertical bundles of dendrites in the neocortex. Z. Anat. Entwickl.-Gesch., 136:213-223, 1972.

Geinisman, Y. and Bondareff, W. Decrease in the number of synapses in the senescent brain: a quantitative electron microscopic analysis of the dentate gyrus molecular layer in the rat. Mechan. Ageing and Develop., 5:11-23, 1976.

Gelfan, S., Kao, G. and Ling, H. The dendritic tree of spinal neurons in dogs with experimental hind-limb rigidity. J. Comp. Neur., 146:143-174, 1972.

Gentschev, T. and Sotelo, C. Degenerative patterns in the ventral cochlear nucleus of the rat after primary deafferentation. An ultrastructural study. Brain Res., 62:37-60, 1973.

Ghetti, B., Horoupian, D. S. and Wisniewski, H. M. Acute and long-term transneuronal response of dendrites of lateral geniculate neurons following transection of the primary visual afferent pathway. In: Physiology and Pathology of Dendrites. (Ed. Kreutzberg, G. W.), Advances in Neurology, vol. 12, Raven Press, New York, 1975.

Globus, A. and Scheibel, A. B. Pattern and field in cortical structure: the rabbit. J. Comp. Neur., 131:155-172, 1967a.

Globus, A. and Scheibel, A. B. Synaptic loci on parietal cortical neurons: terminations of corpus callosum fibers. Science, 156: 1127-1129, 1967b.

Gray, E. G. Electron microscopy of synaptic contacts on dendrite spines of the cerebral cortex. Nature, 183:1592-1593, 1959.

Krieg, W. J. S. Connections of the cerebral cortex. I. Albino rat. A. Topography of the cortical areas. J. Comp. Neur., 84:221-275, 1946a.

Krieg, W. J. S. Connections of the cerebral cortex. I. Albino rats. B. Structure of the cortical areas. J. Comp. Neur., 84:277-324, 1946b.

Kreutzberg, G. W., Schubert, P., Toth, L. and Rieske, E. Intra-dendritic transport to postsynaptic sites. Brain Res., 62:399-404, 1973.

Kreutzberg, G. W., Toth, L. and Kaiya, H. Acetylcholinesterase as a marker for dendritic transport and dendritic secretion. In: Physiology and Pathology of Dendrites. (Ed. Kreutzberg, G. W.), Advances in Neurology, vol. 12, Raven Press, New York, 1975.

Liu, C. N. and Liu, C. Y. Role of afferents in maintenance of den-
    dritic morphology. Anat. Rec., 169:369, 1971.

Mehraein, P., Yamada, M. and Tarnowska-Dziduszko, E. Quantitative
    studies on dendrites in Alzheimer's disease and senile dementia.
    In: Physiology and Pathology of Dendrites. (Ed. Kreutzberg,
    G. W.), Advances in Neurology, vol. 12, Raven Press, New York,
    1975.

Peters, A. and Feldman, M. L. The projection of the lateral genicu-
    late nucleus to area 17 of the rat cerebral cortex. I. General
    description. J. Neurocytol., 5:63-84, 1976.

Peters, A. and Walsh, T. M. A study of the organization of apical
    dendrites in the somatic sensory cortex of the rat. J. Comp.
    Neur., 144:253-268, 1972.

Sadlack, F. J. Environmental influences on the developing visual
    cortex of the kitten. Anat. Rec., 172:397, 1972.

Schober, W. and Winkelmann, E. Der visuelle Kortex der Ratte, Cyto-
    architektonik und sterotaktische Parameter. Z. mikrosk.-anat.
    Forsch. (Leipzig), 89:431-446, 1975.

Schubert, P., Kreutzberg, G. W. and Lux, H. D. Neuroplasmic trans-
    port in dendrites: Effect of colchicine on morphology and
    physiology of motoneurons in the cat. Brain Res., 47:331-343,
    1972.

Scheibel, M. E. and Scheibel, A. B. Structural changes in the aging
    brain. In: Aging. (Eds. Brody, H., Harman, D. and Ordy, J.M.),
    vol. 1, Raven Press, New York, 1975.

Shelanski, M. L. Neurochemistry of aging: Review and prospectus.
    In: Neurobiology of Aging. (Eds. Terry, R. D. and Gershon, S.),
    Aging, vol. 3, Raven Press, New York, 1976.

Sholl, D. A. The Organization of the Cerebral Cortex. Methuen,
    London, 1956.

Siegel, S. Nonparametric Statistics for the Behavioral Sciences.
    McGraw-Hill, New York, 1956.

Terry, R. D. and Wisniewski, H. The ultrastructure of the neuro-
    fibrillary tangle and the senile plaque. In: Alzheimer's Dis-
    ease and Related Conditions. (Eds. Wolstenholme, G. E. W. and
    O'Connor, M.), Churchill, London, 1970.

Valverde, F. Structural changes in the area striata of the mouse
    after enucleation. Brain Res., 5:274-292, 1968.

Walberg, F.   Role of normal dendrites in removal of degenerating ter-
    minal boutons. Exp. Neurol., 8:111-124, 1963.

Wann, D. F., Woolsey, T. A., Dierker, M. L. and Cowan, W. M.   An on-
    line digital-computer system for the semiautomatic analysis of
    Golgi-impregnated neurons. I.E.E.E. Trans. Biomed. Engin., BME-
    20:233-247, 1973.

Woolsey, T. A., Dierker, M. L. and Wann, D. F.   Mouse SmI Cortex:
    Qualitative and quantitative classification of Golgi-impregnated
    barrel neurons. Proc. Nat. Acad. Sci., 72:2165-2169, 1975.

DIFFERENTIAL CHANGES WITH AGING IN OLD AND NEW CORTICES

Madge E. Scheibel and Arnold B. Scheibel

Departments of Anatomy and Psychiatry and Brain Research
Institute, U.C.L.A. Center for the Health Sciences
Los Angeles, CA.

> "But an old age serene and bright
> And lovely as a Lapland night
> Shall lead thee to thy grave."

> Wordsworth

Throughout recorded history, the tragedy of aging has been, not that it comes, but that so often, it brings with it a host of changes in the psychosocial patterns of the individual, changes that may degrade and enfeeble the most gallant and competent. We cannot fail to share, as psychiatrists and as human beings, the pain of subject, family, and friends walking this bitter path together. But we must not lose sight of the fact that where substrate mechanisms can be identified, there is hope, if not of a way back, then at least of a gentler path which may give to more of the aged, some measure of those much-celebrated compensations of age.

Structural changes undergone by the aged and the senile brain have been recognized for over one hundred years but estimates of their significance have varied with the particular zeitgeist. The familiar patterns of intracytoplasmic vacuolization and lipofuscin deposition, plaque formation and neurofibrillary degeneration have seemed alternately significant and trivial to successive generations of clinicians and investigators seeking to establish correlation between human psychomotor performance and postmortem histopathology. It was not until the 1960's that apparently meaningful correlations began to be established between human performance levels and hard counts of histopathological entities (Brody, 1973; Corsellis, 1962; Roth et al., 1967; Simon and Malamund, 1965). Here too, however,

39

the curves were scarcely congruent. The threshold concept of Roth
(1972) attempted to account for the apparent step-wise accession
of psychopathology and remains a useful concept today. Nevertheless
with the exception of Brody's (Brody, 1973) neuron loss data, the
causal relationships tying disordered function to altered structure
remain ambiguous. Even cell loss patterns vary greatly ranging from
50% in superior frontal gyrus (Brody, 1973) to almost total quantitative sparing in the inferior olive. Interestingly, the olive
may show another of the apparent stigmata of aging, lipofuscin
accumulation, as early as the first year of life (Hopker, 1951).

Application of the methods of Golgi to brain tissue from aged
and senile subjects has thrown considerable light on the problem
(Mehraein et al., 1975; Scheibel and Scheibel, 1975; Scheibel et al.,
1975). For the first time, it is possible to visualize directly
the increasing loss of those structures most immediately involved
in the development and maintenance of neural connections. The obvious
loss of dendrite spines associated with progressive attenuation of
dendritic envelopes (figure 1) seems to provide an intuitively more
reasonable pathological substrate for waning psychomotor capacities.
Here in panorama is an overall pattern of progressive attenuation of
neural circuitry, the erosion of redundant systems which, carried
beyond critical thresholds, may be responsible for the observed,
rather sudden stepwise failures in human psychomotor function.
Such data also provide a focus for the electron microscopist who
has already supplied valuable insights into the nature of processes
ongoing within the neural envelope (Wisniewski et al., 1970).

As the Golgi methods are particularly suitable in revealing
changes in the soma-dendrite surface and in the qualitative texture
of most components of neuropil, it is important to evaluate the
nature of these changes in the context of conditions which affect
the original sampling. Human tissue is rarely obtained under ideal
experimental conditions. In the laboratory, animal tissue may be
transfered from the living brain to an initially fixed state in a
matter of seconds by perfusion. Human tissue may have to wait for
many hours before administrative procedures release the remains for
postmortem examination. Inevitably, questions arise regarding
selection of tissue-specific pathology in the larger frame of post-
mortem autolytic changes (Fig. 2). While space does not allow
complete recounting of our control procedures, the following items
may be mentioned. Autolytic changes, when they are present, can be
expected to affect the entire tissue block, resulting in recognizable
patterns of swelling and fragmentation with early loss of small
structures. These would include axon terminals, dendrite spines,
finer dendritic tips, etc. The structural changes with which we deal
are usually cell-specific (e.g. many neurons in the immediate surround
appear intact). Ordinarily, the pathology appears to affect parts of
the cell-dendrite system preferentially, i.e. basilar dendrites,

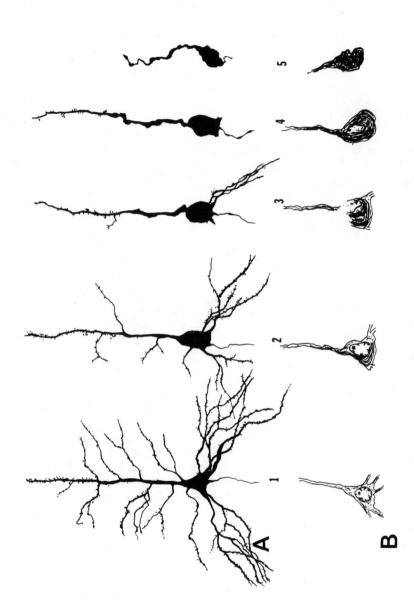

Fig. 1. Summary of progressive changes occurring in neurons of prefrontal neo-cortex with aging and senescence. A, progressive changes as seen with Golgi impregnation methods. B, appearance of neurons stained by a reduced silver method to show neurofibrillary changes of Alzheimer.

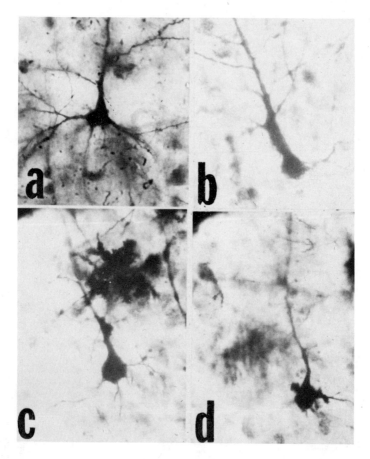

Fig. 2. Progressive changes with aging in neurons of temporal neocortex. a, early changes with some cell body swelling and irregular-
ization of outline in a third layer pyramid (102 yr. old man). b, more
advanced changes with dendrite pathology in third layer pyramid (91
yr. old man). c, similar changes in second layer pyramid (91 yr. old
man). d, far advanced changes in third layer pyramid with total loss
of basilar dendrites (102 yr. old man). Golgi method modifications
X 250.

while leaving other portions relatively or completely intact. Even
the pattern of spine loss and spine sparing show certain regular
features which would be very difficult to explain as a function of the
general process of autolytic deterioration.

    We are presently engaged in companion studies comparing young,
mature, and very old (> 30 months) mice both in terms of possible

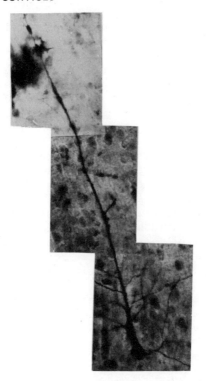

Fig. 3. Photomontage of third layer pyramid in temporal neocortex
of 91 year old man showing loss of dendrite spines, basilar dendrites
and most horizontal branches. Golgi method modification. X 150.

age-related changes and with reference to progressive autolytic
changes (unpublished observations). Under favorable conditions it
has been possible to identify age-related neuronal change throughout
the spinal cord, brain stem, and subcortical nuclei which are similar
to those of human cortex (Fig. 3). Postmortem changes followed on
another graded series with brains fixed at increasingly long periods
after sacrifice have been useful in aiding recognition of the more
generalized effects. Under such conditions, we feel that the results
described as age-related in our blocks of human tissue may be considered valid. Stain methodologies have been described previously
(Scheibel and Scheibel, 1973 and 1975).

THE NEOCORTEX

In previous communications we have described a series of changes
in prefrontal and superior temporal cortex of the aging and senescent
brain. These changes appeared to correlate more closely with the

patient's antecedent level of psychomotor capacities than his
calender age. The changes which we have recently demonstrated
(Scheibel and Scheibel, 1975; Scheibel et al., 1975) include progressive though patchy loss of dendrite spines, changes in the
silhouette of the soma-dendrite complex, and incremental loss of
the entire dendrite domain (Figs. 1-4). Dendritic changes initially
involve horizontal dendritic components and are most obvious in the
basilar dendrite systems.

Progressive loss of this system has been of major interest to
us for several reasons. Earlier work done in our laboratory (Globus
and Scheibel, 1967) indicates that horizontal dendrite systems tend
to become the specific postsynaptic receptor sites for presynaptic
terminals of intracortical derivation. These are presumed to be the
circuit systems most involved with cortico-cortical interactions and
the more subtle aspects of intracortical processing. Our studies
of young and mature cerebral cortex also convince us that the basilar
dendrites, particularly of the large fifth layer pyramidal cells form
dense horizontal plexuses or bundles (Scheibel et al., 1974).
Correlative developmental and histological studies indicate that
such bundles may serve as repository for central programs for the
neuronal systems involved. It follows that the early, selective
loss of these systems, well in advance of similar changes in the
apical shaft, simultaneously disturbs the finer aspects of cortical
function. While eventual total loss of nerve cells becomes an event
of historic and statistical significance, it is equally clear that
the presence of the soma as indicated in any one of a considerable
number of routine histopathological stains is not necessarily in
and of itself the optimal correlate of psychomotor performance.

There seems little doubt that this progressive attenuation in
dendritic neuropil and its eventually resulting neuron loss is a
process ongoing in all neocortical areas, though probably at a pace
specific to the cortical area or zone, and expressed within the
unique genomic pattern of the individual.

THE ENTORHINAL CORTEX

We have had the opportunity of examining several samples of
entorhinal cortex adjacent to the hippocampus proper and structurally
transitional between neocortex and archicortex. While these observations can only be considered preliminary, the results in 3
patients in particular (91, 92, and 102 years old) deserve comment.
In the period before their deaths, these very old individuals showed
what were described as moderate intellectual and emotional changes
commensurate with senility. Two features of the entorhinal cortex
samples from these patients seemed impressive. The first was the
remarkable degree of intactness of the dendritic spine complement

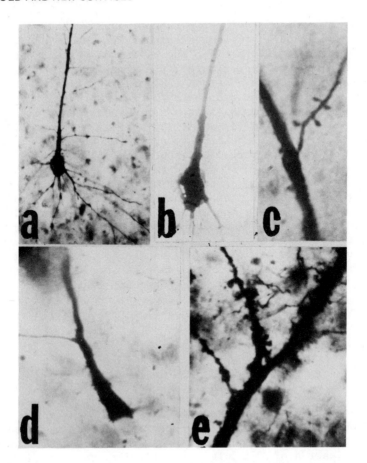

Fig. 4. Various neural elements in the senescent temporal lobe.
a, deep neocortical pyramid showing partial spine loss and attenuation of horizontal dendrite systems. 91 yr. old man X150.
b, same cell photographed at X300 and overexposed to show some
details of surface typography. Somal surface seems rippled and
irregular. c, detail of deep neocortical pyramid showing 4 residual
swollen spines on dendrite branch, 91 yr. old man X600. d,
entorhinal cell of 72 yr. old man showing almost complete loss of
basilar dendrite system, X350. e, detail from CA4 hippocampal
pyramid showing many intact dendrite spines and some attached
mossy tuft terminals, 72 yr. old man, X600.

on a high proportion of the pyramidal cells (pyramids). The second
was the appearance of an unusual histopathological entity along the

apical shaft of many of the deep pyramids which we have not seen
elsewhere. Specifically elongated spindle-like swellings were found
at several different levels along the apical shafts and were often
covered with spines in approximately the same density as the more
normal appearing dendrite shaft on each side. While the majority
of affected entorhinal pyramids bore one such spindle body, some
had two or three. Figure 5a shows a typical deep entorhinal pyramid
with one spindle body located about 150 micra from the cell body.
Note that its dimensions are roughly similar to the soma although
somewhat longer and slimmer, i.e. about 50 micra in length and 10-15
micra in width. Fig. 5b-e shows the partial preservation of spines
along the apical shaft and frequently on the surface of the spindle
body. Figs. 5d and 5e illustrate another interesting feature about
these structures. For any local group of entorhinal pyramids, the
spindle bodies often are located adjacent to each other, at
approximately the same level within the cortex. At the moment, there
is no obvious explanation for this phenomenon although it might
relate either to similarity of gradients in intracellular transport
mechanisms - or lack of them - among adjacent neurons. Alternatively,
the causal process might depend in some manner on an adjacent blood
vessel which would initially affect all of the dendrite systems in
its immediate vicinity.

THE ARCHICORTEX

The hippocampal-dentate complex shares a number of changes with
other cortical areas in the process of aging and senescence. While
some of these changes are routinely demonstrated by the usual
histopathological stains, more dramatic variations can be visualized
through application of the Golgi method. With this technique, a
progressive, perhaps inexorable process which gradually disrupts
the smooth contours of soma and dendrite, can be demonstrated.
Ultimately, this process strips the spine complement from the
dendritic surfaces, and dismembers the dendritic domain, leaving
in the final stages, a swollen or pyknotic cell body surrounded
by neuroglia.

The Hippocampus

A progressive sequence of changes in hippocampal pyramids has
been seen in several of our very old patients (78 - 102 years) as
well as in several who have shown senile dementia changes in their
seventh and eighth decades. The earliest noticeable variations
include irregular swelling of the cell body and of the dendrite
tree, especially at points of bifurcation (Figs. 6c and 11).
Spines are lost in a patchy distribution, often beginning in the
most peripheral portions of the dendrite envelope. Horizontal

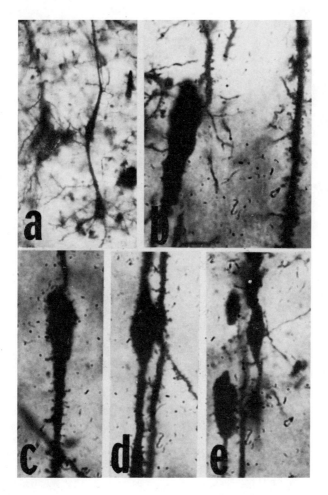

Fig. 5.   Aging changes in pyramids of entorhinal cortex of 102 yr.
old man. a, low power view of pyramidal cell with spindle body
along dendrite about 150 mμ from cell body, X60. b, single spindle
body with broken dendritic stalk and apparently normal adjacent
dendrite shaft with many intact dendrite spines. c, detail of
dendrite shaft with spindle body, both bearing spines. d, details
of 2 adjacent shafts, both spine covered and both apparently bearing
spindle bodies at the same level. e, fragmenting spindle bodies
from several adjacent dendrite shafts.   Stained by Golgi modifications,
X360.

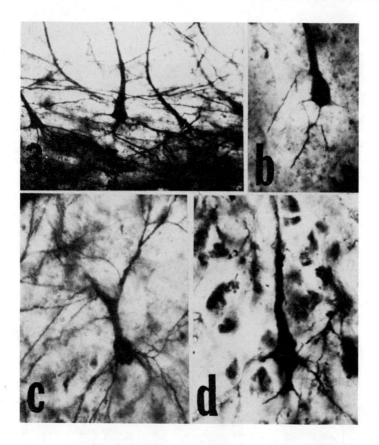

Fig. 6. Changes in hippocampal pyramids in the aging brain. a,
ensemble of hippocampus pyramids in 102 yr. old man showing dendritic
distortions. b, severe loss of basilar dendrites, 91 yr. old man.
c, early changes in CA$_2$ pyramid, 91 yr. old man. d, pigment-filled
cells surround CA$_3$ pyramid losing its basilar dendrites and most
of its spines. Stained by Golgi modifications. a, X150; b, c, d,
X250.

dendrite elements disappear as the process continues resembling
thereby the deterioration pattern of neocortical pyramids. Loss of
basilar dendrites is sometimes dramatic (Figs. 6b and d). In
several of our oldest cases, portions of the apical and basilar
dendrite systems show considerable distortion as if pulled out of
shape by adjacent contracting foci (Figs. 6a and 11). Loss of the
basilar system seems to precede final deterioration of the apical

shafts (Fig. 11) which may have small isolated patches of spines even in very late stages of dissolution.

The Golgi method is not appropriate for quantitative determinations because of the limited and unpredictable nature of its impregnation. This is, of course, simultaneously one of its greatest strengths. We are therefore unable to estimate directly what proportion of the total number of hippocampal pyramids are undergoing this attritional process at any one time, nor the total number of cells which will be affected in some measure in this way. Comparison of Golgi impregnations with Nissl or hematoxylin and eosin controls is not particularly useful here, although some measure of the proportion of neurons involved in some phase of the process of senescence can be gleaned from the number of pigment-filled 'ghost' somata which do show up in Golgi impregnations (Fig. 6d). From these we estimate that by the eighth or ninth decade there is at least minimal involvement of 60-80% of hippocampal somata and progressive dendritic pathology in 20-40%. The first figure is in general agreement with the figures of Tomlinson (Tomlinson, 1972). The second, of course, awaits confirmation from a wider experience with archicortical material.

We are not yet in a position to differentiate clearly among idiosyncratic patterns of soma-dendrite attrition in the various hippocampal subzones. At present we have the distinct impression that dendritic structure and associated components are best preserved in CA_4. Figure 4e is an example of good preservation of pre and postsynaptic structures in this area in a 72 year old man with moderately advanced pathology elsewhere in hippocampus. CA_{1-3} are all capable of showing advanced pathological changes. Our own limited experience indicates the greatest amount of change occurs in CA_3.

The Dentate Gyrus

Progressive changes in the cell body and dendritic complement of dentate granules appears to be a regular feature of the aging brain, although, as in other sites, there is considerable variability of pattern and the extent of change which does not seem closely tied to the chronological age of the individual. In our experience so far, the sequence of change is quite similar to that in other cortical systems, and includes development of swelling and irregularities of outline in soma and dendrite shafts, patchy loss of dendrite spines, and the appearance of nodular enlargements, especially at dendritic terminals and branch points (Figs. 7a-e). Unusually long and/or swollen spines may be left in small individual groups for some time after the majority have disappeared.

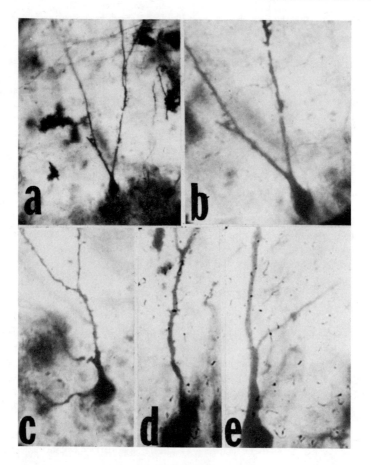

Fig. 7. Changes in dentate granule cells in the aging brain. a
and b, 2 views of dentate granule cell from 72 yr. old man showing
loss of part of the dendrite envelope and almost complete loss of
dendrite spines. c, granule with a few scattered residual spines in
72 yr. old man. d, dendrite shaft of granule with scattered spines
in 102 yr. old man. e, dentate granule in 102 yr. old man with
partial loss of dendrite system and almost complete loss of spines.
Stained by Golgi modifications. a, X150, b, c, d, X350.

     Attenuation of the dendritic domain is also a prominent feature
of the process (Figs. 7c and 7d). Dentate granules have no basilar
dendrite system, and seldom an unpaired apical shaft. The progressive
diminution of the dendrite domain is expressed, rather, in loss of
second and third order dendrite branches (Lindsay and Scheibel, in

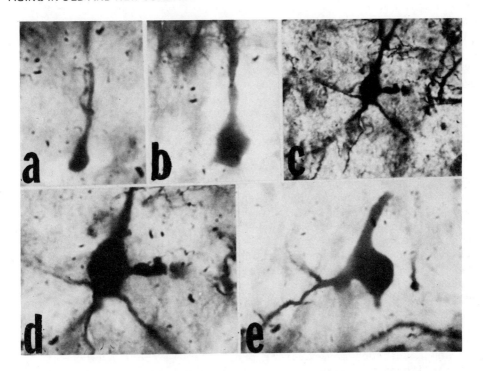

Fig. 8. Changes in hippocampal-dentate complex neurons in 30 month old mouse. a and b, dentate granules showing distortions of soma-dendrite silhouette and loss of dendritic mass. c, CA$_2$ pyramid showing partial loss of basilar dendrites. d and e, CA$_2$ and CA$_3$ pyramids showing swelling of somata and partial loss of basilar dendrite systems. Stained by Golgi modifications. Magnifications: a and c, X600; b and d, X800. (Courtesy of Dr. J. Machado-Salas).

press) and shortening or falling back of the entire bifurcating dendrite apparatus upon the cell body (Figs. 8a, 8b and 10). We are not able to estimate the proportion of dentate granules whose dendrite envelopes follow this degenerative sequence. However, it is worth noting that in most of our Golgi material where the presence of cell body 'ghosts' provides an index as to general configuration of the cell body layer, (and in our aniline stained control material) the layer of dentate cell bodies seems to remain essentially intact. This is so even in the very old and senile, whose dentate gyri show tightly packed somata and relatively modest glial invasion. This is in accord with the relatively greater intactness of the dentate granule population in temporal lobe epilepsy (Scheibel and Scheibel, 1973).

OVERVIEW OF THE DATA

The results of this investigation, taken together with our previous reports indicate an overall pattern of neuronal change proceeding inexorably in both neocortex and archicortex. While the brains of presenile and senile dements serve as the histo-pathological model in its most florid form, it is clear that similar changes, in milder form and to varying degrees, invariably character-ize the aging process. The changes which we have found in old, transitional, and new cortices are, to some extent, idiosyncratic, but the dominant theme appears to consist in progressive restriction of the amount of dendritic surface together with loss of spines. Where the involved neurons have both apical and basilar dendrite systems, the latter developing latest in the course of ontogeny are also the first to be lost (Scheibel and Scheibel, 1975). We have commented previously on the possible functional significance of this type of loss in neocortex where the horizontal systems appear to receive synaptic inputs of intracortical origin (Globus and Scheibel, 1967). Additionally, the basilar dendrite system, especially of fifth layer pyramids, generate densely intertwined bundle systems which have been proposed as repositories for central programs (Scheibel, 1974). A hypothesis would be that the type of dendrite loss which characteristically accompanies the process of aging and senescence may restrict progressively those aspects of cortical circuitry involved in the most subtle types of cortical processing, as well as destroying, incrementally repositories of program storage.

In our present study, emphasis on entorhinal (transitional) cortex and archicortex has revealed several factors worth further comment. The spindle bodies which appear unique to entorhinal deep pyramids constitute, so far as we now know, part of a special degenerative pattern also marked by unusually long maintenance of dendrite spines and less obvious, generalized distinctive dendritic pathology, until the primary dendrite shaft actually begins to fragment (Fig. 9). The significance of the spindle body and its relationship to pathological processes remains to be determined. Electron microscopic evaluation will be needed to determine whether these structures represent areas of enhanced production of abnormal tubulin (Wisniewski et al., 1970) or are more similar to initial segment enlargements of meganeurites as described by Purpura (personal communication) in Tay-Sach's disease, and which also are spine covered.

The fairly precise placement of groups of these spindle bodies at the same height in entorhinal cortex is also of considerable interest and may, in fact, prove of possible etiological significance. If the geographic clustering is related to the position of vascular channels in cortex, this might suggest direct dependence of the

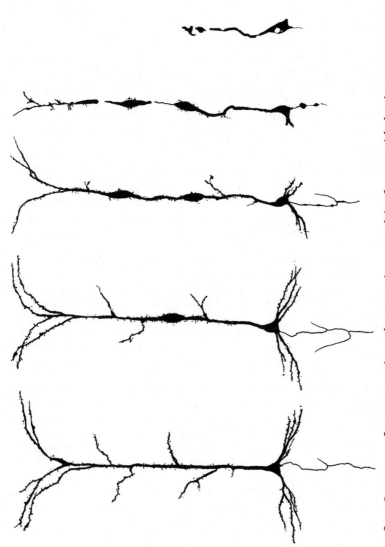

Fig. 9. Summary of progressive changes in entorhinal pyramid during senescence.

pathological element on some factor which arrives via the blood
stream, whether virus, auto-immune bodies or other factors. In
this regard it is interesting that in our Golgi studies of tissue
specimens from patients with temporal lobe epilepsy, we were struck
by the wide range of pathological change from small focal areas of
spine loss and dendritic nodulation affecting only part of a single
dendrite (Fig. 10), to far advanced pathological states resulting
in cell death (Scheibel and Scheibel, 1973). Such findings led us
to the tentative conclusion that temporal lobe epilepsy may constitute
an ongoing, progressive syndrome rather than a clinical monument to
birth trauma. Furthermore, in series of unpublished observations,
we have found that local dendrite pathology such as spine loss and
dendritic nodulation frequently occurs initially in the proximity
of blood vessels, especially abnormal appearing vessels, thereby
raising similar questions of possible infectious or auto-immune
etiology.

The appearance of developing pathological changes in hippocampal
neurons is similar to those we have described in prefrontal, parietal,
and temporal cortices (Fig. 11). We are impressed repeatedly by the
probability that an ongoing process which may produce minimal change
in a nerve cell body when viewed with the usual histopathological
methods, may have already damaged that neuron as a functioning
element in a matrix of neural circuitry, through impairment of the
dendritic domain. Quantitative estimates of the number of senile
plaques, of Alzheimer's neurofibrillary changes, of granulovacuolar
degeneration and of cell body fall out (Brody, 1973; Tomlinson, 1972),
have been used in attempts to establish relationships between
disturbed function and underlying substrate pathology. We suggest
that a more sensitive measure of hippocampal pathology may be found
in the pattern and extent of loss of dendritic surface area.

It is now fairly well recognized that in most spine bearing
cortical neurons, it is the spine itself, rather than the dendritic
surface which receives the great majority of synaptic terminals
(Colonnier, 1966). In the most precise sense, then, it would be
the total number of functioning, residual spines which would constitute the significant variable for correlation purposes.

The functional sequellae of progressive impairment of the human
hippocampus and entorhinal cortex during the process of senescence is
not yet clear. The general relationship between memory function and
the temporal lobe seems established (Milner, 1972) although a precise
localization of function is not known. Recent physiological studies
by O'Keefe (1976) and others seem to provide support for a cognitive
mapping function for hippocampus, where very small cell clusters
encode data for a vast number of identifying characteristics of
'familiar' environments. Granting the problems in cross-species
transposition, if the human hippocampus should share similar functions,

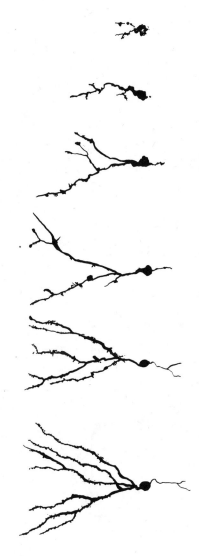

Fig. 10. Summary of progressive changes in dentate granule cell during senescence.

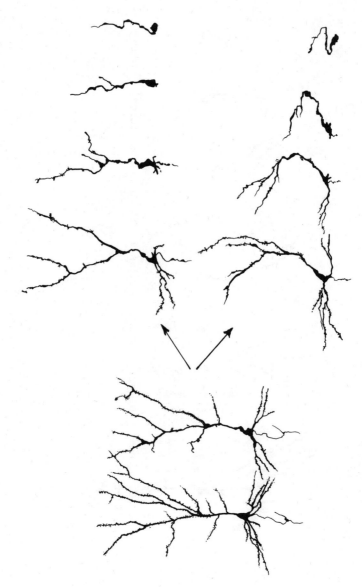

Fig. 11. Summary of progressive changes in the hippocampal pyramid showing two possible sequences of senescent changes.

some degree of 'explanation' might then be at hand for the distressing inability of the senescent individual to maintain his
orientation in space and time. Progressive attrition of the neural
elements and synaptic connections concerned with mapping the time-
space envelope around the individual could render him vulnerable
and unattached, eyless in Gaza, and a stranger in time.

Acknowledgements: This study was supported by USPHS grant
N.S. 10567. Dr. Uwamie Tomiyasu provided the human tissue specimens,
and Mr. Abe Green helped in preparing the histological material.

REFERENCES

Brody, H. Aging of the Vertebrate Brain. In: Development and
    Aging in the Nervous System, (Ed. M. Rockstein), Academic
    Press, New York, pp. 121-133, 1973.

Colonnier, M. In: Brain and Conscious Experience, (Ed. J. C.
    Eccles), Berlin-Heidelberg, N.Y. Springer, pp. 1-23, 1966.

Corsellis, J. A. N. Mental Illness and the Aging Brain, Institute
    of Psychiatry, Mandstey Monograph #9 Oxford University Press,
    London, 1962.

Globus, A. and Scheibel, A.B. Pattern and Field in Cortical
    Structure: The Rabbit. J. Comp. Neurol. 131:155-172, 1967.

Hopker, W. Das Altern des Nucleus Dentatus. Z. Alternforsch. 5:
    256-277, 1951.

Lindsay, R.D. and Scheibel, A.B. Quantitative Analysis of Dendritic
    Branching Pattern of Dentate Granule Cells from Human Dentate
    Gyrus. Exp. Neurol., In Press.

Mehraein, P., Yamada, M. and Tarmowska-Dziduszko, E. Quantitative
    Study on Dendrites and Dendritic Spines in Alzheimer's Disease
    and Senile Dementia. In: Psychology and Pathology of Dendrites,
    (Ed. G. W. Kretzberg), Raven Press, N.Y., pp. 453-458, 1975.

Milner, B. Disorders of Learning and Memory After Temporal-lobe
    Lesions in Man. Clin. Neurosurgery 19:421-446, 1972.

O'Keefe, J. Units in the Hippocampus of the Freely Moving Rat.
    Exp. Neurol. 51:78-109, 1976.

Roth, M. Recent Progress in the Psychiatry of Old and its Bearing
    on Certain Probelms of Psychiatry in Earlier Life. Biol.
    Psychiat. 5:103-125, 1972.

Roth, M., Tomlinson, B.E. and Blessed, G. The relationship between
    Quantitative Measures and Degenerative Changes in the Cerebral
    Grey Matter of Elderly Subjects. Proc. R. Soc. Med. 60:254-260,
    1967.

Scheibel, M.E. and Scheibel, A.B. Structural Changes in the Aging
    Brain. In: Aging Vol. 1, (Eds. H. Brody et al.), Raven Press,
    New York, pp. 11-37, 1975.

Scheibel, A.B., Scheibel, M.E., Davis, T.L. and Lindsay, R.D.
    Basilar Dendrite Bundles of Giant Pyramidal Cells. Exp. Neurol.
    42:307-319, 1974.

Scheibel, M.E., Lindsay, R.D., Tomiyasn, U. and Scheibel, A.B.
    Progressive Dendritic Changes in Aging Human Cortex. Exp. Neurol.
    17:392-403, 1975.

Simon, A. and Malamund, N. Comparison of Clinical and Neuropathologi-
    cal Findings in Geriatric Mental Illness. In: Psychiatric
    Disorders in the Aged, Geigy, Manchester, U.K., p. 322, 1965.

Tomlinson, B.E. Morphological Brain Changes in Non-Dementia Old
    People. In: Aging of the Central Nervous System, (Eds. H. M.
    Van Praag and A. K. Kalverboen), Dr. Envon F. Bohm, N. Y.,
    pp. 38-57, 1972.

Wisniewski, H.M., Terry, R.D. and Hirano, A. Neurofibrillary
    Pathology, J. Neuropathol. Exp. Neurol. 29:163-176, 1970.

EFFECTS OF AGE-RELATED RANDOM AND COORDINATED LOSS OF MEMORY ENGRAMS ON ERROR RATES DURING MEMORY RETRIEVAL

Bernard L. Strehler

Division of Biological Sciences
University of Southern California
Los Angeles, CA.   90007

I.   INTRODUCTION

Age-related memory dysfunction and attendant changes in that curious entity called "self", as well as its perception by other selves and by itself, are among the most distressing of the changes that are intrinsic to the aging process. The amelioration of age related memory defects would seem best based on an understanding of how memory engrams are stored within and retrieved from the remarkable machine, the brain is. This paper briefly presents the essence of a mechanistic theory of memory storage and retrieval within and from the cerebral cortex, outlines potential sources of memory deficits implicit in this model and relates the above to recent anatomical, physiological, and mathematical observations. In particular, the implications of these observations with respect to differential effects between random cell attrition during aging and non-randomized cell loss (localized infarcts, senile dementia, etc.) are considered.

II.   MEMORY STORAGE: A Brief outline of a mechanistic theory

Portions of the theory have been published elsewhere and a comprehensive presentation is being prepared for publication in the near future (Strehler, 1976a,b). The essential components are:
1.   Sensory inputs are transformed into unique patterns of pulses in time by virtue of the transmission of single input pulses to successive neurons over parallel lines of different length (Strehler, 1969).
2.   Such delay line networks in effect generate a coded representation of each separate input source, i.e. the code consists of a pattern of pulses in time unique to each separate input source.

3.   These different pulse patterns are widely distributed within appropriate portions of the brain to matching delay line decoder networks. However, they only cause a response when the several pulses that make up a pattern summate spatially on selected decoding neurons. Generally a decoding neuron will not respond if only a single copy of a pulse pattern is presented to it during its de-coding-integrating time.

4.   Provided that such a decoding network is temporarily or permanently facilitated as a result of the above decoding operations, it will be able, subsequently, to regenerate a pattern of pulses which is complementary to the triggering input in the specific sense that the output will consist of the mirror image (in time) of the input pattern.

5.   A second round of decoding-recoding therefore results in the regeneration of the originally-detected input pattern. This provides a means through which coded representations of past inputs (memories) may be recovered from the system, upon appropriate cueing.

6.   Combinations of coded representations of "simultaneous" inputs to the cortex are stored redundantly in a number of different cortical columns, specifically those that sub-serve the input modality that provided the coded input informational patterns.

7.   Such storage is postulated to involve the facilitation of selected patterns of synapses between recurrent collaterals of layer 5 pyramids and the dendritic spines at the bases, along the vertical shafts and in the regions of the terminal arborizations of layer 3 pyramids that are part of a functional "column" or cortical module (Hubel and Wiesel, 1969; Szentagothai, 1975). In effect, each functional unit or module serves as an address for the storage of related data input patterns.

8.   In addition, it is proposed that patterns of pulses (stand-ing for addresses) are stored in the form of facilitated synapses between the apical branches of layer 3 pyramids and axons derived from associative and callosal fibers traversing layer 1 horizontally as described by Szentagothai. Storage of these addresses also occurs between recurrent axons of layer 3 pyramids and the shafts and apices of layer 5 pyramids. The layer 3 and layer 5 pyramids thus act reciprocally on each other, each decoding messages (data codons or address codons) that are then stored in the other cell type.

9.   Retrieval of such stored coded information may occur in either of two alternative modes: (a) through the input of cueing data which generates the output of addresses corresponding to the cues applied or (b) through the input of addresses derived from other parts of the system, which inputs cause the output of data stored associatively with the addresses addressed. Stated otherwise, such a reciprocal capacity of addresses to generate data as output and of data to generate addresses as output provides a highly efficient means for the storage and retrieval of data because the system can effectively be searched in parallel. This, unlike present day digital machines, permits a whole lifetime of memory to be searched in real time.

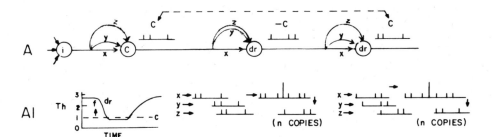

Fig. 1.   Some Elementary Operations Described in Theory.
A: Input at cell (i) results in output of pattern (C); decoding-
recoding of C by dr results in output of anticodon(-C); decoding-
recoding of (-C) yields (C).
Al: Left inset: Facilitation (f) of decoder-recoder (dr) occurs as
result of spatial summation of (C) via paths x,y and z; Threshold
of coder (c) is unaltered.   Right: Indicates mode of spatial
summation via delay-line networks and outputs derived in multiple
copies.

        10.   It should be emphasized that data are not stored in direct
association with each other.   Rather, data points (patterns standing
for particular input combinations) are stored in association with
appropriate combinations of addresses concurrently.   This concept
is in accordance with the experiments and interpretations of Lashley
(1929).
        11.   Retrieval of serial sets of stored data occurs through the
sequential addressing of different combinations of columns (addresses),
the combined outputs of which are "examined", as it were, for data
present in highest redundancy, a process closely reminescent of
contrast enhancement in the visual system and elsewhere, effected
through lateral inhibition (Eccles, 1973).   Such highest redundancy
data outputs are then perceived as the correct "memory traces",
derived directly or indirectly from cueing inputs.
        12.   An advantage of particular significance implicit in the
redundant storage of the same sets of data in different combinations
of addressable columns is that each column may, under these circum-
stances, be used to store many different sets of data, thus enhancing
greatly the efficiency of usage of available "memory space".
        13.   Such increased efficiency of memory space use however occurs
at the expense of memory "ambiguity" errors, errors of a predictable
magnitude.   There is an increasing probability (as the "bins" com-
prising a particular combination of columns become filled to a greater
and greater degree), that random coincidences in particular stored
data points will occur during retrieval and be indistinguishable from

true data. Generally, such storage ambiguity noise will increase as a function of memory filling and decrease as a function of redundancy of storage at any particular level of filling of memory bins.

14. Finally, the items stored in permanent memory are very few compared to the totality of inputs provided to the system during a lifetime. Selective storage occurs through two different kinds of rehearsal. The first of these is caused by the redundant presentation of the same pattern of inputs repeatedly and at different times; the second occurs through unconscious rehearsal (putatively mediated by the amygdala and hippocampus) of data which was presented to the system in an emotionally evocative situation. Stated otherwise, if a particular experience occurs which has a high emotional connotation this experience is stored more indelibly within the cortex than are routine experiences because it is rehearsed unconsciously (i.e. without awareness of the subject's rehearsal process). Such an unconscious rehearsal need only involve the re-presentation of addresses that have recently been used to store data points. Such addresses are perhaps what is temporarily stored in the hippocampus and re-transmitted to the previously active cortical columns if the affect is sufficiently great. However, if the data stored in these address combinations is not to reach the conscious level, the addresses must be re-presented to the cortex in scrambled (randomized) form in time. Otherwise they would interfere with the efficient processing of continuing inputs to the system.

III.   ANALYSIS OF SOURCES OF MEMORY DYSFUNCTION

In general, only three kinds of changes during aging, could be responsible for the gradual failure of memory. These are:
    (1) Changes in the properties of individual neurons;
    (2) Changes in the interactions between neurons; and
    (3) Loss of neurons, either randomly with respect to each others' locations or focally (i.e. concurrent loss of many adjacent neurons). As will be demonstrated in the last part of this paper, the latter would be expected to have much more drastic effects on memory and performance, particularly of serial tasks, either mental or motor. Some of these changes have been discussed more extensively in previous publications (Strehler, 1976a,b). In the following paragraphs some of these concepts will be reviewed, particularly, the differences to be expected from random loss of neuronal elements as compared to those anticipated if many neurons subserving the same group of memory engrams are lost simultaneously, through local infarcts or senile plaque formation.

A.   Changes in Neuronal Properties: There are a number of documented age-changes in neurons: accumulation of Age Pigments (Reichel et al., 1968), accumulation of neurofibrillary tangles in certain locales (Terry et al., 1976) and changes in DNA which strongly suggest that the genes coding for ribosomal RNA are progressively

lost during aging are among the more recent quantitative findings
(Johnson et al., 1972, 1975). While the accumulation of age pigments
and neurofibrillary tangles is not demonstrably harmful during normal
levels of activity, these inclusions very probably decrease the
reserve capacity of neurons to function at maximum rates for extended
periods of time. They therefore probably contribute to the earlier
onset of mental fatigue characteristic of many older persons. It is
unlikely on the basis of first principles that occupancy of up to
75% of perinuclear volume by age pigments as observed by Mann and
Yates (1974) would fail to reduce the cells' content of functional
elements such as mitochondria and Nissl substance (rRNA). In fact,
Mann and Yates observed a reciprocal relationship between lipofuscin
content and rRNA in individual cells in microspectrophotometric
studies. Similarly, whether neurofibrillary tangles are a cause or
an effect of some other pathological process, their presence is both
associated with regions of plaque formation and the latter are clearly
associated with greatly diminished mental ability, afflictions so
marked that they are termed dementia. The evident loss of rDNA
genes during aging in various postmitotic tissues including brain
(dogs) and in human myocardium, implies that the maximum rate of
protein synthesis will decrease, particularly when heavy work demands
are put on the system, (provided, of course, that the transcription
of rRNA limits the availability of ribosomes for synthetic activities).
The decrement of Nissl substance with age and its slower repletion
following depletion under stress (Andrew et al., 1952) is probably
related to the evident loss of rDNA during aging.

     B. Changes in Neuron-Neuron Interactions: This area possesses
many possible, though by and large uninvestigated, sources of memory
dysfunctions during aging. In particular, because neurons not only
transmit information from place to place within the brain, but also
regulate the processing of such information by other neurons, changes
in the efficiency of regulatory functions (such as redundancy detection, address advance, vigilance, attention span, and efficacy of
storage of memories in consolidated form) would all be expected to
decrease the efficiency of processing of information and of recall.
Implicit in the model presented here and elsewhere are certain
predictable decrements. These will not, however, be discussed in
detail at this time. However, it should be pointed out that the
reticular formation, probably involved in EEG control (periodic
stimulation of this system is capable of driving the EEG) has a
certain phase relationship to the firing of individual neurons.
It may well be that the reticular formation's activity is key to the
sorting out of high redundancy engrams from lower redundancy ones
during memory retrieval and (cueing of) memory access, and probably
also this system is involved in the sequential activation of different
combinations of addresses (columns) in an orderly and coordinated
fashion. Therefore, any lesions in this structure or in the diffuse
reticular projection to the cortex would be expected to result in a
decrease in the efficiency of memory retrieval, even in the absence

of pathologies within the engram storage systems themselves.

Implicit in the coding-decoding-coding operations outlined in section II, above, is the concept of a relatively precise match between the delay line networks that generate coded patterns of data and the networks that decode such information (a communication channel). Obviously, it would be of little utility if the number of discriminable channels (represented by discrete, recognizable patterns of pulses) a system could generate and detect were less than the number of separate channels needed to transmit and process coded information. Two factors determine the number of separate channels that can be discriminated from each other: (a) the precision with which the time difference between pulses in a train can be differentiated and (b) the number of pulses used to make up a pattern train. In general, the number of separate channels that can be detected is given by the expression $C_h = \dfrac{X^{(n-1)}}{(n-1)}$ (Equation 1), where X = the number of separate intervals that can be discriminated one from another, where n = the number of separate pulses that make up an individual train (codon), and where C_h = the number of discriminable channels. Examples: if the code is doublet and if x = 500, 500 channels can be discriminated; if the code is triplet (n = 3) and x is 500, C_h = 125,000. If x is only 100 and a quadruplet code is used 166,666 channels may be discriminated. Clearly, such a system of coding makes very economical use of pulses in defining (symbolizing) channels!

The exact match concept (between coder and decoder) is clearly very crucial in the transmission and decoding of coded information and would be expected to be very sensitive to any change in the system which would differentially alter the conduction time (velocity) either in the coder or in the decoder networks. One such important variable during aging, may be "local temperature" within different portions of the brain. Because the local temperature is determined by the balance between heat production within the brain and the rate of its removal by the circulation (assuming that the temperature of blood arriving at the brain is essentially uniform), it follows that any differential change in blood flow within coder and decoder regions will inevitably "detune" coders from their decoders and have dramatic or drastic effects on memory retrieval. Partial occlusion of specific arteries (due to spasms, edema following trauma, emboli, defects in local regulation of blood flow, etc.) will result in temporary and reversible defects in memory or motor functions (e.g. mild strokes). Permanent changes in blood flow in limited regions will permanently detune coders and decoders from each other and result in more or less permanent loss of memory or motor functions dependent on the affected area, with or without cell death.

C. Cell Loss: The death of brain cells during aging appears

to occur through two quite different processes: one of these is a
gradual decrease in brain mass, ascribable, in part, at least to
losses of cells in layer 4 of the cortex. Loss of Purkinje cells
from the cerebellum was reported many years ago by Ellis (1920) and
more recently, careful studies have revealed modest to marked cell
attrition in many if not all brain regions (Brody, 1976; Brizzee
et al., 1976). There is also evidence that the number of synapses
in certain regions of the brains of experimental animals decreases
with age (Bondareff et al., 1976; Terry et al., 1976). The remainder
of this paper will deal with predictable effects of such losses on
memory functions as derived from the basic postulates of the model
presented in part II.

IV.   EFFECTS OF ENGRAM ATTRITION ON MEMORY RETRIEVAL

A detailed discussion of the proposed pathways and functional
interactions between cells within a column will be presented elsewhere. In order, however, to proceed logically in the following
discussion, an elementary relationship presented by Szentagothai (1975)
needs to be reiterated. Four cell types must interact in order to
store an engram (data point vs address) in memory and during retrieval
of this relationship from memory. These cells are: (1) the spinous
pyramids, (2) stellates of upper layer 4, (3) the layer 3 and (4)
layer 5 large pyramids. One group of layer 4 cells transmits
information via recurrent axons to the shafts of layer 5 pyramids;
the other transmits information (probably addresses) to the layer
3 pyramids (See Fig. 2A). As mentioned earlier, each class of
pyramid decodes and inverts (in time) the patterns it receives and
transmits these to the other class of pyramids in whose basal (layer 3
pyramids), shaft and apical branches facilitation occurs--synapses
--via recurrent collaterals of the large pyramids of layers 3 and 5,
reciprocally (See Figs. 1; 2B,C; 3). Should any cell in this ensemble
of 4 making up a sub-part of a functional unit fail to function, the
unit as a whole would cease to function! However, because information
is evidently stored redundantly for reasons of economy the loss of
any single functional unit will not appreciably interfere with memory
function.

A.   Basic Rules Relating Redundant Storage and Storage Noise

1. Advantages of Redundant Storage: The apical branches of
layer 3 and 5 pyramids reportedly possess between 10^4 and 10^6 synapses.
Clearly, if only one pattern of pulses were stored (through synaptic
facilitation) in each pyramid, a vast amount of potentially usable
"storage space" would be wasted. Furthermore, it would be necessary
to provide a separate group of cells in each sensory modality for each
possible instant in time in which memories might be stored. The
number of such units needed for a 100 year lifetime would be about

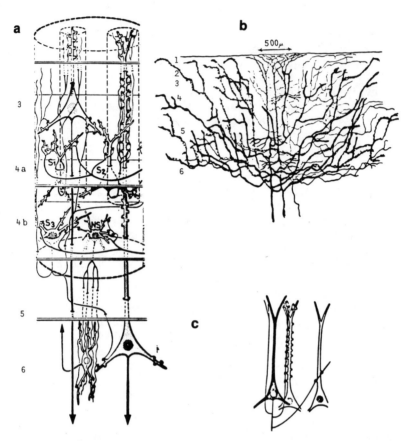

Fig. 2.   Some Elementary Anatomical Relationships between Pyramids and
Layer 4a Stellates and Star Pyramids: A.   The two cell types denoted
S_1 and S_2 receive inputs and transmit excitation to layer 3 and layer
5 pyramids, respectively.   After Szentagothai (1975); B.   Recurrent
collatorals of three pyramidal cells.   The heavy lines represent
collaterals from layer 5 pyramids; the light lines represent collaterals from layer 3 pyramids.   Note that the layer 5 collaterals possess
essentially vertical segments, in most cases, in the vertical shaft
regions of layer 3 pyramids.   Thus these collaterals are suited to
establish the multiple synaptic "bins" as well as the multiple
contacts with the apical branches, as described in the text. (After
Scheibel and Scheibel, 1970); C.   Nature of collaterals between
adjacent pyramidal cells.   According to Szentagothai (1975), there
is a decreasing probability of multiple contacts between recurrent
axons of one cell and its neighbors' dendritic shafts as the distance
between cells increases.   That this may not be the case as suggested
by an examination of Figure 2B.

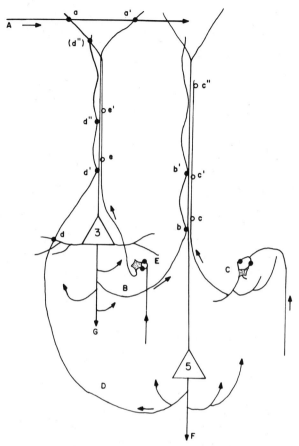

Fig. 3. Basic Neuronal Circuit Which Permits Storage of Data VS
Address in a Cortical Module: An address pattern derived from another
module traverses layer 1 axon at A. This pattern is decoded at a and
a' and causes cell 3 to transmit multiple copies of this pattern via
B to the apical dendrites of cell 5, where this pattern is stored as
facilitated synapses b and b'. Simultaneously, data patterns received
by cell C, a star pyramid, are decoded at c, c' and c'' and cause cell
5 to emit the mirror image of the data pattern which is transmitted
via collateral D to cell 3 where it is stored at synapses d, d' and
d''. (Note: the d'' in parentheses (d'') indicates that portions of
patterns may be stored in the apical dendritic branches of layer 3
pyramids.). To generate the data associated with a particular address
when that address is presented via E, a stellate in upper lamina 4,
the address is decoded (and inverted, if it consists of more than 2
pulses) at synapses e and e', and transmitted via a recurrent axon to
synapses b, b' which, previously facilitated, cause cell 5 to fire
and to generate outputs as synapses d, d' and d'' are traversed when
cell 3 is close to its threshold. The output from this cell and other
cells in the module consists of multiple copies of the various data
points previously stored with that address. Each of the layer 3 and
layer 5 cells make connections with the opposite cell type within a

module via the recurrent axons originating at the base of the pyramids.
Only a single such recurrent axon for each cell type is shown in the
diagram (in the interests of clarity). To generate copies of the
address associated with cueing input data patterns, the data is
presented via cell C, its time inverted pattern is transmitted and
decoded by synapses d, d' and d", and the output of the address
occurs as a pulse traverses previously facilitated synapses b and
b'. The address appears as output at the bottom of cell 5 (at F).
Data patterns appear as outputs at G.

2×10^{10}, a number not dissimilar from the total number of cells in
the CNS. (!!) On the other hand, if only 4000 columns (addresses)
were present and were subdivided into groups of 999,1000,1001,1002,
the number of separate combinations of such columns taken 4 at a time
would be about 10^{12}. Therefore, provided that each recorded instant
is stored redundantly in a different address combination, the system
can provide many times the number of addresses (combinations) needed
to store a whole life-time of memory engrams redundantly. The
surprising conclusion is that redundancy of storage increases the
efficiency with which a given amount of storage space can be utilized
---essentially because each column may participate in the storage of
many different patterns of input combinations. The consequences of
this relationship have been examined mathematically and the conclusions, sans derivations, are presented in the following pages.

     2. Relationship between number of items entered in an address
and number of items stored in such address: If one defines the number
of items (data points) that could maximally be stored in an address
as m(the number of separate "bins" in which data points may be
recorded) and if the number of data items presented for storage is
designated as n, the number of items actually stored will be less
than the number of items presented, because identical data points
will, on a chance basis, be parts of many different combinations of
input patterns. The number of data points actually stored within an
address (or column) may be designated n, and the ratio n'/m in effect
defines the percentage of bins filled in a given address. The equation
that relates the ratio of entries to bins (n/m) to the percentage
occupancy of bins (n'/m) is:
$$n'/m = 1 - \frac{1}{e^{(n/m)}} \qquad \text{(Equation 2)}.$$
When m items have been entered, the value of n'/m = 1 - 1/e = about
63%. At low ratios of n to m, the number of bins occupied is
approximately equal to the number of entries, n, but as the ratio
increases the curve asymptotically approaches 100%. The derivation
of this equation will be presented elsewhere (See Fig. 4A).

     3. Effect of % occupancy of storage bins on the ambiguity noise

levels during retrieval of redundantly stored information: In order
to extract stored information from a system such as that described
in earlier sections of this paper, it is necessary to process
sequentially only the most redundant items generated out of memory
when any particular address (module) combination is addressed. Only
the stored items which are generated in a redundancy equal to the
number of modules addressed represent true stored information. Added
to this will be a certain fraction of "retrieval-ambiguity noise".
When the ratio n'/m is very small, the value of such noise is also
very small, but as n'/m approaches 1, the ambiguity noise level
approaches 100%. Thus, the amount of information that can be stored
within such a system in retrievable form (low noise) increases with
increasing values of n/m and decreases as the redundancy of storage
increases. The average level of redundant storage is defined as R..
In order to evaluate the % of noise present in output (in addition
to signal) at any redundancy level, R, it is necessary to know the
value of n'/m and of R. The general equation which gives the %
noise is:

$$\% \ N \ = \ (1 \ - \frac{1}{e^{\ n/m}})^{\ R} \qquad \text{(Equation 3)}$$

Note that when n=m, the redundancy required to decrease the noise
level by a factor of 10 increases by 5 units of R for each log
decrement in noise level (See Fig. 4B, 5).

4. Relationship between Redundancy of Storeage, % memory filling
and optimum usage of memory space: Even though it is clear that
redundant storage increases the efficiency with which memory bins
may be utilized, it is also intuitively obvious that too great
redundancy of storage will eventually decrease the efficiency of use
of memory space. Stated otherwise, if R is very large, the number of
bins filled in order to store a given memory pattern will be greater
than the advantages gained through redundant storage at somewhat lower
levels of redundancy. This suggests that there is an optimum level
of bin occupancy and redundancy for any given permissable error rate
during memory retrieval. This optimum can be derived by plotting
the values of n/m and R as n/mR vs R (See Fig. 4C).

This plot reveals that the maximum efficiency of use of memory
space occurs at different levels of redundancy according to
intuitively obvious relationships. Clearly the maximum amount of
stored information should be present when the % filling of bins is
50%. The value of n/m to give this % filling is 0.693147. At this
level of filling (50%), the noise level will decrease by a factor of
2 for each unit of redundancy added, and more importantly in the
present context, the ambiguity noise level will double for each
redundant copy of a memory engram lost during aging (if the % filling
is exactly at the optimum...50%). In practical terms, an error rate
of 12.5% requires a redundancy of 3; an error rate of about 1/1000
requires a redundancy of 10, etc. etc. The efficiency of use of
memory space is about 21% for the former error level; it is about

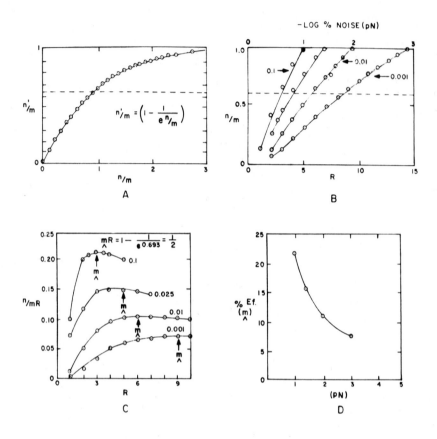

Fig. 4. Memory Capacity and Noise Level Parameters.
A. % of bins filled (n'/m) as a function of number of random entries
(n) in (m) available bins, when m >> 1;   B.   Values of number of
random entries (n) divided by number of available memory bins (m) vs
Redundancy (R) of storage at constant %'s of "Ambiguity Noise" defined
as (Error/(Signal + Error) = -log Noise = "pN";   C.   Efficiency of
Utilization of Total Memory Space (bins) as a function of Redundancy
of storage (R) at various prescribed error rates (0.1, 0.01, etc.).
Note that the maximum efficiency (m) increases rapidly as a function
of R and that m is reached when n/m ≠ 1 - 1/e = .63.....;   D.   Plot
of (m) vs pN.   Note that when (n'/m) = 1 = (1/$_e$0.693) = .4685..,
the efficiency of storage for any redundancy level greater than 1
is optimal for any noise level.   The value 0.4685 is very similar
to the cube root of 0.1 (.464..).   Therefore, an increase in
redundancy by three units will decrease the noise level by a factor
of 10 at optimal filling of bins.

	1	2	3	4	5	6	7	8	9	10	11
A	EI PR	AE O	DN WY	EI SU	DL MN	AD LO	AE G	IM NS	AC N	AT Y	BT Y →TO A1
B	IM R	AE OP	ADI NY	BM UY	ADE NS	DG OW	AE I	LN S	AC LN	TY →TO B1	
C	EIO RY	EL MN	AD LP	AD GU	IMN OY	ADE NS	AS Y	BN T	CEI TW →TO C1		

(A1, B1, C1; A4, B3, C1; A3, B6, C9)

Fig. 5. Example of triply redundant storage of three sequential messages in separate address systems: A(1 to 11); B(1 to 10); and C(1 to 9). Retrieval of stored information requires entry of appropriate address combination, listed below figure. Correct data points will be in each of the addressed boxes (3 copies). To obtain the next sequentially stored data point, the boxes immediately to the right of the previous boxes are examined and the triply redundant letters are noted. This is repeated until 2 or more consecutive address combinations yield no triply redundant outputs. The first message, (Address combination A1, B1, C1) begins "RED......" The other two messages may be retrieved by using the other address combinations listed. The three messages, taken together, may be an apt commentary.

10% for an error rate of 1/100, 7% for an error rate of 1/1000 and still at about 3.5% for an error rate of 10^{-6}. (!) (See Fig. 4D).

5. Relationship between cortical architecture and storage noise:
    The discussion of storage efficiency and storage-retrieval generated ambiguity noise levels presented in the previous sections is based on a system in which the pulse pattern that denotes a particular "bin" is generated unambiguously when memory is retrieved. In this portion of the discussion it is shown that a linear array of facilitatable synapses as previously suggested (Strehler, 1976a) is both anatomically unsound (Szentagothai, 1975) and possesses inherent noise generating characteristics that severely limit the storage capacities when m is large. This follows from the following arguments: If m facilatable synapses arranged linearly receive 0.693 m inputs (50% filling), the number of patterns stored relative to the % filling is derivable from the following equation:
    $n'/m = (1 - 1/e^{ix/m})$ (Equation 4),   where i = number of patterns entered (stored), x = number of pulses/pattern, m = number of occupiable bins. On a random basis, if each bin has the same probability of being occupied, it is clear that the probability of having the "first" and "last" bins occupied in a linear sequence is the product of the probability of having any bin occupied by the probability of having any other bin occupied. Thus, if the percentage of occupancy is n'/m, the probability of having any longest pattern stored is $(n'/m)^2$. However, there are 2 ways that the next longest pattern (m-1 bins in length) could arise and there are m-x ways that the shortest pattern could arise as noise (storage). This means that the probability of obtaining the shortest pattern x pulses long is $(n'/m)^x$. (m-x) (which approximates $(n')^x/m^{(x-1)}$ when m $\cong$ (m-x).

Thus, short patterns (high frequency) are much more probable as noise than long ones are. Specifically, it can be shown that the following equation holds:

$$\% \ N_{r_{max}} \cong m \ (1-1/e^{(n/m)})^x \cong (1-1/e^{\ ix/m})^x \qquad \text{(Equation 5)}$$

where % $N_{r_{max}}$ is the probability that the shortest pattern (x pulses long) will occur when i entries are made.

If we set a noise level of 0.1 for three redundant copies of stored information and set m = 5000, we find that only 75.67 triplets can be stored before the high frequency noise level exceeds about 0.5/ unit which represents an efficiency of space usage of about 4.54%, a value only 10% of the maximum storage efficiency theoretically attainable in a system whose bins are readily identifiable. Elsewhere the alternative solutions to this implied efficiency limit will be dealt with in extenso. Briefly, two alternatives, involving the subdivision of the storage system among multiple lines along a given dendrite permit an increase of storage capacity within permissible

noise levels by a factor of about 2.7. This increases the efficiency
to about 1/5 of the optimum (provided that about 20 lines make
contact with a given dendrite).

An alternative solution, suggested by purely anatomical considerations, is the following: The recurrent axons of the layer 5
pyramids have a low probability of intersecting with the basal dendrites of a layer 3 pyramid (geometrical considerations); they have
a high probability as pointed out by Szentagothai (1975) of contacting the vertical shafts of dendrites of nearby pyramids and have a
reasonable probability of making multiple contacts with the apical
branches. At and near the cell body dendritic spines are very rare
or absent; they appear to be sparse near the branch points at the
apices of the shafts and to be relatively dense in the more apical
portions of these branches. This suggests that the recurrent axons
make three consecutive contacts with a given layer three pyramid's
dendrites (1 or a very few in the basal region, multiple contacts
along the vertical shaft and, after a relatively sparse zone, multiple
contacts along the apical branches). The camera lucida drawings of
Scheibel and Scheibel (1970) which include the recurrent axons of
three adjacent pyramids (2 layer 5 and 1 layer 3 pyramid) are consistent with this anatomical interpretation (See Fig. 2B).

The significance of these findings in the present context, is
that it permits a single axonic recurrent fiber to send pulses
sequentially to three temporally-spatially separated zones of a given
layer 3 cell. Following the first contact, there is an appreciable
period of "silence", followed by a relatively high activity, followed
by a period of relative silence followed by a period of high activity
again. Thus, the cell will be unable to decode closely spaced pulse
patterns; it will, rather, favor the decoding of patterns that correspond to the three zones of spines described above. The result is that
the problem of high frequency noise is eliminated or greatly reduced.

A further implication of these findings is that, given multiple
recurrent axons from different layer 5 pyramids contacting the 3
regions of a given layer three pyramid, there will be a kind of
"tuning" to a most favored pattern of pulses in time. This follows
from the relationships defined in Equation 6:

# of Patterns Decodable = $(X + Y - 1)(X + Z - 1) - (X^2 - X)$,
(Equation 6), where X = number of possible bins in the basal region,
where Y = number of possible bins in the vertical shaft region and
where Z = number of possible bins in the apical branch region.

The values of X, Y and Z can be estimated as follows: The distance*from various parts of the basal dendrites to the portion of
the shaft that possesses spines ranges from about 500 to 1500 μ;
the sahft itself extends about 500-3000 μ, and the apical regions
_____
* In human cortex

extend another 500–1500 μ beyond the branch points。 The diameter of
the fine axons adjacent to the dendritic shaft is as low as 0.1 μ
which gives a conduction velocity of about 0.15m/sec = 150 μ /msec
(Peters and Walsh, 1972). The maximum firing rates we have observed
in large cells in the cat visual cortex are about 1.2 kc. These
values maximally permit about 10–20 bins to be present in the basal
regions; about 20 along the shaft and another 10 along the apical
branches. Fitting these values into equation 6, when X = 1, one
finds that about 200 different patterns of triplets are storable in
a given dendritic shaft /recurrent axon. If X is increased to 10,
the number of decodable triplets turns out to be about 460 and is
ca 750 if X is increased to 20.

Thus, it appears that multiple recurrent axons do not greatly
increase the number of channels that are decodable by a given cell.
However, if as in the example above, the maximum value of X is about
10, when Y and Z are 20 and 10 respectively, the probability of decoding a triplet whose length is determined by the "first bin in X"
and by the middle bins in Y and Z is 50 times greater than the
probability of decoding triplets involving bins at the extreme
positions of Y and Z. What this means is that a particular layer
three pyramid is selectively tuned to decode a particular kind of
triplet and that the probability of decoding and storing a triplet
that varies from this optimum decreases drastically as the triplet
departs from the optimal spacing. Should the patterns of pulses
derived from different portions of the retina, for example, vary in
some systematic pattern that corresponds to the favored decoding
probability in a given column, the spatial representation of visual
field in the primary visual cortex, for example, would be explicable.

To summarize this section, it appears not unreasonable that each
layer 3 pyramid is tuned to be most responsive to a particular pattern
of pulses in time. The local distribution of architectures within a
column of such pyramids would presumably permit selective response to
and decoding of selected groups of patterns corresponding, for
example, to lines of particular orientation, length, color sensitivity,
etc. as demonstrated by Hubel and Wiesel and others. The first pulse
in a triplet of pulses would be stored in the apical dendritic
branches, the second on the vertical shaft and the third on the basal
dendritic branches.

B. Aging and Error Rates in Memory Functions: Functional Loss
Consequent to Increased Noise

A key role of memory in adaptive behavior is its participation in
predictive processes, specifically the predication of which of many
alternative courses of action is most likely to enhance the survival
probability of the individual (or the species). Memory represents a
selective record of environmental patterns, of responses to them

and the past effects of such actions. During maturation and pre-
senility, a normal human being generally improves in the effectiveness with which he responds to environmental challenges and oppor-
tunities because, as memory space becomes more fully occupied with
records of past experiences, the capacity to make valid predictions
regarding the probable effects of actions also improves--a property
sometimes referred to as wisdom.

But as the components in the sensory appendages lose their
acuity and sensitivity, and as components in the brain itself
deteriorate or are lost by death of cells or losses of synapses, a
counter process--decreased effectiveness of response and of predictive
ability--gradually counteracts the benefits implicit in stored,
accrued experience.

Concurrent with aging of other parts of the body, a gradual
atrophy of brain mass, partly due to cell atrophy and partly due to
cell loss in specific areas, leads to an increased error rate---a
debility that is added to the debilities resulting from decreased
effectiveness of interactions of control systems with memory systems.
In the final section of this paper, some quantitative relationships
(due to loss of "memory space" and the probability of errors, some
of which lead to fatal "accidents") will be considered. In particular,
the quantitative effects of cell loss (reduced redundancy of memory
storage) on noise-derived errors in memory, judgment or motor
performance will be evaluated.

Four kinds of memory attrition will be considered briefly.
These are: 1. Memory attrition due to loss of synapses on surviving
cells; 2. Memory attrition consequent to cell atrophy; 3. Memory
attrition due to random loss of cells and 4. Memory attrition due to
patchy, localized degeneration of the cerebral cortex, such as occurs
in Alzheimers disease and, prematurely, in Down's syndrome (Mongolism).

There is evidence both from laboratory animals and (indirectly)
in man that the number of synapses in the brain/cell decreases during
aging (Terry and Gershon, 1976). The Scheibels (personal communication) have observed progressive atrophy of pyramidal cells (retraction
of apical and basal dendritic branches, in particular). Such atrophy
must be accompanied by a decrease in the number of synaptic connections
a given pyramidal cell makes with its neighbors, if only because the
regions of atrophy are heavily populated with dendritic spines and
the axonal presynaptic elements that contact them. Whether such
atrophy is intrinsic to the pyramidal cells proper, or a result of
"disuse atrophy" (well documented by Cowan in developing avian
systems) cannot be stated with any degree of certainty at present.
But because the brain is an integrated-interdependent system,
decreased inputs from or to any portion of it (from sensors to
higher-level-abstraction-processors) may well lead to synaptic loss,

cell atrophy and even death--similar to that observed in developing
nervous systems.

The degree and distribution of neuronal losses through cell
death is still a matter on which workers in various laboratories
disagree in some instances. A summary of recent findings is given
in the recently published symposium volume edited by Terry and
Gershon (1976). Most workers seem to agree that about 20% of the
cells in specific brain regions have been lost by age 80-100. This
loss is particularly notable in layer IV of aged monkey cortex.
The pattern of cell loss in senile and presenile dementia appears
to be quite different from what is observed in aged persons not
afflicted with this unfortunate disease. As will be shown below,
effects on memory and therefore on function would be expected to be
greatly different if cell loss is patchy rather than random. This
is primarily because the loss of a localized group of cells which
carry out related functions will either obliterate that function or
greatly reduce its efficiency, whereas random loss of cells and
synapses will generally produce a more or less equal loss of functions
of different kinds. With respect to error rates due to increased
retrieval-ambiguity noise, the effects of synaptic losses, cell
atrophy and cell death are formally equivalent and the quantitative
projections of such loss will be presented first.

1.   Effects of Random Loss of Memory Engrams:

In part IV/A, above, it was shown that the level of storage
noise is a function both of the % filling of memory bins and of the
redundancy of storage; increasing the former increases error rates,
while increasing the latter reduces them according to the relationship
in Equation 3:

% Errors (Error Rate) = k(% Errors) = $k(1 - 1/e^{n/m})^R$. Now it
is well established that the age specific death rate due to accidents,
like most other causes of death, follows the Gompertz relationship,
$R_m = R_o e^{at}$. More interestingly, in the present context, is the fact
that most accidents that lead to death at any age are the results of
errors either in information processing or in the execution of
specific actions. Both of these procedures usually require the
retrieval from memory of stored sequential memory. Therefore, the
probability of committing a fatal error is a positive function of
2 variables, (a) the probability of error/operation (Error Rate) and
(b) the number of sequential operations required to retrieve a
relevant memory train and/or to put into effect a particular motor
response.

At precisely 50% filling of memory bins, the effect of the loss
of one redundant copy of stored information will increase the, error
rate by precisely a factor of two, essentially because the substitution

of R-1 for R in Equation 3 (see above) doubles the error rate when
the term in the parentheses = 0.5. More generally the average error
rate multiplied by an appropriate constant, K, will be related to the
probability of death due to accidents based on faulty memory processing as follows:

(Equation 7)

$$K\overline{(E.R.)} = K(k) (n'/m)^{R_i(1 - bt)}$$, where n'/m = average percent
filling of memory bins, R_i = initial level of storage redundancy,
t = age in years and b = the fraction of redundancy lost per year.
The above equation can be re-written as: (Equation 8)

$$R_m \text{ (accidental)} = K(k)(n'/m)^{R_i}(m/n')^{R_i bt}) = R_{o(e.r.)} X^{at}.$$

If, as observed, X^{at} increases by a factor of 2 every 8 years or so,
one can calculate the value of n'/m at various values of R_i and b,
using the relationship implicit in Equation 8, $n'/m = 1/(2)(1/R_i bt)$.
The calculated values of n'/m for different values of R and b are
shown in the following tabulation:

b	R	n'/m (when t = 8 years)
0.0025	5	0.1%
"	10	3.13
"	15	9.92
"	25	25.0
"	30	31.5
"	50	50.0
0.005	5	3.13
"	10	17.7
"	15	31.5
"	20	42.0
"	25	50.0
0.008	5	11.0%
"	10	33.8
"	15	48.6
"	20	58.2
"	100	89.7
"	1000	98.9

The above demonstrates that a value of R between 10 and 20 is
sufficient to provide reasonable error rates (10^{-3} to 10^{-6}) at slightly
less than optimum filling. Moreover, this value of R(ca. 15) will
generate a Gompertz doubling time of 8 years, provided that the
actual loss of initial redundancy (R_i) is about 0.8%/yr(b). This is
about 4 times the actual rate of cell loss observed (0.2%/yr.), but
because (as pointed out earlier) at least 4 different cell types
are involved in the storage of a memory engram, the loss (randomly)
of any one of these 4 cells will cause the engram to become un-
retrievable . Using the binomial distribution law, p(X) = N!/X!·
{(N-X)!(p ^{X})(q $^{(N-X)}$)}$^{-1}$, where N = No. of cells in a functional
memory unit = 4, where p = probability that a cell (or functional

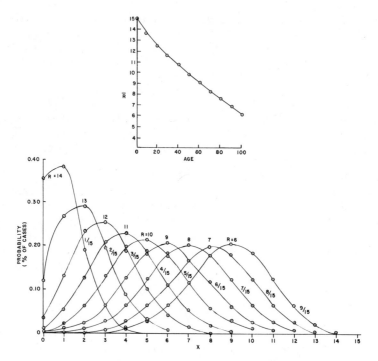

Fig. 6. Upper Graph: Relationship between age and Average Remaining
Redundancy (assuming that loss of any one of the four cells involved
in a storage unit such as depicted in Figure 3 causes loss of one
redundantly stored engram and that the rate of cell loss approximates
0.2%/yr. Lower Graph: R = Remaining Redundancy at various ages.
The X axis gives the actual redundancy remaining. The Y axis gives
the probability (% of cases) of finding a remaining redundancy at
each actual value of precisely X. Essentially the figure demonstrates
that about 50% of the memories stored redundantly will suffer an
attrition greater than the average attrition (R_i less average R lost!).
The plots are derived from application of the binomial distribution
(see text), where N = 15 and p ranges from 1/15 to 9/15. Note that
the distribution is approximately Poisson for small values of p and
essentially Gaussian as p and q approach equality (e.g. R=7 or R=8).

synapse in a memory engram will be lost =0.002/yr. x age, where
q = 1 - p = probability that a functional unit will not be lost,
and solving for X = 0, one obtains p(0) = $(1 - 0.002t)^4$. Assuming
an average initial redundancy, R_i, of 15, the remaining average
redundancy at various ages is as follows: (See Fig. 6, upper inset).
Age: 0   10   20   30   40   50   60   70   80   90   100
R : 15   13.8 12.7 11.7 10.7 9.8   9.0   8.2   7.5   6.8   6.15

     The above figures indicate that between age 0 and age 100 about
9 out of 15 redundant copies of stored information may be expected

to be lost on the average. The error rates for single operations
in a sequence of operations can be calculated from these values,
assuming that the system is nearly optimally (50%) filled. At age
20, for example, the probability of error per operation is about
$1/2^{12} = 1/4096$, whereas at age 100 the rate of errors has increased
to about 1/64, a factor of 64. Using the binomial distribution law
it is possible to calculate the variations of actual redundancy
remaining when the average redundancy is R (remaining redundancy)
(See Fig. 6, bottom). This permits one to estimate the % of serial
operations of different lengths which will involve at least one
error per sequence. For example, at age 72 the probability of
commiting an error in a sequence consisting of 16 steps (a simple
task) is only 0.01 (1%). Therefore, 99 out of 100 such simple tasks
will be successfully completed at this age. At age 100, however,
the probability of an error in such a simple task is about 9% which
means that 1 out of 11 such tasks will be erroneously performed. For
more complex tasks (e.g. 64 or 512 steps) the probability of error
at age 72 is 1/8 and 3/4 respectively; at age 100 the probabilities
are 6/10 and 98/100 respectively. But at age 30 the expected error
rates for tasks of 64 and 512 steps respectively are only about
1/1000 and 1/10 respectively (See Fig. 7).

It is reasonable to assume that complex tasks are less frequently
encountered than simple ones and that the probability of encountering
a task is inversely related to its complexity. This point cannot
be developed in the space available here, but will be fully detailed
elsewhere. Given this assumption, however, it is possible to
calculate the integrated probability of errors in performing tasks
of a great range of magnitudes of complexity. When this is done,
one obtains a Gompertz curve approximation that is essentially
logarithmic between age 30 and 85, as is observed experimentally.
The slope of the curve obtained possesses a doubling time of about
10 years, suggesting that the percent filling of memory bins is
somewhat below 50% in a real system (See Fig. 7).

To summarize this section, the attrition of redundantly stored
memory at the observed rate is able to generate the Gompertz function.
The average redundancy of initial storage is between 10 and 16 and
in keeping with Szilard's theory of mortality, a small number of hits
per functional unit (4 components/unit) is both sufficient to
provide the needed Gompertz slope and to fit the postulates and
data Szilard considered.

2. Effects of Focal Losses of Memory Engrams

The effects of coordinated (rather than random) losses of groups
of neurons that serve related redundantly represented functions will
be considered in this final section. Plaques may account for as
much as 15-25% of the cortical grey matter volume in severely

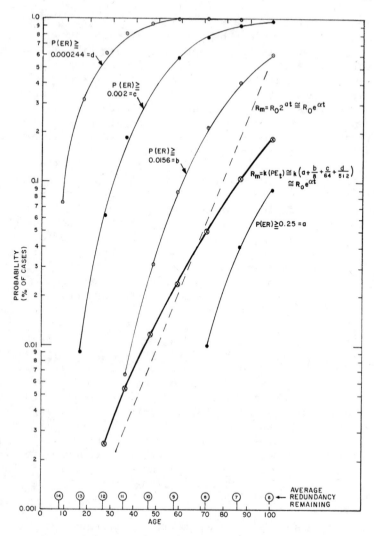

Fig. 7. Plot of Effect of Task Complexity on the probability of error per task (P.E.) vs age (open circles). The heavy line (circles with x's inside them) shows the high degree of approximation to a Gompertz function ($R_m = R_o e^{at}$), if the assumption is made that the frequency with which a task is encountered decreases as an inverse function of the complexity of the task increases linearly. The dotted line depicts a Gompertz plot in which the doubling time is exactly 8 years. The X axis depicts age and remaining redundancy (as derived from Figure 6) and the Y axis is the logarithm of probability of death per unit of time.

affected senile dements. If the cortex were viewed from the surface inward, even a small % volume loss due to plaques would include a substantial fraction of the columns underlying the surface. It is

known that each column has a relatively specific response (and
presumably a specific function) and that it is, in effect, tuned to
a group of related inputs (see discussion above). The loss of a
whole functional column or even a closely adjacent group of columns
would result in the simultaneous loss of a large fraction of identical,
redundant engrams in each plaque. Therefore, any sequential operation
which required the function of the anatomically contiguous cells lost
in a plaque, would be either highly error prone or even obliterated.
If about 10% of such large functional units were deleted from within
a specific cortical region, the effect would be to reduce the # of
sequential operations in the affected area to only about 10 consecutive correct outputs from memory, on the average.

The following tabulation depicts the relationship between %
volume lost as plaques, the complexity of the task (from 2 to 64
operations per task) and the chance that an error will be made
in performing serial tasks of different complexity.

Serial Operations in Task	5% of Columns Lost	10% of Columns Lost	15% of Columns Lost
	(Probability of error per task)		
2	1/10	1/5	3/10
4	1/5	1/3	1/2
8	1/3	4/10	3/4
16	1/2	4/5	9/10
32	4/5	29/30	199/200
64	19/20	499/500	9999/10,000

(Note: The above values represent "rounded fractions" derived
through the application of the binomial distribution.)

In effect, then, patchy cell loss will increase the error rate
(probability of failure to perform tasks) over the error rate calculated
if only random cell loss were to occur by factors of about 500 for a
simple (ca. 8 step) task and about 800 for a somewhat more complex
(64 step) task, respectively. Even if only 5% of the columns were
randomly deleted through Alzheimers or other focal lesions, such a
patients would perform on a 64 step task with the same efficiency
as would a non-dement at an age in excess of 120 years! Even for a
simple, 8-step, task, an Alzheimer's dement with 5% patchy loss of
columns would perform about like a 115 year old non-dement. In
summary, then, the effect of patchy cell loss on performance is
enormously more harmful than is a similar % loss of cells on a
random basis.

SUMMARY

The quantitative effects of cell loss in the cerebral cortex on
memory functions, (particularly on the frequency of errors based
on ambiguities in retrieval of stored memories including learned

motor responses) have been evaluated with respect to the complexity
of the task, the number of copies (redundancy) of stored information
and the patterns of cell loss. Several previous studies indicate
that about 0.2% of the cells in the cerebral cortex (particularly
in layer 4) are lost per year. In the mathematical model of memory
storage and retrieval summarized in this paper, which is consistent
with current neuroanatomical and neurobiological knowledge, 4
different cell types cooperate in the storage/retrieval of a "memory
engram". Thus, random loss of 0.2%/yr. of cells will inactivate
0.8%/yr. of storage units, a rate more in accord with losses of other
physiological functions as defined by Nathan Shock. On the basis
of the probability distribution of challenges of different complexity,
the integrated frequency of error rates as a function of age was
calculated and shown to approximate a Gompertz doubling time of
about 9 years. On the other hand, patchy loss of cells such as
occurs in senile dementia will have much more drastic effects on
the error rates (higher by a factor of 500 to 900) for the same %
loss of neurons. A tentative basis for an understanding of the
gross deterioration of memory functions in aging as well as in senile
and presenile dementia and the need for experimental evaluation in
quantitative terms become evident.

Acknowledgement: Work supported, in part, by a grant from the
L.A. County Heart Assn.

REFERENCES

Andrew, W. Cellular Changes with Age. Charles C. Thomas, Springfield,
     Ill., 74 pp., 1952.

Brizzee, K.R., Ordy, J.M., Hansche, J. and Kaack, B. Quantitative
     Assessment of Changes in Neuron and Glia Cell Packing Density
     and Lipofuscin Accumulation with Age in the Cerebral Cortex of
     a Non-Human Primate. In: Neurobiology of Aging, (Eds. R. D.
     Terry and S. Gershon), Raven Press, N.Y., pp. 229-244, 1976.

Brody, H. An Examination of Cerebral Cortex and Brain-Stem Aging.
     In: Neurobiology of Aging, (Eds. R.D. Terry and S. Gershon),
     Raven Press, N.Y., 1976.

Eccles, J. The Understanding of the Brain. McGraw-Hill, N.Y., 1973.

Ellis, R.S. Norms for some Structural Changes in the Human Cerebellum
     from Birth to Old Age. J. Comp. Neurol. 32:1-34, 1920.

Hubel, D.H. and Wiesel, T.N. An Anatomical Demonstration of Columns
     in the Monkey Striate Cortex. Nature 221:747-750, 1969.

Johnson, L., Johnson, R. and Strehler, B. Cardiac Hypertrophy,
    Aging and Changes in Cardiac Ribosomal RNA Gene Dosage in Man.
    J. Mol. Cell. Cardiol. 7:125-133, 1975.

Johnson, R., Chrisp, C. and Strehler, B. Selective Loss of Ribosomal
    RNA Genes During the Aging of Post-Mitotic Tissues. Mech. Age.
    Dev. 1:183-198, 1972.

Lashley, K. Brain Mechanisms and Intelligence. U. of Chicago Press,
    Chicago, 1929.

Mann, D. and Yates, P. Lipoprotein Pigments--Their Relationship To
    Aging in the Human Nervous System: I. The Lipofuscin Content of
    Nerve Cells. Brain 97:481-488, 1974.

Peters, A. and Walsh, T.M. A Study of the Organization of Apical
    Dendrites in the Somatic Seneory Cortex of the Rat. J. Comp.
    Neur. 144:253-268, 1972.

Reichel, W., Hollander, J., Clark, J. and Strehler, B. Lipofuscin
    Pigment Accumulation as a Function of Age and Distribution in
    the Rodent Brain. J. Gerontol. 23:71-77, 1968.

Scheibel, M.E. and Scheibel, A.B. Elementary Processes in Selected
    Thalamic and Cortical Subsystems--the structural substrates.
    In: The Neurosciences Second Study Program, (F. O. Schmitt,
    Ed. in Chief), The Rockefeller University Press, N.Y., pp. 443-
    457, 1970.

Strehler, B. Information Handling in the Nervous System: An Analogy
    to Molecular Genetic Coder-Decoder Mechanisms. Persp. Biol.
    Med. 12:584-612, 1969.

Strehler, B. Molecular and Systemic Aspects of Brain Aging: Psycho-
    biology of Informational Redundancy. In: Neurobiology of Aging,
    (Eds. R.D. Terry and S. Gerhson), Raven Press, N.Y., pp. 281-311,
    1976.

Strehler, B. Genetic and Neural Aspects of Redundancy and Aging.
    In: Proc. 6th European Congress on Basic Research in Gerontology,
    Weimar, DDR, Apr. 1976, (Ed. U. J. Schmitt), in press.

Szentagothai, J. The "Module-Concept" in Cerebral Architecture.
    Brain Res. 95:475-496, 1975.

CHANGES IN EEG AMPLITUDE DURING SLEEP WITH AGE

I. Feinberg, S. Hibi and V. R. Carlson

V. A. Hospital, San Francisco and Laboratory of
Psychology, NIMH

INTRODUCTION

The literature on changes in human sleep patterns with age was
recently reviewed in detail (Feinberg, 1976). One of the sleep
variables most sensitive to age is the amplitude of the electroencephalogram (EEG), especially that of the phase of sleep characterized by dense, high-voltage slow (delta) waves (stages 3 & 4 in the
Dement and Kleitman (1957) classification system). Here we shall
present hitherto unpublished data which illustrate the increase in
EEG amplitude during infancy and its decline during adolescence, the
periods of most rapid change. In addition, we shall show that these
and other effects of age on delta activity during sleep can be
detected by computer analysis during periods of much slower change,
even when the analysis is restricted to a narrow age range.

In the two studies described below, quite different methods of
measurement were employed. The first study was semi-quantitative
and involved measurement of the ten highest waves on those pages of
the EEG record which had been selected as representative of delta
activity for each S. The second study employed a computer program
for period and amplitude analysis of the sleep EEG. This program,
developed in our laboratory over the past 5 years, provides data
for frequencies, amplitudes, curve length, and various ratios of
these measures, in a wide range of frequency bands.

1. Visual measurement of delta amplitudes

The sleep EEG in the newborn infant is relatively undifferentiated.
Amplitudes are generally low and it is difficult or impossible to

distinguish among waking, active sleep and quiet sleep on the basis
of EEG criteria alone.

EEG development occurs rapidly after birth; sigma spindles,
K-complexes and high voltage slow activity are clearly apparent in
Non-Rapid Eye Movement (NREM) sleep by the middle of the first year
of life (Dreyfus-Brisac et al., 1958; Parmelee et al., 1967).   Here
we shall describe changes in EEG amplitude during NREM sleep (denoted
as "quiet" in the neonate, NREM subsequently) across the human life
span.

Method

Data for visual analyses were selected from ongoing studies in
two laboratories.   In one, the principal investigator, Dr. A.
Parmelee, of the Department of Pediatrics at UCLA, is concerned with
sleep patterns in infancy and the early years of life; in the other,
the principal investigator (IF) is studying sleep patterns from
childhood to old age.

Pilot studies showed that the number of EEG pages required to
obtain representative results would be prohibitively large if purely
random selection was employed.   Consequently, one of us (SH) scanned
ink-written EEG records of subjects between the ages of 4-96 years,
choosing for measurement those pages which seemed typical of the high
amplitude activity of each subject; Ms. E. Stern in Dr. Parmelee's
laboratory selected typical samples of records from quiet sleep in
normal subjects aged 3 mos. to 4 yrs.   From these segments 5 consecutive 20-sec. artifact-free epochs were chosen for measurement.
The ten highest waves in each epoch were measured and the average
amplitude of each wave (long + short sides/2), scaled according to
the amplitude calibration, was determined.   The averages of these
50 waves provided the score for each subject.

The two laboratories employed different recording techniques.
Recording was bipolar (left frontal-left central) for Dr. Parmelee's
Ss (aged 3 mos. - 4 yrs.), and monopolar (left central-mastoid) for
our Ss (aged 4 - 96 yrs.).   In principle, the bipolar recordings
should produce lower amplitudes.   Actually, the few points of overlap
at age 4 years showed similar values.   In any event, the data of
greatest interest are those which represent the main periods of
amplitude growth and decline.   These maximal rates of change occur
during infancy and adolescence; the data for each of these periods
were drawn from a single laboratory.

Results

The results are illustrated in Fig. 1.   A sixth-order polynomial
provided a significant fit (F = 16.0; p < .001) for the overall curve,

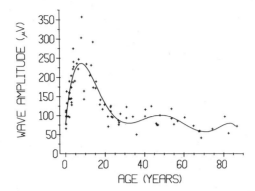

Fig. 1.   Average amplitude of EEG slow waves during sleep in normal
subjects between the ages 0.25 and 86 years.   Each point represents
the mean of 50 waves for one subject selected as described in the
text.   The curve is a 6th order polynomial which significantly
improves goodness of fit over lower-order functions.   The main
points of interest in this curve are the marked increase in amplitude
during infancy and the marked decline during adolescence.   The later
fluctuations are of doubtful significance.

but the higher orders, required for the apparent fluctuations in
middle and old age, seem to us of doubtful significance.   Of greater
importance is the clear-cut growth in amplitude during infancy and
early childhood.   Some extraordinarily large waves (up to and sometimes exceeding 1 mV) were recorded from the scalp in subjects around
age 4-5 yrs.   The marked decline which occurred in adolescence was
equally impressive.   Separate linear regressions for the age range
3 mos. - 10 yrs. and 10 - 26 yrs. were highly significant (F = 28.4
and 44.4 resp.; p <.005 for both).   The slope for the ascending limb
of the curve was 17.1 μV/yr.; for the descending limb it was -11.8
μV/yr.   While the absolute values of the data points are probably
of limited significance, the rates of change may ultimately provide

clues to the nature of the underlying physiological processes.

    2. <u>Computer analysis of sleep EEG.</u>

      Sleep stage scoring is highly dependent upon pattern recognition. We therefore apply both visual and computer methods to our sleep records. We visually distinguish among REM and NREM and waking states on the basis of the ink-written record. The NREM segments are indexed with a time code, and then subjected to computer analysis.

      We have devised a method of period and amplitude analysis for the sleep EEG which utilizes a PDP-12 computer. Using this method, EEG (analog) signals are played back at 4 times recorded speed into the A-D converter of the computer. The signal analysis program, PANV 35, operates as follows. The signal is divided into half-waves, and each half-wave is classified as falling into one of a number of specifiable frequency bands. For each frequency band, the number of half-waves, the total time occupied by such waves, the total integrated amplitude of these waves, and their curve length is summed over each consecutive epoch of specifiable length. The sums for each epoch are stored on digital tape for subsequent computer analysis. In addition, a similar analysis of the time between zero values of the first derivative of the input signal is performed, and the results stored. The last occurring time code is also stored with each 20-second epoch to permit comparisons between the ink-record and the computer measures.

      The PANV 35 processed data is then transferred to IBM 9-track tape. The IBM tape is then processed by an IBM 360/50 computer. The data are printed out and also stored on a disc by a series of PL/1 ("PANAL") programs. The final printed output contains the following information for each S: For each night in each condition, for each NREM period, and for all NREM sleep during the night, for the frequency bands 0-1, 1-2, 2-3, 0-2, 0-3, 3-4, 4-8, 8-12, 12-15, 15-23, 0-23, >23 Hz, the following variables are computed:

    1) Integrated amplitude (μV sec.)
    2) Curve length (μV)
    3) Time in band (sec.)
    4) Number of baseline crossings
    5) Average integrated amplitude per wave (μV sec.)
    6) Average sample rectified amplitude (μV)
    7) Average curve length per wave (μV)
    8) Average wave slope (μV/sec.)
    9) Average wave frequency (Hz.)
  10) Average wave frequency, weighted by wave duration (Hz.)
  11) Average curve length per wave/sample amplitude

For the first four variables, values are also computed:

    a) for the average 20-second epoch
    b) as a percentage of 0-3 Hz for the first 5 frequency bands
    c) as a percentage of 0-3 Hz for the first 3 frequency bands

These data are also stored on discs and are used to plot histograms and graphs or are retrieved for various statistical tests.

Amplitude Calibration

Since amplitude measures are crucial to the data we present, we shall briefly describe our calibration procedure. A calibration signal of 200 μV, 0.5 Hz positive square waves was played through the data recording system prior to each nights recording. The high pass filter (time constant 0.3 sec.), caused the calibration signals to be recorded as alternating positive and negative 200 μV "spikes". The calibration source (Grass square wave calibrator) has a nominal accuracy of 2%.

Prior to off-line analysis of the NREM EEG, the calibration signal is analysed by the PANV 35 program. During the actual EEG analysis, all amplitude measures are scaled according to the calibration measurement before being stored on tape. Integrated amplitude is measured with a resolution of 0.2 μV x sec.; curve length is measured with a resolution of 2 μV.

A report based upon data from a preliminary version (PANV 33) of the signal analysis program was recently published (Church et al., 1975). Here we shall describe correlations between age and computer-derived, as well as visually scored sleep variables in 20 young normal adults ranging in age from 18 to 22.5 yrs. These data were taken from a study of the effects of exercise on sleep (J. Walker et al., in preparation). In this investigation, 10 Ss who ran an average of 6.3 miles daily were matched with non-runners from the same college for height, weight, age and estimated sleep length. The matching was satisfactory except for weight. The non-runners weighed significantly less than the runners (146 vs 139 lbs.; p < .01). Ss were recorded for 4 consecutive nights. On the first 3 recording days, the runners and non-runners engaged in their usual activities. On the fourth day, these activities were reversed: the runners did not run and the non-runners ran 1.5 mi. Sleep EEGs and eye movements were recorded for 7.5 hrs/night with time in bed carefully controlled. Our methods for recording sleep have been previously described (Feinberg et al., 1967). "Blind" scoring was carried out for NREM stages classified according to the Rechtschaffen and Kales (1968) criteria and for REM periods according to the methods described by Feinberg et al., 1967).

The first night was an adaptation night and its data were not analysed. Here we shall present data from the second and third nights, which represent the habitual activity levels of the two groups. In the analysis below, data for each S represent the mean values for these two nights.

Analysis of the data from the entire study revealed no effects of exercise on stage 3-4 sleep. This result is consistent with the bulk of observations in the literature, notably the findings of Webb and Agnew (1974), Horne and Porter (1975; 1976) and Zir et al. (1971). Accordingly, the data for the entire group were combined (N=20) and a correlation matrix including age was computed for the main visual and computer-derived sleep measures.

RESULTS

The format of this volume did not permit inclusion of the entire correlation matrix. Table 1 lists the main correlations for visually scored NREM sleep variables and for computer measures of delta activity, as well as the means and standard deviations of these measures.

Total sleep time showed a statistically significant negative correlation with age, as did total delta sleep (stages 3 + 4). NREM duration was not significantly correlated with age. Measures of REM sleep (not shown) were not correlated with age or with NREM or delta measures.

Delta EEG waves are usually considered those in the 0-2 or 0-3 Hz frequency band. We computed the correlation matrix for each of these bands separately and obtained highly similar results. Here we present only the 0-3 Hz data, as these are the more comprehensive.

Although NREM duration was not significantly correlated with age (r = -.29), the weak relationship present might have acted to inflate spuriously the other correlation coefficients. To evaluate this possibility, the NREM-age correlation was partialled out from each of the other age-correlations in Table 1. In every instance, these partial correlations remained statistically significant at the same confidence levels.

The correlations between age and computer measures of 0-3 Hz activity were remarkably high, considering the narrow age range involved. For all NREM sleep, total mean values/night for integrated amplitude and time in 0-3 Hz showed significant negative correlations with age and mean frequency, a highly significant positive correlation. For the average 20-sec. epoch of NREM sleep, integrated amplitude and time in band also showed significant negative correlations with age. The correlation with age of the number of baseline crossings

Table 1. Pearson correlation coefficients among age, delta sleep stages and computer measures 0-3 Hz activity in NREM sleep. N = 20; age range is 18-22.5 yrs.

	Mean	(SD)	Age	Correlation with: Stages 3 + 4	Mean freq.
Total sleep	450.9 min	(21.9)	-46*	16	-28
Total NREM	322.5 min	(28.9)	-29	25	-38
Stages 3 + 4	84.9 min	(25.2)	-48*	--	-60**
Int. amp./nt(night)	272767.5 uv·sec	(57986.0)	-58**	70***	-67**
Time in band/nt.	12223.9 sec	(1536.0)	-55*	47*	-74***
BL crossings/nt.	36222.5	(3560.0)	-42	40	-51*
Mean freq./nt.	1.74 Hz	(0.06)	64**	-60**	--
Ave. int. amp./wave·nt.	14.95 uv·sec	(2.36)	-59**	76***	-65**
Ave. sample amp./nt.	22.2 uv	(3.0)	-48*	73***	-45*
Int. amp./20-sec. epoch	280.8 uv·sec	(51.1)	-59**	75***	-65**
Time in band/20-sec. epoch	12.6 sec	(0.88)	-66**	58**	-90***
BL crossings/20-sec. epoch	37.43	(1.51)	-43	43	-41

*p<.05   **p<.01   ***p<.001 (two-tailed tests).

in 0-3 Hz did not reach statistical significance.

To evaluate further these unexpectedly strong correlations of computer sleep measures with age, scattergrams for each relationship were plotted. None of the correlation coefficients was found to depend upon extreme values.

Mean frequency within 0-3 Hz has not previously been reported as a delta sleep measure. It is of interest that this variable was not only strongly related to age, but also showed highly signi- ficant negative correlations with amplitude within this narrow frequency band.

A number of computer variables showed statistically significant correlations with measures of delta sleep. While quite substantial, these relations were not in themselves sufficiently strong to permit prediction of sleep stages.

In summary, our data indicate that the decline in visually-scored delta sleep over the range 18 - 22.5 yrs. is associated with a reduction in amplitude and in time occupied by 0-3 Hz activity and with an increase in the average frequency of waves in this band. The actual number of waves (baseline crossings) showed a substantial negative correlation with age which just fell short of statistical significance. However, as noted above, we computed the same correla- tion matrix for 0-2 Hz activity. For this frequency band, baseline crossings (BLX) showed statistically significant negative correlations with age: $r = -.57$ for total BLX/night and $r = -.65$ for BLX/20 sec. epoch ($p < .01$ for both). These correlation coefficients remained at the same significance levels with the NREM-age correlation partialled. Thus, the number of delta waves in the 0.2 Hz band is negatively correlated with age. The difference in results for 0-2 and 0-3 Hz bands may be an indication of two opposing processes on the BLX measure: average frequency increases with age while the number of waves decreases.

DISCUSSION

It is of interest to compare the age-changes in EEG amplitudes during sleep with those observed during waking. Matousek and Petersen (1973) have presented the most extensive data on amplitude changes during waking. They studied 401 normal subjects without mutual kinship who ranged in age from 1 to 22 yrs. Activity in six frequency bands was measured for several bipolar EEG derivations. In contrast to the growth in amplitude we observed for delta activity during sleep in the first 5 years of life, Matousek and Petersen found a monotonic decline between ages 1 and 15 yrs. The decline measured in their delta band (1.5 - 3.5 Hz) for the F3-T7 derivation was from

23.6 uV at 1 yr. to 8.7 uV at age 15 yrs. (r = -.63, p<.001). The correlation between delta amplitude during waking and age over the range 16-21 yrs. did not reach significance (r = -.14).

In contrast to these findings, we observed an increase in delta amplitudes during sleep from age 3 months to a maximum at about age 5 yrs. and then a steep decline between ages 10-20 yrs. Our manual measurements of the ink-written records are admittedly far more crude than the computer measures of Matousek and Petersen, but this difference could not account for the entirely different shape of the amplitude trend over the first 5 years of life. It therefore appears that EEG amplitudes during sleep and waking evolve differently with age during the first 5 years of life. The existence of these differences would seem to rule out the possibility that the age changes in amplitude are due to extracerebral factors, such as skull-conductivity, for such factors would exert the same effects during sleep and waking.

In contrast to the early years, the rates of decline of EEG delta amplitudes over the age range 10-21 yrs. were proportionally similar during sleep and waking, although the absolute decline was much greater for sleep. Matousek and Petersen reported a change from 14.6 to 6.8 uV, or 53% over this range; the curve in Fig. 1 shows a decline from about 225 uV to about 125 uV, or about 45%.

We noted above that we place little weight on the apparent amplitude fluctuation in the older age ranges shown in Fig. 1. These doubts are partly based upon the data of Agnew (1973), which suggest instead a curvilinear decline. Agnew reported changes in sleep EEG amplitude from a mean nightly value of 23 uV x min. at age 25 yrs. to 22 uV x min. at mean age 35 and then to 16 uV x min. at mean age 65 yrs. Agnew's study, which constitutes the most extensive available description of the effects of age on sleep EEG amplitude, also demonstrated high night-to-night reliability for amplitude measures within Ss.

Turning now to the results of our second study, we were surprised to observe the significant negative correlation between age and total sleep time; such a result has not previously been reported for Ss in this age range. This finding may be a chance result. An alternative possibility is that a decline in TST is, in fact, measureable over this age range but can only be detected if time in bed is rigidly controlled, as was done in the present experiment.

The substantial correlations between computer measures of activity in 0-3 Hz. and amount of visually scored stage 4 EEG should come as no surprise. Neither, however, should they encourage the use of these methods for sleep stage scoring. Measures of amplitudes and frequencies within the delta band in epochs visually classified as

NREM sleep can be expected to correlate well with visual scoring of NREM sleep stages 2-4 only in subjects with broadly similar EEGs. When sleep EEG tracings are obtained from Ss whose records are more heterogeneous as a result of a wider age span, brain pathology, or experimental (e.g., pharmacologic) manipulations, human scorers invoke pattern recognition responses for sleep stage scoring which are difficult to mimic with computer programs.

We are impressed to find that our computer measures had sufficient resolution to detect amplitude and frequency changes in 0-3 Hz activity during sleep within the narrow age range of 18 - 22.5 yrs. These relations were independent of variations in total NREM sleep. In addition to the decline in amplitude, we found that the number of delta waves and the time occupied by these waves were negatively correlated with age. Thus, it appears that the decline in visually scored stage 4 sleep with age is associated with changes in total amplitude, number and time occupied by delta waves, and with the density of these waves during NREM sleep, and that these different contributions can be distinguished with computer techniques.

What mechanisms might underlie the pronounced changes in sleep EEG amplitude with age? It is generally accepted that the high voltage, slow fluctuations in potential recorded at the scalp are generated by synchronous potential changes in large pools of cortical neurons controlled by subcortical (thalamic?) pacemakers. A reduction in the amplitude of these EEG waves might therefore result either from reductions in the number of neurons within the pools or from a decrease in their average response to the synchronizing pacemaker, or from changes in the intensity or distribution of pacemaker output.*

With respect to the age changes in sleep EEG amplitude described above, it seems possible that alterations both in size of pool and in average neuronal response occur at different points in the life cycle. The rapid and striking growth in delta amplitude during the first years of life may be an electrophysiologic correlate of the vastly increased connections within the cortex associated with post-natal maturation and development (Conel, 1939-1963); these connections could make possible synchrony in larger neuronal pools. However, it seems unlikely that the equally striking decline in amplitude of delta sleep during adolescence presents a converse decrease in size of the responding pools. It is more plausible that this latter change stems from a decline in the average neuronal response to the sleep

---

*It is also possible that the cortical rhythms are "endogenous" and not dependent upon subcortical input. Endogenous rhythms would vary in amplitude according to the size of the pool or of the average neuronal change.

pacemaker or from a narrower distribution of the pacemaker output, although the biophysical bases for such changes are entirely unknown. We previously hypothesized that the striking fall in duration of stage 4 sleep during adolescence may be related to the decline in brain plasticity which occurs at this time (Feinberg and Carlson, 1968; Feinberg and Evarts, 1969). The reduction in amplitude found here may be an additional reflection of this change; the product of the fall in duration and amplitude may together reflect the magnitude of this reduction in plasticity.

The pathological changes in the brain in old age might produce both a reduced neuronal pool and a decrease in average neuronal response to the synchronizing pacemaker. The size of the pool could be diminished by interruption of cortical circuits by senile plaques and by cell loss. A diminution in average neuronal response might be produced by the several varieties of intra-neuronal pathology described elsewhere in this volume. Both of these changes might combine to produce the amplitude decrements in late life. If these factors are indeed responsible, amplitude of delta activity should correlate with cognitive impairment in the elderly. However, in seeking such correlations, one must control for the contribution of delta EEG of pathological origin which is often of relatively high amplitude (Feinberg et al., 1967) and which may represent a different physiological process.

Elsewhere, we put forward the hypothesis that it is NREM sleep which reverses certain of the effects of waking on brain (Feinberg, 1974). We proposed that this reversal takes place at an intense rate early in the night, when the concentration of "substrates" produced by waking is high, and more slowly as sleep progresses. We suggested that the decline in density of delta EEG across the night reflects the kinetics of this process. It is of interest to note, in the present context, that amplitude as well as the abundance and duration of delta decline systematically across the night (Church et al., 1975; Feinberg and others, unpublished observations). It seems possible that this within-night change represents a reduced response of neurons to the synchronizing pacemaker as the substrates for sleep processes are consumed.

SUMMARY

We carried out manual measurements of amplitude of delta waves during sleep on ink-written EEG records from Ss aged 3 mos. to 96 yrs. We observed marked growth (17.1 uV/yr.) in delta amplitude during infancy and a pronounced decline (-11.8 uV/yr.) during adolescence. A second study involved computer analysis of delta activity during NREM sleep in 20 Ss who ranged in age from 18 to 22.5 yrs. This analysis revealed strong negative correlations of

amplitude and strong positive correlations of frequency with age for
EEG activity within the 0-3 Hz. band. In addition to the decline
in amplitude of delta activity, our data revealed negative correlations with age for the number of delta waves and for time occupied
in delta waves.

These results supplement those obtained with visual scoring of
the sleep EEG. The age changes in computer EEG measures are consistent with the decline in time occupied by visually scored stage
4 over this same range. The amplitude change could be interpreted
as suggesting that the intensity of the stage 4 activity, as well
as its duration, declines with age.

We speculated that, at different points in the lifespan, changes
in amount of delta sleep might reflect alterations in the size of
the pool, or in average neuronal response within the pool, of neurons
whose synchronous potential changes are recorded as EEG slow-waves.
We reiterate our previous suggestions that changes in delta sleep
with age may be correlated with changes in brain plasticity.

Whatever the merits of these speculations, it is an empirical
fact that the EEG of NREM sleep changes markedly in frequency and
amplitude with age and that computer analysis can detect these changes
over a remarkably narrow age range. These findings give grounds for
optimism that application of these computer methods to the sleep
EEG over a wider age-range, carried out in conjunction with measures
of other biopsychological changes in the same subjects, might yield
data of considerable interest to those concerned with aging in the
central nervous system. Such studies are being actively pursued in
our laboratory as is the application of these techniques to stage 4
changes induced by drugs and psychopathology.

REFERENCES

Agnew, H.W., Jr. Integrator Analysis of the sleep electroencephalo-
    gram. Electroenceph. Clin. Neurophys. 34:391-397, 1973.

Church, M.W., March, J.D., Hibi, S., Benson, K., Cavness, C. and
    Feinberg, I. Changes in frequency and amplitude of delta
    activity during sleep. Electroenceph. Clin. Neurophysiol. 39:
    1-7, 1975.

Conel, J.L. The post-natal development of the human cerebral cortex.
    Vols. I-VII, Harvard University Press, Cambridge, MA., 1939-1963.

Dement, W.C. and Kleitman, N. Cyclic variations in EEG during sleep
    and their relation to eye-movements, body motility, and dreaming.
    Electroenceph. Clin. Neurophysiol. 9:673-690, 1957.

Dreyfus-Brisac, C., Samson, D., Blanc, C. and Monod, N. L'electro-encephalogramme de l'enfant normal de moins de 3 ans. Etudes neo-natal. 7:143-175, 1958.

Feinberg, I. Changes in sleep cycle patterns with age. J. Psychiat. Res. 10:283-306, 1974.

Feinberg, I. Functional implications of changes in sleep physiology with age. In: Neurobiology of Aging, (Eds. R.D. Terry and S. Gershon), Raven Press, New York, pp. 23-41, 1976.

Feinberg, I. and Carlson, V.R. Sleep variables as a function of age in man. Arch. Gen. Psychiat. 18:239-250, 1968.

Feinberg, I. and Evarts, E.V. Changing concepts of the function of sleep: discovery of intense brain activity during sleep calls for revision of hypotheses as to its function. Biol. Psychiat. 1:331-348, 1969.

Feinberg, I., Koreski, R.L. and Heller, N. EEG sleep patterns as a function of normal and pathological aging in man. J. Psychiat. Res. 5:104-144, 1967.

Horne, J.A. and Porter, J.M. Exercise and human sleep. Nature 256:573-575, 1975.

Horne, J.A. and Porter, J.M. Time of day effects with standardized exercise upon subsequent sleep. Electroenceph. Clin. Neuro-physiol. 40:178-184, 1976.

Matousek, M. and Petersen, I. Frequency analysis of the EEG in normal children and adolescents. In: Automation of Clinical Electroencephalography, (Eds. P. Kellaway and I. Petersen), Raven Press, New York, pp. 75-143, 1973.

Parmelee, A.H., Jr., Wenner, W.H., Akiyama, Y., Stern, E. and Flescher, J. Electroencephalography and brain maturation. In: Regional Development of the Brain in Early Life, (Ed. A. Minkowski), Blackwell: Oxford, pp. 459-476, 1967.

Rechtschaffen, A. and Kales, A. (Eds.) A Manual of Standardized Terminology, Techniques and Scoring System for Sleep Stages of Human Subjects. Public Health Service, U.S. Govt. Printing Office, Washington, D. C., 1968.

Webb, W.B. and Agnew, H.W., Jr. Sleep and waking in a time-free environment. Aerospace Med. 45:617-622, 1974.

Zir, L.M., Smith, R.A. and Parker, D.C. Human growth hormone release
    in sleep: Effect of daytime exercise. J. Clin. Endocr. 32:
    662-665, 1971.

BIOCHEMICAL SIGNIFICANCE OF AGE PIGMENT IN NEURONES

A. N. Siakotos[1], D. Armstrong[2], N. Koppang[3], and J. Muller[1]

[1]Indiana University School of Medicine, Indianapolis, Indiana; [2]University of Colorado School of Medicine, Denver, Colorado; and [3]National Veterinary Institute, Oslo, Norway

The progressive intracellular accumulation of age pigment or lipofuscin granules in non-dividing cells is generally taken as one hallmark of cellular aging. The relationships of the intracellular lipofuscin concentration with the reduction of cellular efficiency in senescent tissues is not clear. In fact, there has been very little speculation, let alone solid evidence, on how these accumulating lipofuscin bodies interfere with and/or alter the metabolic economy of the aging cell. The presence of lipofuscin granules in the central nervous system of very young children or newborn infants has been, at times, in dispute. The reason for this uncertainty is not clear. It may on the one hand be due to the lack of specificity of histological techniques employed to detect lipofuscin or, on the other, to the extraction of the early lipid-rich precursors of age pigment by the solvents used for the dehydration of tissue specimens. Although the observations on the presence of lipofuscin in brains of children within the first year of life are very few, some authors have observed lipofuscin granules in the spinal cord of human fetuses (Humphrey, 1944 and Chu, 1954). Brody (1960) first reported the absence of lipofuscin in newborn to two month old human brain, but later (Brody, 1974) observed lipofuscin in the inferior olive of a three-month-old child. In his earlier study, Brody (1970) used dioxane dehydration and paraffin embedding in his tissue preparations. As will be pointed out later in this report, the extraction and concentration of trace quantities of lipofuscin by subcellular fractionation techniques is a more efficient technique for the detection of low concentrations of lipofuscin granules and lipofuscin-like particles from large samples of human brain. In any event, the relative paucity of lipofuscin granules in normal human infant brains is apparent in an electron micrograph of cortical

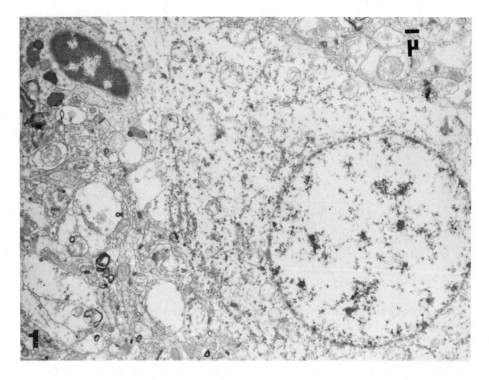

Fig. 1. An electron micrograph of a cortical biopsy of human brain,
5 years old. There are no lipofuscin granules to be noted. (11,500X)

biopsy of a 5 year old brain shown in Figure 1. In contrast, two
electron micrographs (Figures 2 and 3) of an autopsy specimen of
normal human brain of 53 years of age reveals many lipofuscin granules.
In Figure 3, the massive intraneuronal accumulation of lipofuscin
appears to have displaced normal cellular organelles such as the
mitochondria, to the periphery of the cell. In addition, Figure 3
reveals extensive clumping of the rough endoplasmic reticulum. The
age-related accumulation of intraneuronal lipofuscin has been well
documented in animal studies (Brizzee et al., 1974). In man, large
amounts of lipofuscin may accumulate in some neuropathologic conditions,
especially Huntington's Chorea (Telez-Nagel et al., 1973), and
Alzheimer's disease (Wisniewski and Terry, 1973). Similar accumulations may be seen in the brains of patients with long-term epilepsy,
possibly secondary to drugs or anoxia, and also in patients with
chronic alcoholism (Siakotos, unpublished data).

     The lipopigments, in general, have been reviewed by Porta and

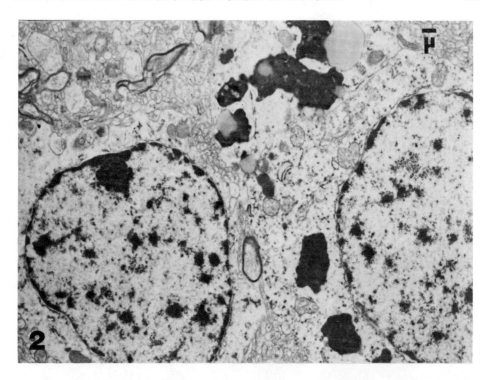

Fig. 2.   An electron micrograph of human brain, 53 years old, obtained
at autopsy.   This electron micrograph reveals a number of electron
dense lipofuscin granules.   (9,750X)

and Hartroft (1969) and the biochemical properties of lipofuscin, in
particular, have been reviewed by Siakotos and Koppang (1973); Siakotos
and Armstrong (1975).   Recently Csallany and Ayaz (1976) have described
the fluorescence emission spectrum of lipofuscin and its spectral
peak which is reduced to 435 mμ when interfering vitamin A or vitamin
A degradation products are first removed by column chromatography.
Tissue extracts prepared under these conditions exhibit identical
excitation-emission fluorescence spectra, with another autofluorescent lipopigment, ceroid.   The significance of this report remains
uncertain since the authors used only tissue extracts, rather than
extracts of pure lipofuscin.   Taubold et al. (1975) have shown that
extracts of a highly purified sample of human brain lipofuscin
exhibit a fluorescence emission peak at 495 mμ.   Thus the fluorescence spectra of age pigments isolated from brain tissue remain
uncertain.

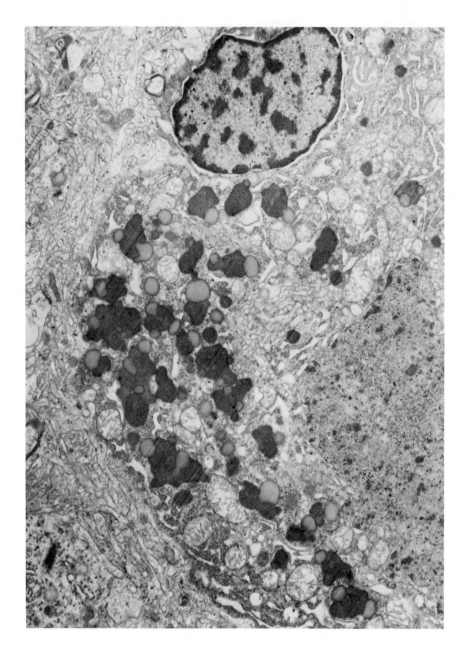

Fig. 3. A different area of the same specimen as in Figure 2. Note
the large mass of lipofuscin granules within the neurone cell body
has displaced many mitochondria to the periphery of the cell.
The smooth endoplasmic reticulum shows marked dilatation with
clumping of the ribosomes in the rough endoplasmic reticulum.
(9,750X)

The genesis of lipofuscin has been widely debated. Some investigators have proposed a lysosomal origin, others favor a mitochondrial origin of the pigment. Still others suggested that golgi and/or
other subcellular organelles are involved in the formation of lipofuscin. Nearly all of these conclusions are based on morphological
studies with no chemical evidence to support these radically differ-
ing views. Our interests lie in the isolation and biochemical
characterization of subcellular organelles from brain and other
organs. It is from this line of investigation that the data reported
in this paper are derived.

Our earlier studies (Siakotos et al., 1970; Siakotos et al.,
1972; and Siakotos et al., 1973) have focused on the subcellular
isolation of lipofuscin, lipid globules and ceroid from tissues.
In 1970, Siakotos, et al. showed that isolated pure preparations of
lipofuscin exhibited a variety of morphological forms when viewed
at the ultrastructural level. Figure 4 is taken from an earlier
publication (Siakotos et al., 1970) and shows at least five distinct
morphologic types of lipofuscin, including many globular lipid-rich
areas in an isolated preparation of lipofuscin obtained from a pooled
sample of 10 normal human brains (age 40-60 years). The classical
granular lipofuscin granules (G) present a fine structure of convoluted
rods with inclusions of lipid globules. Type GL (granulolinear)
lipofuscin shows a fine granular matrix with an occasional linear
structure in parallel arrays. Type L consists of amorphous lipid
globules which may be unique, e.g. lipid filled lysosomes, or be
derived from the fragmentation of granular lipofuscin (G). Macrogranular bodies (MG) are also seen. Generally all particles in such
preparations are associated with some form of electron-dense pigment.
The systematic application of the subcellular approach to the study
of large samples of human brain from newborn to the 80th year should
provide some pertinent information on the developmental changes
observed in lipofuscin and lipofuscin-like subcellular particles.
Neurones are post mitotic cells. Therefore, neuronal organelles,
present early in life may be expected to remain or be altered by
anabolic or catabolic process during the life span of the individual.
In the present study, a new approach has been taken to isolate and
purify lipofuscin and lipofuscin-like particles from samples of
pooled human brains, taken from persons 1 month to 80 years of age.
The quantitative yield of such organelles and the nature of their
ultrastructure should provide a new approach to the study of the
developmental changes in lipofuscin and lipofuscin precursors from
the human brains.

MATERIALS AND METHODS

Sucrose (special enzyme grade) was purchased from Leon Labs,
St. Louis, Missouri. Other chemical reagents were obtained from

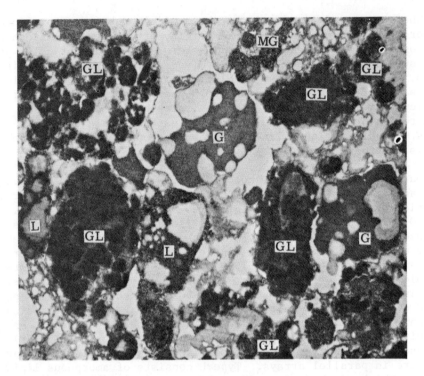

Fig. 4. Isolated lipofuscin fraction from normal human brain.
Classical granular lipofuscin bodies (G) with a granular matrix and
light areas of lipid. The remaining three types of lipofuscin are
associated with a large amount of vacuolated lipid material,
presumably neutral lipid. The granulolinear bodies (GL) show areas
of different densities due to varying compaction of the granular
matrix, and multilamellar areas. Another particulate (L) consists
of globules of various sizes. The macrogranular bodies (MG) contain
coarse granular material. Reprinted by permission of Biochem. Med.
4:361-375 (1970). (14,500X)

commercial sources. For electron microscopy, samples of lipopigments
were fixed in 2% osmium tetroxide, washed, and dehydrated as described
previously (Siakotos et al., 1970).

Preparative Isolation of Human Brain Lipofuscin

An outline of the mass isolation procedure for lipofuscin is
given in Figure 5. All post-mortem human brain samples were examined
as fresh coronal sections by a pathologist. Wherever necessary,
appropriate sections were taken for formalin fixation and the
remaining brain was frozen at -25°C until five brain samples were
collected for each decade. Prior to fractionation the frozen brain

Briefly blend brain in Solution 1 (a,b,c), pass through a Parr bomb at 900 psi(d), centrifugations as follows:

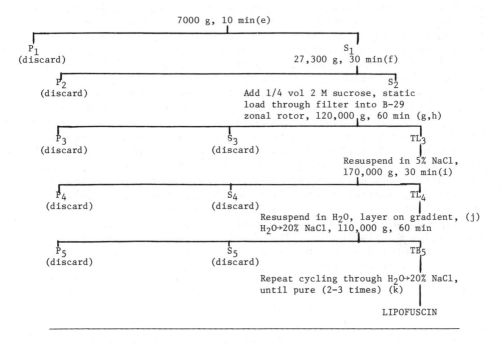

Fig. 5.   Flow diagram for the mass isolation of lipofuscin from brain. Letters in parenthesis refer to the text.

samples were thawed overnight at 4°C. The tissue was then blended for 5-10 seconds in a one-gallon Waring blendor with solution 1 (0.4 M sucrose, containing 0.05 M Tris base) in the ratio of 0.6 Kg brain per liter of solution 1 (a,b,c). Next the homogenate was further disrupted by treatment with nitrogen at 900 psi in a Parr cell decompression bomb. After 10 minutes the pressure was released, the homogenate collected (d) and centrifuged at 7000 g, 10' in a Sorvall RC-3 centrifuge with an HG rotor (e). The result was a pellet (P_1) and supernatant (S_1). At this point the pellet was discarded and the supernatant centrifuged at 27,300 g for 30 minutes in the SGA rotor (f). Again, the supernatant and light brown floating (S_2) layer of fat was resuspended in 0.4 M sucrose and a

1/4 volume of 2.0 M sucrose added to increase the medium density.
The preparation was static-loaded under gravity into an IEC B-29
zonal rotor (g), through a 420 mesh nylon filter in a 142 mm disc
filter holder (Millipore YY-22) and finally accelerated briefly
to completely fill the rotor. The rotor was sealed and accelerated
to 120,000 g for 60 minutes (h). At that time, the rotor was
stopped, disassembled, and the center core removed. The packed
lipofuscin concentrate (TL$_3$) was then scraped with a plastic spatula
into a beaker. The concentrate (TL$_3$) was resuspended in 5% NaCl
in a 200 ml PoHer-Elvehjem homogenizer (1200 rpm) and centrifuged
at 170,000 g for 30 minutes in an IEC A-170 rotor (i). The resulting
packed brown top layer (TL$_4$) was collected by aspiration and purified
further by centrifuging on freshly prepared continuous gradients of
H$_2$0 to 20% NaCl at 110,000g for 60 minutes in an IEC SB-110 rotor
(j). After each pass through the gradient the top brown band was
collected by aspiration and recycled through the H$_2$0 to 20% salt
gradient until only one uniform brown band was obtained. Examination
of the preparation by phase contrast microscopy revealed a pure
preparation of lipofuscin. The sample of lipofuscin was then dialysed
against distilled water in the cold overnight. Aliquots of the
dialysed sample were then taken for dry weights at 90°C.

RESULTS

     The yields of isolated purified preparations of lipofuscin and
lipofuscin-like suspensions are given in Table I and are also
plotted in Figure 6. Table I shows that the concentration or poolsize
of lipofuscin or lipofuscin material per brain was relatively uniform
up until 16.8 years of age. At that point, 16.8 years, the poolsize
of lipofuscin per brain increased with age. By contrast, when the
data were calculated on a dry weight concentration of lipofuscin per
100 grams of dry weight of brain then a very high value of 0.051%
was observed within the first three months of life. This neonatal
concentration of "lipofuscin" then dropped dramatically to roughly
1/4 of this value at 8.60 years of age and continued to decrease to
1/5 of the 0.36 year value at 16.8 years of age. At that point
(16.8 years), the concentration of age pigment per gram of brain
(on a dry weight basis) progressively increased with age. In the
last column of Table I, the dry weights of normal human brain for
these same ages are presented. As can be seen at 0.36 years of age,
the neonatal brain is 88.79% water, in contrast to the 8.6 year
sample which was only 77.87% water.

     Electron micrographs of the isolated preparation of lipofuscin
are shown in Figures 7 through 12. The 0.36 year old sample (Figure
7) shows a large number of lipid bodies or lipid-filled lysosomes
enclosed by a membrane with occasional electron dense lipofuscin-like
areas relative to the globular granules. As brains of progressively

Table I. Yields of lipofuscin and lipofuscin-like material from normal human brain.

	Age (mean)*	Concentration of lipofuscin per brain	Percent lipofuscin per 100 gm dry weight of brain	Dry weight of brain**
1	0.36	34.59	0.051	11.21
2	8.60	35.96	0.015	22.13
3	16.80	25.06	0.010	22.13
4	45.60	50.67	0.019	21.75
5	66.80	88.37	0.036	21.20
6	78.80	72.00	0.030	20.90

*Mean age in years of pooled sample of five normal human brains.

**Calculated from data of Rouser and Yamamoto (1966).

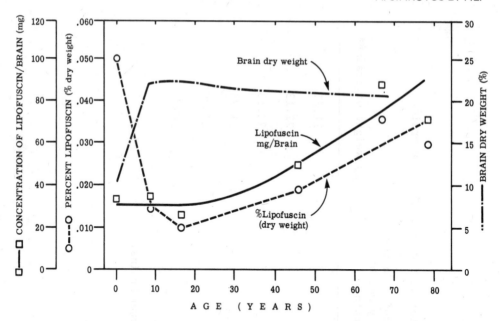

Fig. 6. The concentration of lipofuscin in human brain with age.
The concentration of lipofuscin (dry weight) is given per brain in
the solid line. The percentage of lipofuscin (dry weight) relative
to brain, dry weight is given by the dashed line, while the remaining
curve is the calculated brain dry weight for normal human brain.

older individuals were used to prepare lipofuscin, the isolated
preparations showed a relatively higher proportion of electron dense
lipofuscin. In addition, there is an increase of the granulolinear
macroglobular forms with age (Figures 11 and 12).

DISCUSSION

    An open question has been whether lipofuscin or lipofuscin-like
intracellular organelles occur in brains of young children. The
application of a subcellular fractionation technique to concentrate,
purify, and measure quantitatively such isolated preparations yields
data that seem to indicate that lipofuscin-like particles (lipid
filled lysosomes or lipid globules) exist in the neonatal human brain.
A careful study of the electron micrographs (Figures 6 and 7) of neonatal or 8.6 year old brains reveals many lipid globules or lysosomes
filled with material which does not stain intensely with osmium
tetroxide. Occasional electron dense areas are seen in the "globule"

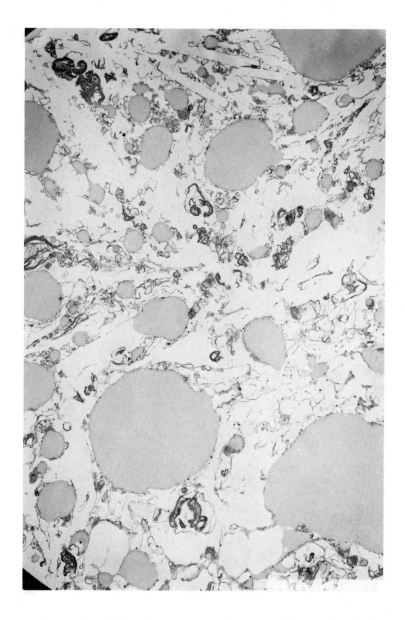

Fig. 7. Lipofuscin fraction from five normal human brains with a mean age of 0.36 years. Note the globular structures with some electron dense areas. (8000X)

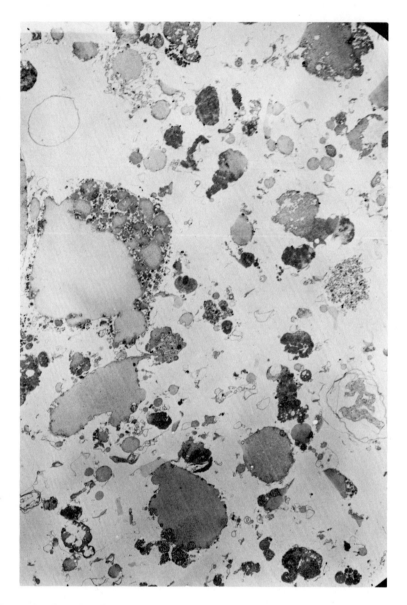

Fig. 8. Lipofuscin fraction from five normal human brains with a
mean age of 8.6 years. Note the appearance of macrogranular areas
on the globules and the appearance of electron dense granulolinear
particles. (8000X)

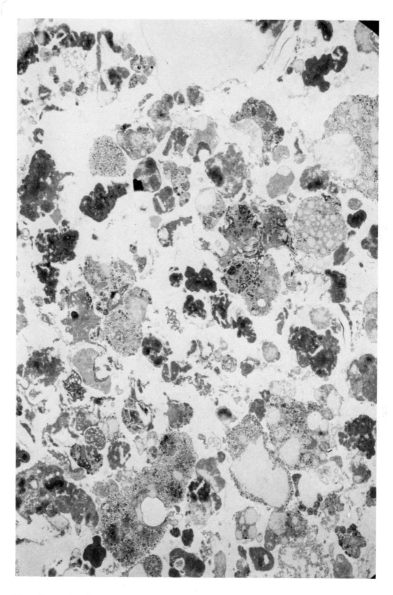

Fig. 9. Lipofuscin fraction from five normal human brains with
a mean age of 16.8 years. Many electron dense structures are
present. (8000X)

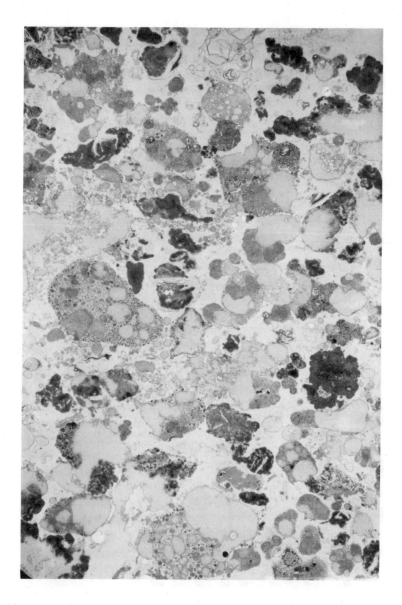

Fig. 10.   Lipofuscin fraction from five normal human brains with
a mean age of 45.6 years.   All four types of lipofuscin are seen.
(8000X)

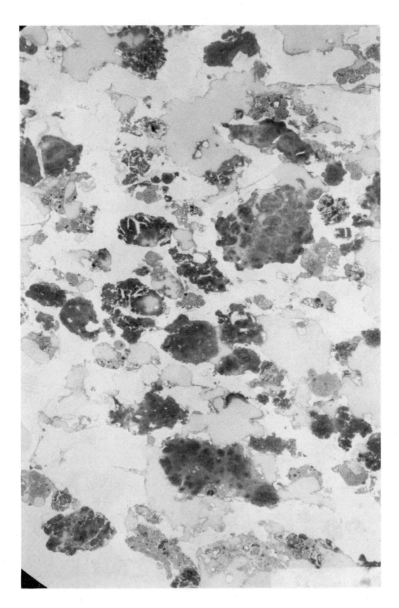

Fig. 11. Lipofuscin fraction from five normal human brains with a mean age of 66.8 years. (8000X)

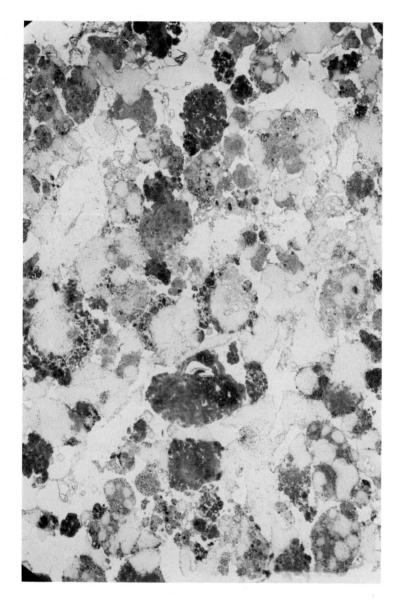

Fig. 12.   Lipofuscin fraction from five normal human brains with a
mean age of 78.8 years.   (8000X)

membrane. Therefore, we assume these globular structures are
lipofuscin precursors. Studies in liver (Siakotos et al., 1973)
indicate such particles contain acid phosphatase only in the limiting
membrane or "globule" edge. In addition, the pool of these
lipofuscin-like organelles remains constant on a mg/brain basis
over the first 16.8 years of life (Figure G, Table I). However,
the amount of lipofuscin-like fraction when calculated as lipofuscin
content per unit dry weight of brain, is significantly higher
during the first three months of life, and decreases rapidly
during the next 8.6 years of life to reach a minimum at 16.8 years.
It is well known that the human brain reaches a maximum size at
ages 18-25 years (Ordy et al., 1975). The data in Figure 6 and
Table I indicate there is a pool of subcellular organelles, lipofuscin or lipofuscin-like material, even in early life. Moreover,
this "age pigment" pool size remains relatively constant per brain,
despite rapid developmental changes, such as growth during the
first year of life. What is the source of this pool of organelles?
Does this fraction represent an intracellular pool of detritis in
the lysosomes derived from the remodeling of intracellular and
cellular structures during the prenatal and neonatal periods in
brain? Or do these lipofuscin-like structures represent storage
depots for surplus or toxic materials released during normal
metabolic cellular processes during the life of the neurone? If
the latter proposition is true, then the size of the available
storage depots early in life may determine the damage potential of
toxic and surplus products of metabolism produced later in life.
Our initial reports (Siakotos et al., 1972), have shown that lipofuscin
accumulates, and binds or stores very high titers of lysosomal
hydrolases. The present study provides preliminary evidence that
the autofluorescence of the fractions isolated and shown in Table
I increase with age. The proposition is advanced that the maturation
and sequential formation of age pigment or lipofuscin in human brain
occurs by the scheme given in Figure 13. This figure was adapted
in part from Goldfisher et al. (1966) and Novikoff et al. (1973)
and was presented in an early form in a previous paper (Siakotos
and Armstrong, 1975). In this scheme the "lipid globule" or cyto-
lysosome continues to fuse with lysosomes and microperoxisomes to
form an early prelipofuscin granule which matures with age by the
constant addition of lysosomal and peroxisomal enzymes to form a
final mature lipofuscin granule. The cytolysosomes probably ingest
large quantities of neutral lipids found in the neonatal brain
(Rouser and Yamamoto, 1968). The rate of formation of lipofuscin
granules may then be governed by: a) the availability and size of
the initial neutral lipid and cytosome pool; b) the rate of lysosome and microperoxisome biogenesis; and c) the intracellular
accessibility of lysosomes and microperoxisomes. The production
of secondary autofluorescent products within the maturing lipofuscin
granule would be of a secondary nature and should not affect the
rate of formation. These latter changes are part of the maturation

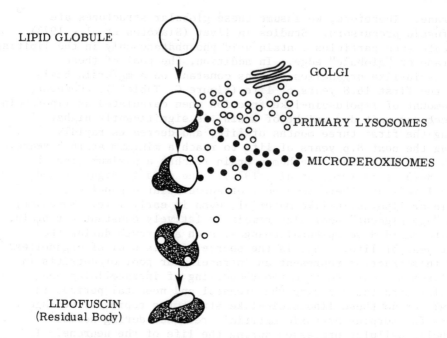

Fig. 13. The development sequence for lipofuscin in brain. The
particle marked lipid globule may be a lipid globule or a lipid
filled lysosome. Maturation occurs by the continuous fusion of
lysosomes and microperoxisomes with the addition of acid hydrolases,
cation, etc. and production of brightly fluorescent polymeric
compounds.

process. The last condition would be totally dependent on the
availability and accessibility of peroxisomes and catalase to
oxidants, such as hydrogen peroxide or other peroxides. In the
past, most studies designed to establish or verify theories on
the genesis of age pigment have remained close to areas well known
to cell biologists, such as well defined organelle systems. In our
view, the time has come to bury these restrictions, and to consider
in a new light, the initial lipofuscin precursors along with the
sequential development and maturation lipofuscin.

    Acknowledgements: The authors wish to thank Drs. Gary Mierau,
Ghildren's Hospital, and Michael Norenberg, Veterans Administration
Hospital, Denver, Colorado, for the brain specimens and Dr. Bernardino
Ghetti for the lipopigment electron microscopy. This study was
supported by the National Retinitis Pigmentosa Foundation, the
Childrens Brain Disease Foundation, and by USPHS grants RR 5371 and
NS 09760.

REFERENCES

Brizzee, K.R., Ordy, J.M. and Kaack, B. Early appearance and regional differences in intraneuronal and extraneuronal lipofuscin accumulation with age in the brain of a non-human primate (Macaca mulatta). J. Gerontol. 29:366-381, 1974.

Brody, H. The deposition of aging pigment in the human cerebral cortex. J. Gerontol. 15:258-261, 1960.

Brody, H. Personal communication Brizzee, K.R., J.C. Karkin, J.M. Karkin, J.M. Ordy and B. Kaack (1975). Accumulation and distribution of lipofuscin, amyloid, and senile plaques in the aging nervous system. In: Aging, Vol. I, (Eds. H. Brody, D. Harman, and J. M. Ordy), Raven Press, New York, pp. 39-78, 1974.

Chu, L. A cytological study of anterior horn cells isolated from human spinal cord. J. Comp. Neurol. 100:381-413, 1954.

Csallany, A.S. and Ayaz, K.L. Quantitative Determination of Organic Solvent Soluble Lipofuscin Pigments in Tissues. Lipids 11:412-417, 1976.

Goldfischer, S., Villaverde, H. and Forschirm, R. The demonstration of acid hydrolase, thermostable reduced diphosphopyridine nucleotide tetrazolium reductase and peroxidase activity in human lipofuscin pigment granules. J. Histo. and Cytochem. 14:641-652, 1966.

Humphrey, T. Primitive neurones in the embryonic human central nervous system. J. Comp. Neurol. 81:1-45, 1944.

Novikoff, A.B., Novikoff, P.M., Quintana, N. and Davis, C. Studies in microperoxisomes IV. Interrelations of microperoxisomes, endoplasmic reticulum and lipofuscin granules. J. Histo. and Cytochem. 21:1010-1020.

Ordy, J.M., Kaack, B. and Brizzee, K.R. Lifespan Neurochemical changes in the human and non-human primate brain. In: Aging: Clinical, Morphological and Neurochemical Aspects in the Aging Central Nervous System, (Eds. H. Brody, D. Harmon, and J.M. Ordy), Raven, Press, New York, Vol. I, pp. 133-189, 1975.

Porta, E.A. and Hartroft, W..S. Lipid pigments in relation to aging and dietary factors (lipofuscin). In: Pigments in Pathology, (Ed. W. Wolman), Academic Press, New York, pp. 192-235, 1969.

Rouser, G. and Yamamoto, A.   Curvilinear regression course of human
    brain lipid composition changes with age.   Lipids 3:284-287, 1968.

Siakotos, A.N. and Armstrong, D.   Age pigment, a biochemical indicator
    of intracellular aging.   In: Neurobiology of Aging, (Eds. J.M.
    Ordy and K.R. Brizzee), Plenum Press, New York, pp. 369-399, 1975.

Siakotos, A.N. and Koppang, N.   Procedures for the isolation of lipo-
    pigments from brain, heart and liver, and their properties: A
    review.   Mech. Aging and Develop. 2:177-200, 1973.

Siakotos, A.N., Watanabe, I., Pennington, K. and Whitfield, M.
    Procedures for the mass isolation of pure lipofuscin from normal
    human heart and liver.   Biochem. Med. 7:24-38, 1973.

Siakotos, A.N., Watanabe, I., Saito, N. and Fleischer, S.   Procedures
    for the isolation of two distinct lipopigments from human brain:
    lipofuscin and ceroid.   Biochem. Med. 4:361-375, 1970.

Siakotos, A.N., Goebel, H.H., Patel, V., Watanabe, I. and Zeman, W.
    The morphogenesis and biochemical characteristics of ceroid
    isolated from cases of neuronal ceroid-lipofuscinosis.   In:
    Sphingolipids, sphingolipidoses and allied disorders, (Eds.
    B. W. Volk and S. M. Aronson), Plenum Publications, New York,
    pp. 53-61, 1972.

Taubold, R.D., Siakotos, A.N. and Perkins, E.G.   Studies on chemical
    nature of lipofuscin (age pigment) isolated from normal human
    brain.   Lipids 10:383-390, 1975.

Telez-Nagel, I., Johnson, A.B. and Terry, R.D.   Ultrastructural and
    histochemical study of cerebral biopsies in Huntington's Chorea.
    Adv. Neurology I:387-398, 1973.

Wisniewski, H.M. and Terry, R.D.   Reexamination of the pathogenesis
    of the senile plaque.   Prog. Neuropath. II:1-26, 1973.

CHROMATIN IN AGING BRAIN

F. Marott Sinex

Boston University School of Medicine
80 East Concord Street
Boston, MA.   02118

Dementia is a major problem for the Veterans Administration and will become more so as the World War I veterans enter their seventies and eighties. Dementia and confusional states may occur for a number of reasons. However, in a large number of cases, perhaps half of those with severe memory loss show a pathology similar to that first described in patients with pre-senile dementia by Alzheimer, namely cortical atrophy, neurofibrillary tangles and senile plaques. For want of a better name, one is tempted to call dementia in the elderly with this type of pathology an Alzheimer's type senile dementia, even though by definition Alzheimer's disease is a pre-senile dementia. We may need a better name. Euphanisms cannot hide a problem on which little research is being done, which is costing more and more money, and placing more and more patients in chronic care institutions.

The incidence increases from 45 onward until it is a severe threat to the well being of those over ninety. There are no really satisfactory studies in the United States on the incidence of dementia of defined types. In the English Newcastle study (Kay et al., 1964; Kay, 1972) the prevalence of Alzheimer's type senile dementia in men over 75 was nine times that of those between 65 and 75. Dementia is a problem of staggering proportions, and the linear projections for the incidence of dementia based simply on the numbers of veterans entering the over sixty age group on VA extended care are obviously inadequate in anticipating the impact of this cohort when it reaches advanced old age. One must consider increased utilization of VA facilities by the older post-retirement veterans, and the remarkable increased incidence in the very old as well.

The percent of senile or Alzheimer's type dementia compared

TABLE I

Percent of Chronic Brain Syndrome by Sex and Age

	Senile		Vascular		Other		Total	
	M	F	M	F	M	F	M	F
65 - 75 :	0.5	1.0	2.0	0.3	1.0	1.0	3.5	2.4
75 & over:	4.4	9.3	6.7	2.3	1.1	1.2	12.2	12.7

to other types of chronic brain syndrome is shown in Table I prepared from Newcastle data.

One may attempt to analyze dementia in terms of penetrance and expression. Would everyone get dementia if they lived long enough or is only about 5 per cent of the population at risk? What factors other than aging play a role in the expression or is the aging of the brain the primary factor? If dementia is genetic in origin is dementia a Garrod type inborn error in metabolism with a specific biochemical lesion or are the injuries to the genome in dementia random.

Our approach is to consider the dementia lesion the result of fairly random genetic events involving many genes and their control. We consider almost everyone to be at risk, and the expression to be strongly age dependent. The opposite can be argued, that of those at risk, most become demented, and that relatively few genes are involved, perhaps only one for the most common type of dementia. Finally, one might contend that genetic analysis is futile, and that dementia results from some other cause.

There are a number of analogies between dementia and mental retardation. Many elderly show a relatively benign loss of memory which does not interfere with daily living. They can care for themselves, as can a slightly retarded person, with minimal support. In both cases, psychological difficulties may mimic physiological problems, or a patient may be troubled with both. However in both the elderly and in children there are syndromes of lost cortical function which are severe and progressive. These may have a number of biochemical causes. Although dementia is associated with neurofibrillary tangles and senile plaques, these changes may be merely concomitant rather than causative and expressions of a loss of particular types of cell function.

Scheibel et al. (1975) have described some of the progressive

dendritic changes which occur in both aging and the brains of victims
of dementia. In Golgi stained preparations the extension of the
dendrites from cell body and their branching decrease. Indeed
elements of the pathology of dementia, dendritic change, proliferation
of neurofilaments and the appearance of plaques are found in almost
all older brains, the difference being one of degree.

Ideally we would like to know what causes dementia, how to
prevent it and how to treat it. This requires the development of
some testable hypothesis, and if possible, the development of an
animal model. Dr. Martin Feldman has described (see Dr. Feldman's
chapter) silver stained apical dendrites of neurons in the cortex
of rats and quantitative data on how dendritic extensions decrease
with age. The lost synapses primarily maintained connections among
clusters of neurons in the cortical architecture. The loss of
synapses with age must appreciably reduce the fine tuning in neuronal
function.

We do not know how much biochemical information is required to
establish synapses. The specific recognition signals of the brain
may require both anatomical and biochemical information as well as
stimulation. We believe that the brain would respond to altered or
decreased coding in any proteins required for the formation of
synapses by showing decreased neuronal interaction, and reduced
dendritic extension. Unfortunately, we do not know whether or not
synapses continuously form and disappear in the mature brain since
our electron microscopic pictures represent an instant in time.
Broadly speaking alterations in the proteins required for neuronal
recognition could arise from either mutation or altered control of
genes. We will now discuss some experiments which bear on the
question of the control of genes in the aging brain.

Our first study showed that the melting temperature and hyper-
chromicity of mouse brain chromatin correlated with the amount of
protein present. The amount of protein decreased from birth through
maturity, but in the case of the mouse brain increased somewhat in
senescence (Kurtz and Sinex, 1967).

O'Meara and Herrmann (1972) studied chromatin from liver of
aging C/57 black mice extracting the chromatin with gradually increasing concentrations of salt. They studied the protein removal
and the activation of the chromatin as a template for RNA polymerase
(Figures 1 and 2). Relatively little protein is removed from the
chromatin in low salt concentrations in older animals and in general
it requires a higher concentration of salt to dissociate the protein
from the chromatin (Figure 1). Figure 2 shows the effect of this
protein from young animals is more effective in activating transcription in the chromatin in young livers than in old. The observation of O'Meara and Herrmann (1972) that there is increased interaction

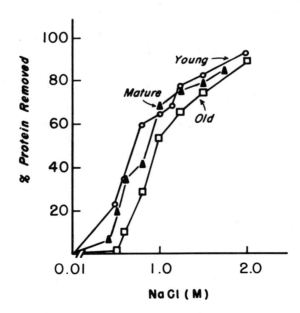

Fig. 1.   The removal of protein as a function of salt dissociation
of mouse liver chromatin from young, mature and old mice.
0-0, young (3.25 months): ▲-▲ , mature (13.75 months):□-□, old
(21 months).

between DNA and protein in aging has recently been confirmed by
Cutler (1975).

In a subsequent study, Kurtz et al. (1974) interfaced a PDP-8
computer with a spectrophotometer to do differential melting curves
on mouse brain chromatin. When DNA passes from a double stranded
state, its ability to absorb light at 260 nanometers substantially
increases since individual bases no longer interfer with each other's
absorption when unstacked. The computer plots a differential of
this curve making repeated measurements at each temperature interval
as the temperature is raised. That is to say it plots whether the
absorption is increasing or decreasing against temperature.

Derivative melting curves for young, mature and old animals
are shown in Figures 4, 5 and 6. In younger animals, as shown in
Figure 4, within the temperature range of 50-60° in which free DNA
or DNA complexed to readily dissociable protein melts, there is

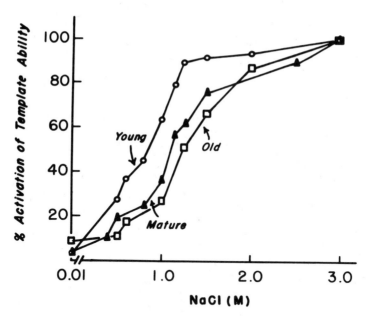

Fig. 2.   Activation of template ability as a function of salt
dissociation of liver chromatin from young, mature and old mice.
The ability of the liver chromatin to serve as a template for RNA
synthesis was assayed by the method of Chamberlin and Berg (1962).
The percentage activation refers to the ratio of cpm of ^{14}C ATP
incorporated into RNA to the cpm incorporated in the presence of
calf thymus chromatin at a similar DNA concentration.

little melting. This is not the case for mature animals, the
derivative melting curve for which is shown in Figure 5. There is
considerable chromatin melting within a temperature range of 50-64°.
Older animals shown in Figure 6 resemble younger animals in showing
less freely melting DNA.

     We interpreted the experiments of O'Meara and Herrmann (1972)
and Kurtz et al. (1974) as indicating that in young animals the
protein which prevents melting at lower temperature dissociates
readily in salt. In the mature animals the open segments would
appear to be clearly delineated but not as active in transcription
as in the young. In the older animals these open sites again become
restricted. We believe this is because the associated protein
becomes altered or denatured or because the state of aggregation

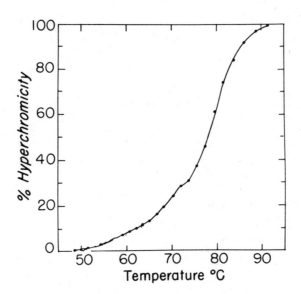

Fig. 3. This is not a derivative melting curve but simply plots increased absorbance versus temperature of a sample of chromatin from the brain of a 12 month old mouse. The measurements were made in 2.5 mM Na of citrate.

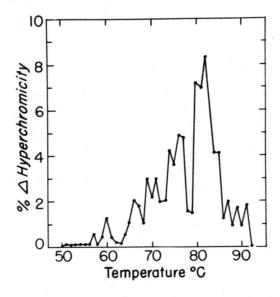

Fig. 4. The averaged derivative melting curve of mice, 3 day, 3, 4, 5 and 6 months in 2.5 mM NaCl and 0.25 mM Na citrate.

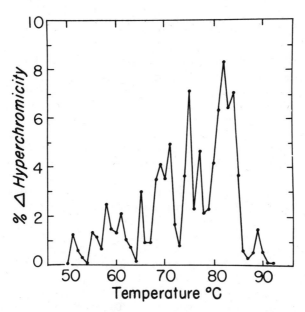

Fig. 5. The averaged derivative melting curve of mice, 10, 12 and 13 months (6 experiments) in 2.5 mM NaCl and 0.25 mM Na citrate.

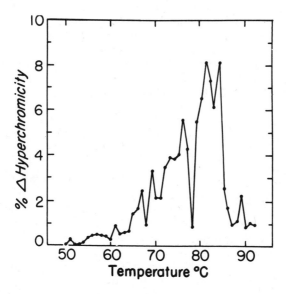

Fig. 6. The average derivative melting curve of mice, 14, 15, 16 and 30 months (8 experiments) in 2.5 mM NaCl and 0.25 M Na citrate.

of the chromatin again changes. State of aggregation includes many possibilities such as crosslinkage of DNA to protein or of DNA with itself (Freese and Castel, 1964) or simply less transcribable genome.

Direct evidence for an increased interaction between DNA and protein in old brain was obtained by Herrmann et al. (1975). They found that the amount of rapidly reannealing or permanently annealed DNA increased in both brain and liver of older mice. The rate of reannealing or the reformation of double stranded DNA from single strands after denaturing is expressed in terms of Cot. This refers to the time required for reannealing under specified standard conditions of concentration and temperature. A small Cot value indicates rapid reannealing. The most rapid reannealing occurs in the situation where the base sequences are such that within a single strand a complimentary sequence or palindrome occurs which is capable of forming an internal loop. The techniques involve a cycle of denaturation and renaturation, with the renatured fraction being removed on hydroxyapatite. The per cent of DNA recovered in the Cot 10^{-5} fraction increased from 0.6 to 1.8 per cent between the ages of 2 months and 27 months. This DNA was prepared by a chloroformisoamyl alcohol procedure which precipitates protein. If this 2-3 per cent protein is reduced to 0.5-0.8 per cent by digestion with pronase, the difference between young and old animals in Cot disappears.

When these rapidly annealing or permanently annealed fractions were denatured with foramide and examined under an electron microscope, the fractions from old animals were found to contain what Herrmann called "hairpins", in which a single strand of DNA loops back upon itself. These structures are presumably stabilized by protein. Such a "hairpin" is shown in Figure 7. Such preparations are heavily shadowed for study by electron microscopy and single and double stranded regions cannot be distinguished.

Supporting the concept that with time the DNA of brain becomes less available for transcription are the experiments of Cutler (1975) in Dallas.

Brain has more open genome available for RNA transcription than any other tissue in the body. In Figure 8 brain and liver are contrasted. Open genome is indicated by the thinner line, non-transcribed genome by the heavy line. The genome is divided into two parts, one dealing with single copy, and the other with multiple copy messenger. It can be seen quite clearly the transcribable message is being shut off with age. The reduction in transcribable message in aging may arise from mutation of DNA or altered control of genes.

The extreme longevity of the human species would tend to favor the contributions of chemical events occurring at a relatively fixed

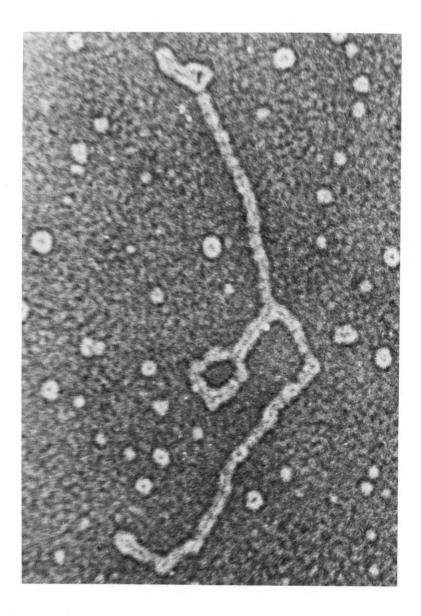

Fig. 7. Electron microscograph of a "hairpin" from spontaneously associating DNA of Cot 10^{-5} isolated from a 28 months old mouse deproteinized in chloroform - isoamyl alcohol, heat denatured and treated with 82 percent formamide. Magnification 380,000x.

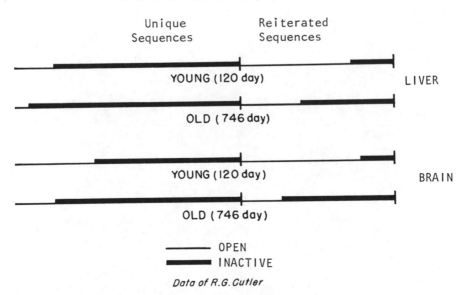

Fig. 8. This figure represents as bars, the data of Cutler (1975).
The thin lines indicate transcribable genome and the heavier lines
nontranscribable genome. The unique and reiterated sequences of
both liver and brain are presented separately. The unique sequences
generate single copies of messenger RNA coding specific proteins.

rate in all species so that the relative importance of different
types of alterations need not be identical in mice and men even
though both age.

We might review briefly evidence for and against somatic mutation
and altered differentiation as a cuase of aging (Sinex, 1977 and
Burnet, 1974).

Some arguments in favor of somatic mutation are as follows:

1. Increased levels of chromosomal aberrations may be demonstrated cytologically in aging animals. While aging injury to DNA
may not be predominantly of this type, there may well be a correlation
(Curtis, 1966, 1971).

2.   The pathology of aging resembles, at least superficially, the pathology of chronic low level radiation injury (Upton, 1957).

3.   Long-lived animals seem to have exceptionally efficient endonucleases for the repair of thymidine dimers induced by ultra-violet light (Hart and Setlow, 1974).

4.   The frequency of mutation in cell culture would suggest that somatic mutation could indeed be significant in an intact animal (Sinex, 1974, 1977).

Evidence against somatic mutation as a cause of aging might be summarized as follows:

1.   Relatively limited studies with bifunctional alkylating agents by Alexander and Connell (1960) failed to show any geromimetic effects.

2.   Aging is not correlated with ploidy.   Extra chromosome sets do not protect against aging, nor does a haploid state make an individual aging prone (Sinex, 1977).

3.   Some other explanation may be more plausible.   The argument we will explore is that aging results from an altered state of differentiation.

We have tried to visualize the type of point mutation that would contribute to aging.   We would suggest that aging mutations are first of all not readily repaired, for the most part because they are not recognizable and in some instances because they are not repairable. If on the other hand a mutation is so trivial that it does not lead to any coding error in DNA replication or RNA transcription or change in DNA protein interaction, then it should not lead to aging.   Certain simple substitution mutations raise the question as to how a repair endonuclease would know which strand to correct, presumably a 50-50 proposition.

Arguments favoring changes in the state of differentiation as a cause of aging include:

1.   Changes in the state of differentiation as a cause of aging includes the production of:
      a) socially undesirable cells which multiply but whose
      function is not in the best interests of the host.
      b) cells fated to die.
      c) more variant cells.

2.   Very short-lived species which would not seem to have much opportunity to accumulate somatic mutations also age.   This implies

aging by a more directed mechanism.

3.   Exceptionally long-lived species would have time to accumulate modified proteins in their chromatin. The most likely change to occur would be the spontaneous hydrolysis of amide nitrogen (Sinex, 1977). Other possibilities include modification of SH groups on nonhistone protein (Tas, 1976), or the crosslinkage of protein to DNA.

4.   The placement of the protein which specifies the differentiated state in the replication of chromatin may be just as or more susceptible to error than DNA replication.

5.   In the tissue culture model cells do not drop out of the cycle on an all or none basis, but seem to move in and out, the number not cycling over a particular period of time increasing with age (Absher et al., 1975).

6.   In culture while the longevity of the culture is relatively fixed, it can be altered, for example, by glucocorticoid hormones (Cristofalo, 1970).

7.   Ploidy experiments may be interpreted as showing not that aging mutations are dominant but that a concept of somatic mutation need not apply (Sinex, 1977).

Let us now return to the point about time dependent chemical change, being favored by the extreme age of human neurons formed before birth and postmitotic for life.

Spontaneous hydrolysis of the phosphate diester of the DNA backbone undoubtedly must occur but should be readily repairable. Of particular interest to us are those reactions which might result in the crosslinkage of protein to DNA. One way this might occur is through the transfer of a deoxyribosyl residue from a purine to the epsilon amino group of lysine during depurination of DNA. We are studying this possibility in model systems and observing the products produced for indications of what to look for in enzymatic hydrolysates of older nucleoprotein as evidence of crosslink formation.

While other crosslinking reactions are possible, involving free radicals, SH or other functional groups the Maillard reaction, as the reaction between reducing sugars and amino acids is called, is readily demonstrable in most nonliving tissue, Gottschalk (1972). Depurination is known to be catalyzed by protons or trace metals (Lindahl and Myberg, 1972).

Pyrimidine elimination from DNA is catalyzed by bisulfite and oxygen (Hayatsu, 1976). SO_2 is a common air pollutant.

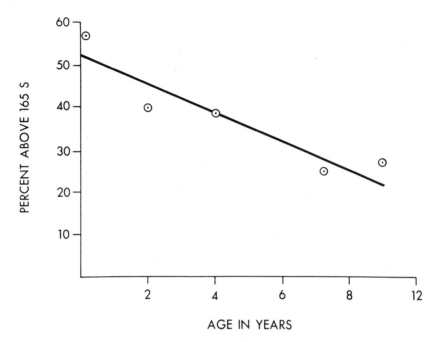

Fig. 9. A plot of data from the paper of Wheeler and Lett (1974). Lysates from the internal granular-layer neurons of the cerebellum of beagles were lysed on an alkaline sucrose gradient and sedimentation profiles prepared. The amount of material sedimenting with a constant above 165 S is plotted against age in years.

Apurinic or apyrimic sites which are not stabilized would eventually undergo spontaneous hydrolysis and repair. There is some evidence that the incidence of single strand breaks in neurons increase with age, namely the studies of Wheeler and Lett (1974), on the cerebellar neurons of aging dogs.

Using a zonal rotor in an ultracentrifuge, Wheeler and Lett lysed a cell suspension on an alkaline sucrose gradient. As the lysis proceeded the DNA separated from other nuclear constituents and became single stranded. The single stranded DNA then broke into segments sedimenting about 165 S. Such segments, although relatively large, are much smaller than the DNA of chromosomes. Wheeler and Lett have observed the amount of DNA sedimenting with a sedimentation constant greater than 165 S immediately following lysis. They feel that this represents the single stranded DNA of chromosomes. These are difficult experiments in which to control all the variables.

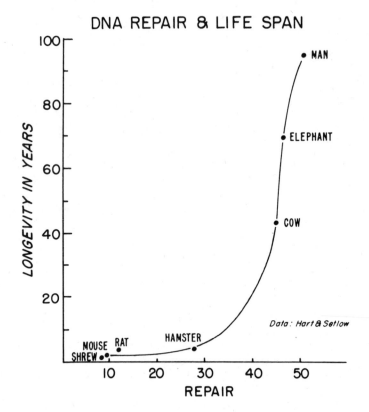

Fig. 10. A plot of grain counts over hydroxyurea inhibited fibroblasts of different species exposed to 10 V/m² of ultraviolet light and labeled with tritiated thymidine.

The results of Wheeler and Lett are shown in Figure 9. We have plotted the fraction of DNA sedimenting over 165 S against the age of dogs. The decrease in sedimentation constant with age might be taken to indicate increasing strand breakage in DNA of old brains or an increased association of DNA with larger protein aggregates which interfere with the release of single strands.

Now let us consider the possibility that individual variation in repair capability could account for some individuals being at risk for dementia and others not. First let us review the Hart and Setlow (1974) data that establishes that there is at least species variation in unscheduled DNA synthesis after irradiation of cells with ultraviolet light.

That longevitous animals have exceptionally good repair is illustrated in Figure 10 prepared from data from Hart and Setlow (1974). Grain counts of unscheduled DNA synthesis following a standard dose of ultraviolet irradiation were made. Longevitous animals had a higher incorporation of tritium labeled thymidine.

All repair processes for DNA share some common features, gap enlargement, activation of nucleotides, filling of the gap and the action of ligase for the final closing. They differ in the types of mutation repaired, and in the size of the excision. We need not consider post replication repair because neurons are postmitotic.

Repair of thymidine dimers is one specific type of endonuclease repair. Its neurological analogue is the retardation associated with xeroderma pigmentosa (Cook and Brazell, 1976).

Repair of x-ray induced injury utilizes another endonuclease system, short patch instead of long patch repair, and removes the products of rather simple alkylations and hydroxylations (Grossman et al., 1975). The neurological analogue is ataxia telangistasia (Hoar and Sargent, 1976).

A third type of repair is through clipping off bases followed by hydrolysis of the apurinic site. An endonuclease catalyzing hydrolysis of apurinic sites has been reported by Lindahl and Anderson (1972) in bacteria and in mammalian liver, (Verly and Parquette, 1973) and thymus, (Ljungquist and Lindahl, 1974). No neurological analogue has been reported.

The removal of purines is interesting in that it represents a process for both repair and injury. N alkylated purines depurinate faster than the purines of normal DNA. The depurination is catalyzed by protons and should be catalyzed by heavy metals as well, since both withdraw electrons (Lindahl and Anderson, 1972; Glassman et al., 1973).

Simple mismatch, as for example after nitrous acid mutations, is at least partly repaired, but the system is unknown.

Ionizing radiation does not produce an Alzheimer type syndrome and would not seem a good model for aging injury. The most important chemical result of ionizing radiation is the addition of hydroxyl free radical to pyrimidimes. Adult neurons are relatively insensitive to radiation, and consequently the more terminal portions of the repair system must be intact. The brain neurons seem less sensitive than the microcirculation. Radiation to the brain induces an inflammatory response with deterioration of myelin (Clemente and Holtz, 1954). The deterioration of cell nuclei which also occurs does not trigger neurofilament formation.

The increased incidence of dementia in women is consistent with the inhibition of DNA repair by estrogen found in a number of tissues. This inhibition is now, however, considered highly specific (Gauden et al., 1972).

We will now consider another topic, the possible role of trace metals in the etiology of senile dementia and their relationship to other types of dementia.

Various relationships can be postulated between abnormal neurofilaments, genetic injury and metals. It has been shown that injection of aluminum salts causes abnormal neurofilaments to appear after a number of days. For example, the production of neurofibrillary tangles, and injury has been reported by Wisniewski and Terry (1970) through injection of aluminum salts into the lateral ventricles or cisterna magna. The system is quite sensitive, a cysterna magna injection in a rabbit requiring 0.1 ml of a 1 per cent solution AlCl3 (Liwnicz et al., 1974). The response in terms of neurofilaments is impressive.

The effects of AlCl3 injection are expressed after a period of time beginning in 48 hours and becoming well established 10 to 20 days after injection, when animals begin to show neurological symptoms. The development of the neurofibrillary tangles would seem to require new protein synthesis. In contrast to the human disease, there are no amyloid plaques. The lesion can be produced in rabbits, cats and monkeys. Mice and rats are resistant.

Spindle inhibitors such as colchicine also produce a proliferation of neurofilaments, (Wisniewski and Terry, 1967). This occurs in less than 24 hours in vivo and in 30 minutes in neuroblastoma cells in culture. The relationship between 10 nanometer neurofilaments, the Alzheimer twisted double filament, tubulin and microtubules remain controversial and is an active field of investigation. Wisniewski and Terry stated that it is not possible to distinguish by electron microscopy, in terms of ultrastructure, between the filaments of injured animals, and animals injured by spindle inhibitors. In the case of spindle inhibitors, a case can be made for at least some filaments forming from depolymerized tubules. Sensitivity of microtubule assembly to Al^{+++} ions would not be surprising considering the importance of GTP and GMP in microtubule polymerization and stabilization (Weisenberg and Deery, 1976), and the possibility that aluminum salts might complex with such cyclic nucleotides at a binding site.

The current literature on neurofibrillary tangles may be summarized as follows (Terry and Wisniewski, 1975; Iqbal et al., 1975). In Alzheimer's presenile and senile dementia the silver staining fibrillary tangles appear to be formed from a pair of helically wound 10 nm filaments. Similar filaments are found in the brains of normal aged humans, as well as in mongolism, the Guam-Parkinsonism dementia complex, postencephalitic Parkinsonism and tuberous sclerosis. The monomer associated with neurofibrillary pathology runs slightly ahead of the fast moving component of tubulin and of human neurofilament protein on SDS acrylamide gels (Iqbal et al., 1974).

The neurofilament monomer of calf brain, while similar to tubulin in amino acid composition and molecular weight, does not bind colchicine or guanosine triphosphate and is a distinct species by electrophoresis.

The neurofilaments induced by aluminum and spindle inhibitors cannot be distinguished morphologically. They have not been characterized chemically.

Thus, neither aluminum nor spindle inhibitors produce the twisted tubules of Alzheimer's type senile dementia. They do however form neurofibrillary tangles of the fibrillary type characteristic of the neurofilaments of the species in which they are produced. Thus Al^{+++} toxicity in rabbits may either produce a characteristic lesion unrelated to a human dementia or be a model for dementia in which the human species forms a twisted filament while a rabbit does not.

There is yet another category of filaments present in cells and in nervous tissue. There are actin filaments (LeBeux and Willemot, 1975). The actin monomer is slightly smaller than tubulin and forms twisted double filaments which give tight complexes with heavy metals such as lanthanum.

Now let us return to chromatin. Crapper et al. (1973) has found that the chromatin of Alzheimer's type senile dementia brains contains significantly more Al^{+++} than normal elderly brains. The localization of Al^{+++} in metaphase chromosomes can be demonstrated histochemically (DeBoni et al., 1974). It is of interest that Douvas et al. (1975) have claimed that both actin and tubulin are major constituents of the nonhistone component of chromatin, actin constituting 7.6 per cent of the nonhistone protein and tubulin 12.9 per cent. Sheets of actin filaments can be demonstrated in the cytoplasm of several non-muscle cell types (Sauger, 1975). Crapper's observation can thus be interpreted in two ways. Either environmental exposure to Al^{+++} or metabolic idiosyncrasies affecting Al^{+++} metabolism occur in certain individuals causing them to suffer chronic brain injury, or that the brain or the brain chromatin of Alzheimer's type senile dementia victims is altered so that there is more binding of a universal probe, Al^{+++}. It is possible that the

binding of Al^{+++} to chromatin and the proliferation of filaments
are related phenomena.

The effect of trace metals on DNA mutations and nucleoprotein
is of particular interest in that such approaches might well lead
to specific preventive and therapeutic strategies to reduce exposure
and protect the brain.

The final subject I wish to consider is the capability which a
post mitotic cell has for the repair of injury to protein components
of their nueleoprotein.

The repair of injured DNA may require the removal of much of
the protein at the site of injury (Wilkins and Hart, 1974).   In
addition spontaneous chemical changes such as the loss of amide
nitrogen, altered disulfide linkages (Tas, 1976) and crosslinkage
of deoxyribose to protein in unstable depurinated sequences may lead
to eventual proteolysis.

The repair capability of the cell in terms of replacing protein
is limited.   In young animals we find Hl associated with the polysome
fraction.   In the case of Hl histones in mature tissue, we have found
that Hl is replaced by another protein which closely resembles Hl,
F_1^0 which is predominately found in cytoplasm and possibly is not
able to undergo the same type of acetylation and phosphorylation as
Hl in the nucleus.

The substitution of Hl by F_1^0, we believe, reduces plasticity
of older tissue for altered transcription and replication.   The net
effect of such a substitution on the brain would depend somewhat
on anatomical variations, rate and genetic susceptibility and the
true significance of Hl.

Decreasing the content or accuracy of coded genetic information
is likely to reduce communcation between neurons by interfering with
the formation of correct synapses.   The appearance of amyloid in the
peculiar pathology of the lesions in Alzheimer's type senile dementia,
we believe, is due to a failure in the suppressive function of T-
lymphocytes on antibody producing cells, relating a nuclear phenomena,
in this case recognition of histocompatability loci, to pathology.
We thus postulate a dual failure for similar biochemical reasons,
one in the nuclei of the neurons of the cortex and the other in the
nuclei of the lymphocytes.   These two combined produce an Alzheimer's
like-senile dementia with fewer synapses, cell loss and amyloid
plaques.

Our speculation suggests some questions that might be asked
about dementia victims; their exposure to mutagens, particularly
heavy metals, their immunocompetence particularly in relation to

suppressive function in T cells, their history of infectious illness (since viruses induce DNA strand breakage), and their estrogen history.

There is no reason why senile dementia should not be a preventable and treatable illness. Effective therapy will be found as it has for other illness' through studying epidemiology, the pathology and the biochemistry. There are rational experimental approaches. I have discussed some involving DNA and chromatin. There are others. Dementia is now one of the more challenging problems in medicine.

REFERENCES

Absher, P.M., Absher, R.G. and Barnes, W.D. Time lapse cinemicro-photographic studies of cell division patterns of human diploid fibroblasts (WI-38) during their in vitro lifespan. Advan. in Exp. Med. and Biol. 53:91-105, 1975.

Alexander, P. and Connell, D.I. Shortening of the lifespan of mice by irradiation with x-rays and treatment with radiomimetic chemicals. Radiation Res. 12:38-48, 1960.

Burnet, Sir MacF. "Intrinsic Mutagenesis: A Genetic Approach to Aging". Wiley, New York-Toronto, 1974.

Chamberlin, M. and Berg, P. Deoxyribonucleic acid directed synthesis of ribonucleic acid by an enzyme from Escherichia coli. Proc. Natl. Acad. Sci. USA 48:81-94, 1962.

Clemente, C.D. and Holst, E.A. Pathological changes in neurons neuroglia and blood-brain barrier induced by x-irradiation of heads of monkeys. A.M.A. Arch. Neuro. Psych. 71:66-79, 1954.

Cook, P.R. and Brazell, I.A. Detection and repair of single strand breaks in nuclear DNA. Nature 263:679-682, 1976.

Crapper, D.R., Kushinan, S.S. and Dalton, A.J. Brain aluminum distribution in mouse liver and brain tissues as a function of age. Trans. Amer. Neurol. Assoc. 98:15-20, 1973.

Cristofalo, V.J. Metabolic aspects to aging in diploid human cells. In: Aging in Cell and Tissue Culture, (Eds. V. J. Cristofalo and E. Holeckova), Plenum Press, New York, pp. 83-120, 1970.

Curtis, H., Jr. "Biological Mechanisms of Aging", Thomas, Springfield, 1966.

Curtis, J.M. and Miller, K.   Chromosomal aberrations of liver cells
    of guinea pigs.   J. Gerontol. 26:292-293, 1971.

Cutler, R.G.   Transcription of unique and reiterated DNA sequence
    in mouse liver and brain tissues as a function of age.   Exp.
    Gerontol. 10:37-59, 1975.

DeBoni, U., DeScott, J.W. and Crapper, D.R.   Intracellular aluminum
    binding, A histochemical study.   Histochemistry 40:31-37, 1974.

Douvas, A.S., Harrington, C.A. and Bonner, J.   Major nonhistone
    proteins of rat liver chromatin: preliminary identification of
    myosin, actin, tubulin and tropomyosin.   Proc. Natl. Acad. Sci.
    USA 72:3902-3906, 1975.

Freese, E. and Castel, M.   Crosslinking of deoxyribonucleic acid by
    exposure to low pH.   Biochim. Biophys. Acta 91:67-77, 1964.

Gaudin, D., Gregg, R. and Yielding, K.   Inhibition of DNA repair
    by co-carcinogens.   Biochem. Biophys. Res. Commun. 48:945, 1972.

Glassman, T.A., Klopman, G. and Cooper, C.   Use of the generalized
    perturbation theory to predict the interaction of purine nucleo-
    tides with metal ions.   Biochemistry 12:5013-5019, 1973.

Gottschalk, A.   Interaction between reducing sugars and amino acids
    under neutral and acidic conditions.   Glycoproteins 5(part A):
    144-157, 1972.

Grossman, L., Brawn, A., Feldberg, R. and Mahler, I.   Enzymatic
    Repair of DNA.   Annual Rev. Biochem. 44:19-43, 1975.

Hart, R.W. and Setlow, R.B.   Correlation between desoxyribonucleic
    and acid excision repair and lifespan in a number of mammalian
    species.   Proc. Natl. Acad. Sci. USA 71:2169-2173, 1974.

Hayatsu, H.   Bisulfite modification of nucleic acids and their
    constituents.   Progress in Nucleic Acid Res. 16:75-124, 1976.

Herrmann, R.L., Bick, M.D., Dowling, L. and Russell, A.F.   Age-related
    changes in a spontaneous reassociating fraction of mouse DNA.
    Mech. Age and Dev. 4:181-189, 1975.

Hoar, D.I. and Sargent, P.   Chemical mutagen hypersensitivity in
    ataxia telangiectosia.   Nature 261:590-592, 1976.

Iqbal, K., Wisniewski, H.M., Shelanski, M.L., Brostoff, S., Liwnicz,
    B.H. and Terry, R.D.   Protein changes in senile dementia.
    Brain Res. 77:337-343, 1974.

Iqbal, K. Wisniewski, H.M. and Grundke-Iqbal, I., et al. Chemical
    pathology of neurofibrils. Neurofibrillary of Alzheimer pre-
    senile dementia. J. Histochem. Cytochem. 23:563-569, 1975.

Kay, D.W., Beamish, P. and Roth, M. Old age mental disorders in
    Newcastle-Upon-Tyne, Part I (A study of Prevalence). Brit.
    J. Psychiat. 110:146-158, 1964.

Kay, D.W. Epidemiological aspects of organic brain disease in the
    aged, Age and the Brain. Adv. Behav. Biol. 3:15-28, 1972.

Kurtz, D.I., Russell, A.P. and Sinex, F.M. Multiple peaks in the
    derivative melting curve of chromatin from animals of varying
    age. Mech. Age and Dev. 3:37-49, 1974.

LeBeux, Y.J. and Willemot, J. An ultrastructural study of the micro-
    filaments in rat brain by means of E-PTA staining and heavy
    micromyosin labeling, I. Cell Tissue Res. 160:1-36, 1975.

LeBeux, Y.J. and Willemot, J. The perikaryon, the dendrites and
    the axon, II. Cell Tissue Res. 160:37-68, 1975.

Lindahl, T. and Myberg, B. Rate of depurination of native deoxy-
    ribonucleic acid. Biochemistry 11:3610-3618, 1972.

Lindahl, T. and Anderson, A. Rate of chain breakage at apurinic
    sites in double straned desoxyribonucleic acid. Biochemistry
    11:3618-3623, 1972.

Ljungquist, S. and Lindahl, T. A mammalian endonuclease specific
    for apurinic sites in double stranded desoxyribonucleic acid.
    J. Biol. Chem. 249:1530-1535, 1974.

Liwnicz, B.H., Kristensson, K., Wisniewski, H.M., Shelanski, M.L.
    and Terry, R.D. Observations on axoplasmic transport in rabbits
    with aluminum-induced neurofibrillary tangle. Brain Res. 80:
    413-420, 1974.

O'Meara, A.R. and Herrmann, R.L. A modified mouse liver chromatin
    preparation displaying age-related differences in salt dissociation
    and template ability. Biochim. Biophys. Acta 269:419-427, 1972.

Sauger, J.W. Presence of actin during chromosomal movement. Proc.
    Natl. Acad. Sci. USA 72:994-998, 1975.

Scheibel, M.E., Lindsay, R.D., Toiyasu, V. and Scheibel, A.B.
    Progressive dendritic changes in aging human cortex. Exper.
    Neurol. 47:393-403, 1975.

Sinex, F.M. The mutation theory of aging. In: Theoretical Aspects
    of Aging, (Ed. M. Rockstein), Academic Press, New York, pp. 23-31,
    1974.

Sinex, F.M. Molecular genetics of aging. In: Handbook on the
    Biology of Aging, (Eds. C. Finch and L. Hayflick), Van Nostrand
    Reinhold, New York, 1977 (in press).

Tas, S. Disulfide bonding in chromatin proteins with age and a
    suggested mechanism for aging and neoplasia. Exper. Geront.
    11:17-24, 1976.

Terry, R.D. and Wisniewski, H.M. Structural and chemical changes of
    the aged human brain. In: Aging, Vol. 2, (Eds. S. Gershon and
    A. Raskin), Raven Press, New York, pp. 127-141, 1975.

Upton, A.C. Ionizing radiation and the aging process. J. Gerontol.
    12:306-313, 1957.

Verly, W.G. and Paquett, Y. An endonuclease for depurinated DNA in
    rat liver. Canadian J. of Biochem. 51:1003-1009, 1973.

Wheeler, K.T. and Lett, J.T. On the possibility that DNA repair is
    related to age in nondividing cells. Proc. Natl. Acad. Sci. USA
    71:1862-1865, 1974.

Wilkins, R.J. and Hart, R.W. Preferential DNA repair in human cell.
    Nature 247:35-36, 1974.

Wisenberg, R.C. and Deery, W.J. Role of nucleotide hydrolysis in
    microtubule assembly. Nature 263:35-36, 1976.

Wisniewski, H. and Terry, R.D. Experimental colchicine encephalopathy.
    Induction of neurofibrillary degeneration. Laboratory Investiga-
    tion 17:577-587, 1967.

Wisniewski, H. and Terry, R.D. An experimental approach to the
    morphogenesis of neurofibrillary degeneration and the argyrophilic
    plaque. In: CIBA Foundation Symposium on Alzheimer's Disease and
    Related Conditions, (Eds. G.E. Wolstenholme and M.O. O'Connor),
    Churchill, London, pp. 223-240, 1970.

EFFECTS OF CHRONIC DOSAGE WITH CHLORPROMAZINE AND GEROVITAL H3 IN THE AGING BRAIN

T. Samorajski[1], Albert Sun[2] and C. Rolsten[1]

[1]Neurobiology of Aging Section, Texas Research Institute
of Mental Sciences, Houston, Texas 77030
[2]Sinclair Comparative Medicine Research Farm, University
of Missouri, Columbia, Missouri 65201

Aging may be considered a progressive deterioration of an organism after maturation that leads to physiological decline, increasing incidence of pathological lesions, and death. The rate of aging and duration of life appear to result from an interaction between the genetic program in the cell and influences from the external environment. While the causes of aging are unknown, there is evidence that the rate of aging may be mediated by the brain, especially by the hypothalamus and the closely linked pituitary and peripheral endocrine system (Everitt, 1976). Disproportionate changes in this system may result in "disregulation" of the organism (Frolkis, 1976), or an elevation of hypothalamic threshold to feed back control (Dilman, 1971), which in turn cause the development of age-related pathology.

Disruption of cell and organelle membranes by lipid peroxidation and other means has been postulated to account for much of the decline in physiological function with age (Kohn, 1971; Gordon, 1974). Nerve cells that may last as long as the lifetime of an individual without dividing may be particularly susceptible to membrane damage. Loss of or change in normal function of post-mitotic cells in the hypothalamus might have serious consequences for aging.

Considerable interest has been aroused recently by reports that the life span of some animals may be influenced by a number of drugs that are known or suspected stabilizers of cellular membranes. The dimethylaminoethyl moiety is the common structural feature of these drugs and, presumably, that portion of the molecule responsible for life span extension (Hochschild, 1973). Of additional significance

141

is the fact that injections of meclofenoxate (p-chlorophenoxyacetate coupled with 2-dimethylaminoethyl) and chlorpromazine (also with a dimethylaminoethyl side-chain) substantially reduced age pigment concentration in the neurons of senile animals (Nandy, 1968; Samorajski and Rolsten, 1976). Both drugs manifest antipsychotic properties.

Clinically, the most important of the antipsychotic drugs are the phenothiazines, particularly chlorpromazine and its analogues. Chloropromazine (CPZ) has attained extensive clinical use for tranquilizing emotionally disturbed patients and controlling a wide range of anxiety symptoms in adult and elderly subjects. A major effect of CPZ is to hinder the binding of monoamines (particularly dopamine) to their receptors either by interacting with a particular enzyme system or by altering the permeability of biological membranes. Its tranquilizing properties have been attributed to a depression of the reticular formation and sympathetic activity of the hypothalamus (Himwich, 1962; Killam, 1962).

In spite of the potential significance for aging of chlorpromazine (CPZ) and other antipsychotic agents, the long-term effects of these drugs are essentially unknown for several reasons: the relatively recent introduction of these agents into clinical practice, the variable response of patients to long-term treatment, methodological difficulties with research using human subjects, and the complicated mode and unknown site of drug action. This chapter is a report on a study of some effects of long-term dosage of chlorpromazine (CPZ) in mice, with correlated studies of Gerovital H_3[3] (GH3; 2% procaine hydrochloride, 10.16% benzoic acid, 1.14% potassium metabisulfite, buffered to pH3). The dimethylaminoethyl (or the closely related diethylaminoethyl) moiety is the common structural feature of chlorpromazine and procaine, respectively (Fig. 1).

Dimethylaminoethyl (DMAE) synthesized in the animal body is a precursor of acetylcholine (the mediator of nerve impulses) and phosphatidyl choline, an important constituent of cellular membranes (Hochschild, 1975). These two pathways for DMAE may account for its reported antidepressant effects (Pfeiffer and Murphree, 1958; Murphree et al., 1960) and suggest a role for DMAE in the biosynthesis and repair of membranes. In contrast, diethylaminoethyl (DEAE) has no known functions in nature. Procaine, on the other hand, has been shown to displace membrane-bound calcium (Seeman, 1972) and at higher concentrations, to alter osmotic fragility and specific gravity in nematodes (Zuckerman et al., 1971; Zuckerman et al., 1972). It has also been demonstrated that procaine (GH3) may be efficacious in the treatment of elderly depressed patients (Zung, 1975). If

---

[3]Kindly supplied by Rom-Amer Pharmaceuticals, Ltd., Beverly Hills, CA.

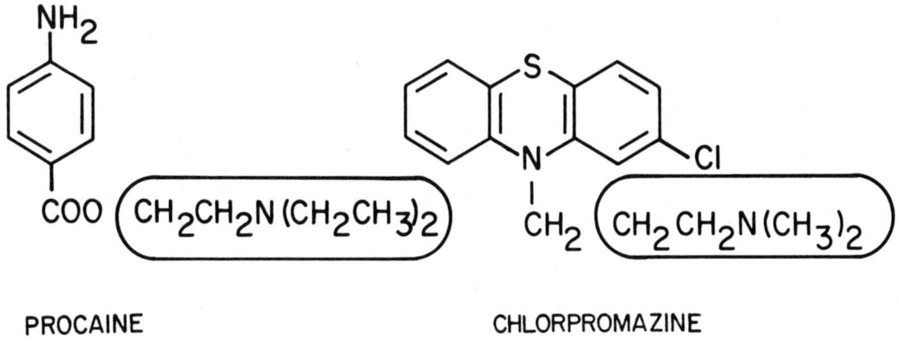

Fig. 1. Procaine and chlorpromazine. The common fragment in the oval (diethylaminoethyl and the closely related dimethylaminoethyl moiety, respectively) may account for the ability of these drugs to stabilize membranes.

membrane damage is associated with aging, agents that damage or
repair cellular membranes might be expected to alter age-related
physiological and pathological processes.

METHODS

Female (retired breeder) mice of the $C_{57}BL/10$ strain obtained
from the Jackson Laboratories at the age of nine months were used
in the study. They were housed in a carefully regulated environmental chamber until 11 months of age when they were matched for
size, weight, and general health, and randomly assigned to six
groups of 15 mice each. All animals were regularly weighed and
inspected for abnormalities for the next three weeks and tested
for locomotor activity in the fourth week. Drug treatments were
initiated at 12 months of age. Figure 2 represents our experimental
procedure for long-term evaluation of mice exposed to placebo, CPZ
(5 and 10 mg/kg) and GH_3 (25 and 50λ/Ss). Various aging parameters
were evaluated during the 11th, 15th, 19th and 23rd months of
the animals' life span. The mice did not receive either drug or
placebo during the test periods. Neurochemical and neuroanatomical
procedures were done at 25 months of age to compliment functional
findings. All of the animals used for the neurochemical and
morphological studies appeared to be healthy at the time of sacrifice.
A summary of some of these findings is presented below. The
deatiled methodology and results are described in separate reports
(Sun, 1974; Sun and Samorajski, 1970, 1975; Samorajski and Rolsten,
1976).

RESULTS

Body Weight and Survival

Body weight changes and survival data are shown in Figure 2.
Both CPZ groups showed a significant weight loss compared to the
matched placebo group. In contrast, the GH_3- and placebo-treated
mice showed no significant difference in body weight until 20
months when there was a significant weight loss among the surviving
GH_3-treated animals. This result may be due to differences in
mortality rates among the various groups. The 50% mortality occurred
at 21.6 and 23.0 months for the two GH_3 groups (25 and 50λ/Ss,
respectively), 22.3 months for both the 5 and 10 mg/kg CPZ groups,
and 23.5 and 24.3 months for the two placebo groups. At 25 months,
survival in the CPZ experiment was 45% for the 5 mg/kg CPZ group,
30% for the CPZ placebo group, and 16% for the 10 mg/kg CPZ group.
Survival in the GH_3 experiment was 33% for the 50λ/Ss GH_3 group.
There were not survivors in the 25λ/Ss GH_3 group and the GH_3 placebo
group.

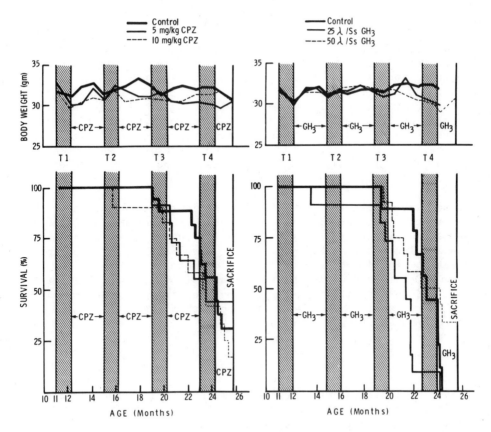

Fig. 2. Effects of placebo (PLAC), chlorpromazine (CPZ), and Gerovital H$_3$ (GH$_3$) on body weight and percentage of survivors of female mice. Placebo, CPZ and GH$_3$ were administered three times per week to mice for three consecutive periods, each consisting of three months of drug treatment followed by a drug-free month for functional and behavioral testing (T). Following the last test period, the surviving animals were again placed on the treatment schedule for one month and finally sacrificed at 25 months of age.

A number of other findings should be pointed out. First, 19 months of age appears to be the critical time for age-induced mortality in this study. Second, both CPZ- and GH$_3$-treated animals began to die at an earlier age. All groups showed a linear mortality rate with age, although the slope of the line appeared less steep among the two CPZ groups and one GH$_3$ group treated with 50λ/Ss. The largest percentage of survivors at 25 months were among the 5 mg/kg CPZ group and the 50λ/Ss GH$_3$ group.

Behavioral Deviations

Spontaneous locomotor activity was assessed before and during drug treatment in an attempt to further elucidate how long-term GH_3 and CPZ exposure may affect post-reproductive aging. Our objective was to determine if behavioral deviations as measured by locomotor activity scores were detectable in aging mice exposed to nine months of treatment. Spontaneous locomotor activity is an effective, simple, and widely used instrument for quantifying basic behavior. Mice readily learn to run in activity wheels, and deviations in daily scores may be taken as an indication of their health (Ordy et al., 1968).

A summary of the results is shown in Figure 3. Spontaneous locomotor activity significantly decreased with age in all of the groups tested. Drug treatment had no differential effects on spontaneous locomotor activity until the 23rd month. At that time, there was a significant decline in the locomotor activity of the 10 mg/kg CPZ compared with 5 mg/kg CPZ and placebo groups. Treatment with GH_3 had an opposite effect; the four surviving $50\lambda/Ss$ GH_3 mice had a higher mean locomotor activity score than the four placebo and one $25\lambda/Ss$ GH_3 treated survivors.

Barbital Narcosis

Since barbital is not extensively metabolized in the body, a change in the duration of its action can be due either to an enhanced penetration into the brain or to an alteration of neuronal sensitivity (Shah and Lal, 1971). The effect of age and treatment with GH_3 and CPZ is shown in Table 1. Age had no significant effect on the onset of barbital action in the placebo-(control), GH_3-, or CPZ-treated mice. There was a slight but not significant increase with age in the duration of narcosis of the control and GH_3-treated mice. Pretreatment with CPZ, however, significantly decreased the duration of barbital narcosis at both the 20th and 24th drug-free test months.

These data suggest that chronic treatment with CPZ may induce functional changes in the mouse brain that may persist even after cessation of treatment. CPZ-induced changes in combination with other drugs may cause adverse reactions as suggested by the barbital test results of this study.

Neuronal Lipofuscin Age Pigment

The accumulation of lipofuscin age pigments with increasing age is one of the most consistent morphological alterations in neuronal

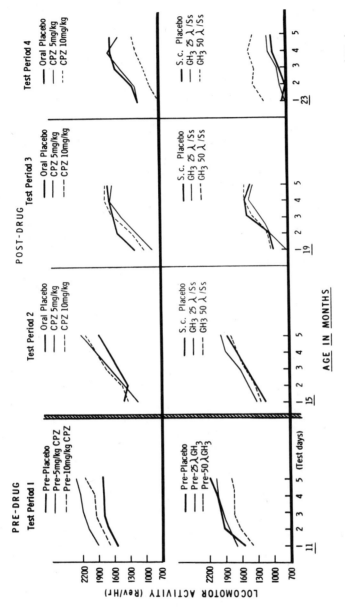

Fig. 3. Effects of placebo (PLAC), chlorpromazine (CPZ) and Gerovital H₃ (GH₃) on locomotor activity scores of female mice at 11, 15, 19, and 23 months of age.

Table 1. Effect of Gerovital H$_3$ (GH$_3$) and chlorpromazine (CPZ) on barbital narcosis in female mice at intervals of 16, 20, and 24 months of age.

AGE	PLAC	GH$_3$, (50 λ/Ss)	CPZ, (10 mg/kg)	P
		Min		
Onset of narcosis				
16 Months	39.8± 1.9 (20)	36.2± 1.8 (12)	36.3± 1.1 (8)	NS
20 Months	31.0± 2.2 (12)	36.1± 3.2 (10)	43.4± 1.9 (10)	NS
24 Months	36.7± 3.6 (6)	43.2± 6.5 (6)	42.3± 2.6 (4)	NS
Duration of narcosis				
16 Months	139.0± 18.2	130.9± 29.1	133.8± 39.8	NS
20 Months	153.0± 25.0	151.4± 29.3	123.4± 29.0	0.025
24 Months	179.5± 74.9	194.2± 78.3	67.3± 6.7	0.01

Each value is the mean ± S.E. Number in parentheses represents the number of animals used.
Values underscored are significantly different by analysis of variance (ANOVA).
NS = not significant.

Narcosis was determined by 250 mg/kg, i.p. of barbital sodium at 23°C. ambient temperature.

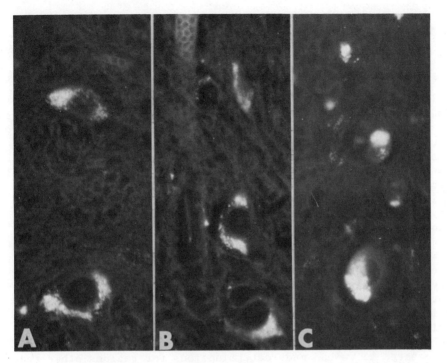

Fig. 4. Comparison of intraneuronal lipofuscin (age) pigment in
fluorescent preparations in the nucleus reticularis gigantocellularis
of 25-month-old female mice. (A) control - shows numerous fluorescent
intraneuronal granules. (B) 10 mg/kg CPZ - lipofuscin is less
noticeable in the lower neuron. (C) 50λ/Ss GH$_3$ - note clumped
lipofuscin bodies in the neuron, X250.

and glial cells in all mammalian species. The rate and degree of
accumulation may be influenced by a wide variety of conditions including drug treatment (Nandy, 1968; Samorajski and Rolsten, 1976).
The accumulation of pigment may be detrimental to the functional
capacity of the neurons (Zeman, 1974).

    The general morphology of the lipofuscin pigment granules in
neurons of the nucleus reticularis gigantocellularis of representative placebo-, CPZ-, and GH$_3$-treated mice is shown in Figure 4.
Two main types of changes were discernible. In agreement with our
earlier findings (Samorajski and Rolsten, 1976), the pigment granules
in the CPZ animals decreased in number and size compared to those in
the control animals. Some of the neurons of the GH$_3$-treated animals
contained unusually large pigment granules, but this was not a consistent finding, and two of the five GH$_3$ samples examined were not
distinguishable from the controls. Thus, the relationship between

CPZ and GH_3 treatment, pigment accumulation, and cell function remains unknown.

Neurochemical Analysis

In an attempt to correlate the observed behavioral differences at 25 months of age with the possibilities of cell death and changes in membrane properties due to drug treatment effects, various neuro-chemical determinations were conducted on portions of the brains from the surviving mice. An analysis of variance was done for each of the following parameters: body weight; telencephalic-diencephalic (forebrain) weight; cerebellar weight; brain stem weight; total protein, DNA and RNA in the cerebellum; and Na-K ATPase activity, norepinephrine and calcium uptake by synaptosomes isolated from the forebrain.

No significant alteration was found in any of the brain weight parameters between placebo-, CPZ-, and GH_3-treated mice (Table 2). Further, there was no significant difference among the three groups in total protein, RNA and DNA in the cerebellum (Table 2). These data indicate that no major changes occurred in glial neuronal relationships in the cerebellum as the result of 10 months of GH_3 and CPZ administration. Perhaps cellular differences would have been detected if we had made determinations for regions other than the cerebellum, or if we had made microscopic comparisons.

Some of the changes in the synaptosomes isolated from the forebrain of 25-month-old placebo, CPZ and GH_3 treated mice are shown in Table 3. There was a significant increase in synaptosomal Na-K ATPase activity in the GH_3 treated mice compared with the control group. There was no significant difference between CPZ and placebo treatment. The increase in enzymatic activity of the GH_3 group may represent an adaptive change in response to 10 months of treatment with GH_3.

Since Na-K ATPase has been associated with neurotransmitter membrane-dependent processes, another experiment was conducted to study in vitro uptake of norepinephrine (NE-^{14}C) and calcium (Ca-45) by nerve terminals. Statistical analyses revealed that uptake of NE-^{14}C was significantly higher for both the GH_3 and CPZ groups compared to controls. There was no significant difference in Ca-45 uptake, although the higher value for the CPZ group approached statistical significance.

Changes in Na-K ATPase activity and NE uptake may indicate that the structural integrity of the membrane may have been altered by treatment with GH_3 and CPZ. It has been proposed that the cell membrane in the brain may be the primary source of aging. If so, these results may have important implications for identifying

Table 2. Summary of body and regional brain weight and cerebellar protein, RNA and DNA values of 25-month-old $C_{57}BL/10$ female mice after 10 months of treatment with placebo (PLAC), chlorpromazine (CPZ), and Gerovital H_3 (GH_3).

Observation on:	Experimental groups			Analyses	
	PLAC N=5	CPZ, 10 mg/kg N=7	GH_3, λ50 /Ss N=4	ANOVA units	P
Body weight	29.8 ± 0.99	29.2 ± 1.53	28.1 ± 0.96	g	NS
Regional brain weight					
Forebrain	310.0 ±10.0	308.4 ± 7.0	304.0 ± 6.4	mg	NS
Cerebellum	53.9 ± 4.4	54.9 ± 2.4	50.0 ± 1.3	mg	NS
Brain Stem	68.3 ± 5.1	71.3 ± 1.6	69.0 ± 9.8	mg	NS
Protein, RNA and DNA of Cerebellum					
Total Protein	119.09± 3.90	108.15± 3.66	107.03± 2.64	mg/g	NS
DNA	6.38± 0.23	6.31± 0.23	6.16± 0.14	mg/g	NS
RNA	5.18± 0.09	4.57± 0.18	4.82± 0.31	mg/g	NS

Each value is the mean ± S.E. N = number of animals in each group; NS = not significant.

Table 3. Summary of neurochemical changes in synaptosomes of 25-month-old $C_{57}BL/10$ female mice after 10 months of placebo (PLAC), chlorpromazine (CPZ), or Gerovital H_3 (GH_3).

Observation on:	Experimental groups			Analyses
	PLAC (N=5)	CPZ, 10 mg/kg (N=7)	GH_3, $\lambda 50$ /Ss (N=4)	P
Na-K ATPase (μmoles P_i/10 min/mg)	3.27 ± 0.40	3.71 ± 0.29	4.06 ± 0.13	0.05
NE-^{14}C uptake (TDPM/μgm)	2482 ± 184	3109 ± 207	3529 ± 264	0.05
Ca -45 uptake (TDPM/μgm)	4103 ± 407	4673 ± 305	4149 ± 338	(PLAC vs GH_3; 0.01) NS

Each value is mean ± S.E. Values underscored are significantly different by analysis of variance (ANOVA); NS = not significant.

molecular mechanisms in membranes and the role of drug treatment in modifying membrane deterioration during aging.

GENERAL SUMMARY AND CONCLUSIONS

From the experimental findings presented in this report, it can be concluded that chronic treatment with CPZ and GH_3 results in significant changes during aging. Some of the conclusions can be summarized as follows:

1. Survival and body weight. The 50% mortality occurred at 21.6 and 23.0 months for the 25 and $50\lambda/Ss$ GH_3 groups, respectively; 22.3 months for both the 5 and 10 mg/kg CPZ groups; 23.5 and 24.3 months for the two placebo groups. Treatment with CPZ resulted in significant weight losses.

2. Locomotor activity. Declined with age for all groups. At 23 months, activity was lowest for the 10 mg/kg CPZ group and highest for the $50\lambda/Ss$ GH_3 group.

3. Barbital narcosis. Pretreatment with CPZ significantly decreased the duration of barbital narcosis at 20 and 24 months.

4. Lipofuscin age pigment. The pigment granules decreased in number and size in the neurons of the CPZ-treated animals. Neurons of three of the five GH_3-treated animals contained unusually large pigment bodies compared to the controls.

5. Body and brain weight; total protein, DNA and RNA of cerebellum. There was no significant difference among the three groups in any of the body and brain weight parameters and total protein, DNA, and RNA in the cerebellum.

6. Na-K ATPase. Prlonged treatment with GH_3 increased synaptosomal Na-K ATPase activity.

7. Uptake of NE-^{14}C and Ca-45. Uptake of NE-^{14}C in nerve ending fractions was significantly higher for both the GH_3 and CPZ groups compared to the control animals. There was no significant difference in Ca-45 uptake among any of the groups.

There are a number of possible interpretations of the experimental findings. Evidently, both Gerovital H_3 and chlorpromazine produce alterations at the membrane level that, quantitatively at least, may be correlated with changes in rodent life span. The amount of drug administered may also be a significant factor in altering the rate of aging as inferred from the difference in the mean life span in response to the two different doses of GH_3. The

causes of death in these experiments are unknown, and the differences between drug toxicity and time pathology in organs other than
the brain need to be considered.

The brain plays a unique role in responding to environmental
challenges through reflexes, conditioning, learning, and feedback
regulation. With increasing age there may be a decline in the
capacity of the brain and other organs to respond, which may
accelerate aging throughout the body and the subsequent production
of age-related disease. That the rate of aging was altered by CPZ
and GH_3 may be inferred from changes in the mean life span of these
animals. However, with advancing age the CPZ- and GH_3-(50λ/Ss)
treated animals as a group died at a slower rate than the controls.
In fact, the highest number of survivors at 25 months of age occurred
among animals treated with 5 mg/kg CPZ or 50λ/Ss of GH_3. Evidently,
these mice were able to adapt to treatment in ways that may have
insured their survival. In this regard, it is interesting to note
that the surviving mice treated with 50λ/Ss of GH_3 had significantly
higher locomotor activity scores compared to placebo- and CPZ-treated
animals. Nerve endings isolated from the GH_3 animals also revealed
the highest Na-K ATPase activity. Na-K ATPase is known to be located
in or on the membrane, providing further evidence that a membrane
change was induced by GH_3 and, to a lesser extent, by CPZ as well.
It is in this context that drug therapy intervention may prove to
be an effective way to influence the rate of aging.

Acknowledgements: The authors are indebted to Dr. Grace Sun
and Dr. Richard Seeman for their assistance in these studies. The
skilled technical assistance of Katherine Pratte and Linda Harvey
is also gratefully acknowledged.

REFERENCES

Dilman, V.M. Age-associated elevation of hypothalamic threshold to
     feedback control and its role in development, ageing and disease.
     Lancet 1:1211, 1971.

Everitt, A.V. The nature and measurment of aging. In: Hypothalamus,
     Pituitary and Aging, (Eds. A.V. Everitt and J.A. Burgess),
     Charles C. Thomas, Springfield, Ill, p. 5, 1976.

Frolkis, V.V. The hypothalamic mechanisms of aging. In: Hypothalamus,
     Pituitary and Aging, (Eds. A.V. Everitt and J.A. Burgess),
     Charles C. Thomas, Springfield, Ill., p. 614, 1976.

Gordon, P. Free radicals and the aging process. In: Theoretical
     Aspects of Aging, (Ed. M. Rockstein), Academic Press, New York,
     p. 61, 1974.

Himwich, H.E. Tranquilizers, barbiturates, and the brain. J.
     Neuropsychiat. 3:279, 1962.

Hochschild, R. Effect of dimethylaminoethanol on the life span of
     senile male A/J mice. Exp. Geront. 8:185, 1973.

Hochschild, R. Effects of DMAE on depression, on in vitro cell
     survival and on animal life span. In: Procaine and Related
     Geropharmacologic Agents - The Current State-of-the-Art,
     (Eds. A. Cherkin and M.A.P. Sviland), VA GRECC Monograph No. 1,
     p. 27, 1975.

Killam, E.K. Drug action on the brain-stem reticular formation.
     Pharmacol. Rev. 14:175, 1962.

Kohn, R.R. Aging of animals: Observations and questions. In:
     Principles of Mammalian Aging, Prentice-Hall, Englewood Cliffs,
     New Jersey, p. 105, 1971.

Murphree, H.B., Pfeiffer, C.C. and Bakerman, I.A. The stimulant
     effect of 2-dimethylaminoethanol (deanol) in human volunteer
     subjects. Clin. Pharmacol. Ther. 1:303, 1960.

Nandy, K. Further study on the effects of centrophenoxine on the
     lipofuscin pigment in the neurons of senile guinea pigs. J.
     Geront. 23:82, 1968.

Ordy, J.M., Samorajski, T., Horrocks, L.A., Zeman, W. and Curtis,
     H.J. Changes in memory, electrophysiology, neurochemistry, and
     neuronal ultrastructure after deuteron irradiation of the brain
     in C57 BL/10 mice. J. Neurochem. 15:1245, 1968.

Pfeiffer, C.C. and Murphree, H.B. Stimulant effect of 2-dimethyl-
     aminoethanol in human subjects. J. Pharmacol. Exp. Ther. 122:
     60A, 1958.

Samorajski, T. Age-related changes in brain biogenic amines. In:
     Aging Vol. 1, (Eds. H. Brody, D. Harman and J.M. Ordy), Raven
     Press, New York, p. 199, 1975.

Samorajski, T. and Rolsten, C. Chlorpromazine and aging in the brain.
     Exp. Geront. 11:141, 1976.

Seeman, P. The membrane actions of anesthetics and tranquilizers.
     Pharmacol. Rev. 24:583, 1972.

Shah, H.C. and Lal, H. The potentiation of barbiturates by desipramine
     in the mouse: Mechanisms of aging. J. Pharmacol. Exp. Ther. 179:
     404, 1971.

Sun, A.Y.   The effect of phospholipases on the active uptake of
    norepinephrine by synaptosomes isolated from the cerebral cortex
    of guinea pig.   J. Neurochem. 22:551, 1974.

Sun, A.Y. and Samorajski, T.   Effects of ethanol on the activity of
    adenosine triphosphatase and acetylcholinesterase in synaptosomes
    isolated from guinea pig brain.   J. Neurochem. 17:1365, 1970.

Sun, A.Y. and Samorajski, T.   The effects of age and alcohol on
    Na-K ATPase activity of whole homogenate and synaptosomes pre-
    pared from mouse and human brain.   J. Neurochem. 24:161, 1975.

Zeman, W.   Presidential address: Studies in the neuronal ceroid -
    lipofuscinoses.   J. Neuropath. Exp. Neurol. 33:1, 1974.

Zuckerman, B.M., Himmelhoch, S., Nelson, B., Epstein, J. and
    Kisiel, M.   Aging in Caenorhabditis briggsae.   Nematologica 17:
    478, 1971.

Zuckerman, B.M., Nelson, B. and Kisiel, M.   Specific gravity increase
    of Caenorhabditis briggsae with age.   J. Nematology 4:261, 1972.

Zung, W.K.   Treatment of depression in the aged with Gerovital H3:
    Clinical efficacy and neurophysiological correlation.   In:
    Procaine and Related Geropharmacologic Agents - The Current State-
    of-the-Art, (Eds. A. Cherkin and M.A.P. Sviland), VA GRECC
    Monograph No. 1, p. 53, 1975.

AGING OF NEURONS IN CULTURE

F. Howard Schneider, Suzanne G. Rehnberg and Mark P. Bear

Geriatric Research, Educational and Clinical Center
Veterans Administration Hospital
Bedford, MA.   01730

INTRODUCTION

Valuable information about cellular and biochemical aspects of aging has been obtained from studies with human and non-human dividing diploid cells in culture (see reviews by Hay, 1970; Hayflick, 1974; Littlefield, 1976 and Orgel, 1973). However, less work has been done using in vitro models to study cellular mechanisms of aging in post-mitotic differentiated cells, such as muscle and nerve. Varon (1975) has recently reviewed the nerve tissue preparations availabe which could possibly be used to study neuronal aging, including organ cultures, nerve tissue explants and reaggregating and dispersed cell cultures. These preparations are especially useful for morphological and electrophysiological studies, but are not as satisfactory for biochemical studies since they consist of a complex mixture of cell types. Furthermore, preparations obtained from mature or very old animals are less likely to yield functionally intact preparations since with age there is an increase in the difficulty of dissociating neuronal tissue into single cells. In view of the difficulties in obtaining preparations of pure nerve cells from animals, we have considered the possibility of using continuous lines of neuroblastoma cells for studies on neuronal aging.

Neuroblastoma cells in culture meet several important requirements which a model for neuronal aging should satisfy in order to be used profitably for biochemical, morphologic and pharmacological studies. It should be possible to obtain relatively large numbers of cells of a single type, to easily manipulate the environment in which the cells are maintained, and to prepare the cells for treatment and analysis without having to resort to traumatic isolation procedures. Further-more, the cells used must be in a postmitotic non-dividing state, and be maintained in this state for periods of time long enough to insure the occurrence of age-related cellular changes.

Mouse neuroblastoma cells were established in culture in 1969 from a murine solid tumor (Augusti-Tocco and Sato, 1969) which had previously been identified as a neuroblastoma by Dunham and Stewart (1953). A characteristic feature of this cell type is that in culture the rapidly dividing tumor cells can be converted into non-dividing cells with many properties similar to those of mature nerve cells. The question to be considered in this paper is whether relatively mature, non-dividing neuroblastoma cells can be used to study cellular events associated with neuronal aging.

I.   Properties of Mouse Neuroblastoma Cells in Culture

Mouse neuroblastoma cells in log growth, with generation times generally around 24 hours, are round or slightly irregularly shaped, with diameters of approximately 25 to 40µ. Usually less than 10 to 20% of a population of cells in log growth possess neurite-like processes. The processes which do occure in growing cultures are for the most part rather short, not exceeding 3 to 4 cell diameters in length (Fig. 1C and 1D).

Inhibition of cell division with a wide variety of agents or conditions can cause neuroblastoma cells to become what is generally referred to as "differentiated" (see review by Prasad, 1975). Typical neurite-like processes are shown in the phase contrast micrographs in Fig. 1A and 1B for cells which have been either exposed to medium with a pH of 6.6 (1A) or which have been treated with 10^{-5}M papaverine (1B), conditions which are known to stimulate process formation (Prasad, 1975; Bear and Schneider, 1975). These processes are morphologically similar in several ways to nerve axons in vivo. Hinkley and Telser (1974) reported that the neurites frequently contain long 250-Å diameter microtubules, an axial bundle of 100-Å filaments and numerous microfilaments of 40-80 Å in diameter. The neurites also contain clusters of 400-600 Å diameter vesicles which are morphologically similar to synaptic vesicles.

The cells which have formed neurites are also biochemically and physiologically similar to mature nerve cells in a number of ways. Cells with neurites are capable of expressing increased activities of acetylcholinesterase, tyrosine hydroxylase, dopamine-β-hydroxylase and choline acetyltransferase (Kates et al., 1971; Anagnoste et al., 1972; Furmanski et al., 1971 and Amano et al., 1972). The cells are also capable of accumulating and metabolizing neurotransmitters (Breakefield, 1976). Electrophysiological and biochemical studies have shown that neuroblastoma cells possess neurotransmitter and hormone receptors which lead to electrical changes and to alterations

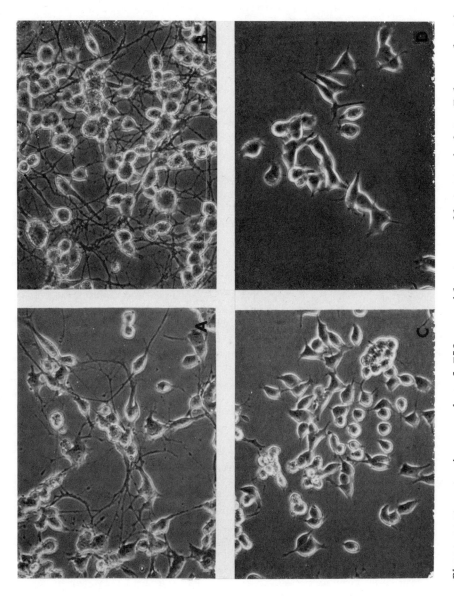

Fig. 1. Phase contrast micrographs of T59 neuroblastoma cells attached to Falcon plastic tissue culture flasks: A, maintained in culture medium with a pH of 6.6 for 5 days; B, treated with 10^{-5}M papaverine for 14 days; C and D, untreated, 3 days after initial seeding. X160.

in cyclic nucleotide levels (Harris and Dennis, 1970; Peacock et al.,
1973; Nelson et al., 1971 and Simantov and Sachs, 1973. Also, see
Prasad, 1975 and Breakefield, 1976). The studies have shown that
there are a variety of receptor types on neuroblastoma cells, such
as those for nicotinic and muscarinic cholinergic agents, α-
adrenergic drugs, dopamine and morphine. Changes in cyclic nucleotides and in the enzymes responsibe for their synthesis offer a
means of monitoring receptor stimulation and blockade, although the
cellular mechanisms involved in inhibition of cell division and
development of characteristics indicative of mature neurons are not
understood. The mouse neuroblastoma cell culture system provides
a valuable model for investigating neuronal differentiation and
function. However, much work will be required to show whether or not
this system can provide relevant information about changes in long-
term nondividing cultures, and whether or not such changes are
analogous to alterations which occur in aging neurons in vivo. This
question is the subject of the remainder of this paper.

II.   Effects of low pH on neuroblastoma cells

The data in Table 1 show that the growth rate decreases and
neurite formation and acetylcholinesterase activity increase when
cells are maintained for 72 hrs. in medium in which the pH had been
reduced to 6.6-6.8 from the normal pH of 7.4 (Bear and Schneider,
1976). The increase in acetylcholinesterase activity reflects an
increase in enzyme specific activity since cell protein increased
only 10% at the lower pH. Neurite formation and enzyme activity
at pH 7.0-7.2 were intermediate between the values for the high and
low pH ranges. Cell viability and detachment of cells from the
growing surface were unaltered at the lower pH ranges even after
120 hr. Returning cells to pH 7.4 after their maintainence in the
low pH showed that the changes at the low pH were completely
reversible within 24 to 48 hr.

Analysis of cell DNA content indicated that T59 cells at low
pH (13 ± 1 pg DNA/10^6 cells; n=3) have less than the DNA complement
for cells in log growth (21 ± 1 pg/10^6 cells; n=3). Since cell
division is unsynchronized in these populations of cells in log
growth, their DNA content should reflect an average of that for cells
spread over the cell cycle, with half of the cells having pre-S
phase DNA content and half with S or post-S phase DNA content.
Therefore, the amount of DNA in the cells at pH 6.6-6.8 indicates
that this population of cells is probably inhibited in the G_1 stage
of the cell cycle. Furthermore, thymidine kinase activity, an
enzyme involved in the utilization of exogenous thymidine for DNA
synthesis, in cells at pH 6.6-6.8 is only 10-15% of the activity
for cells in log growth at pH 7.4 (Bear and Schneider, unpublished
observation). Thus, it appears from these results that populations

Table 1.   Effects of environmental pH on T59 neuroblastoma cell
           growth, neurite formation and acetylcholinesterase
           activity.

PH	Cell Number+	Neurites	Acetylcholinesterase
7.4–7.6	1.46±.43(6)	8.7±3.(6)	1.1±.14(5)
6.6–6.8	.37±.06(6)	70±5.5(6)	5.9±1.1(5)

Cells ($.3 \times 10^6$) were seeded in 25 cm^2 Falcon plastic flasks in
5 ml of GIBCO F12 medium containing 10% newborn calf serum, and
were maintained for 72 hr. at 36° in a moist atmosphere of 95% air/
5% CO_2. Medium was changed every 24 hr. Cell numbers are expressed
as million cells, neurite formation is expressed as the percent of
attached cells which have processes longer than the diameter of the
cell body and acetylcholinesterase activity is expressed as nmoles
of product formed/min/10^6 cells. Acetylcholinesterase activity was
measured in 0.1% Triton–X100 cell extracts by the procedure of
Ellman, Courtney, Andres and Featherstone (1961). Differences
between values for 7.2–7.4 and 6.6–6.8 were significant at p<.05
or better.

of viable, nondividing neuroblastoma cells, arrested in G_1, can be
obtained by lowering the culture medium to pH 6.6–6.8. The use of
low pH to arrest cell growth can be added to the list of agents and
conditions which reduce neuroblastoma cell division and induce
differentiation, and is a potential method for obtaining populations
of nondividing cells for studies on cellular aging.

III.   Potential problems related to inhibition of cell division
       for aging studies

Any method selected for obtaining populations of nondividing
cells for aging studies can potentially produce effects of its
own on the cells, effects which are not directly related to aging
but that are characteristic of the particular agent or condition.
Two such possibilities will be discussed in this section.

A.   Multiple effects of drugs

Cells in culture are not exceptions to the generality that drugs
can produce more than one effect in biological systems. Frequently,
the various effects have different concentration-response relationships, and, therefore, are produced in varying degrees at different

drug concentrations. Butyric acid, which can be produced in cells
from dibutyryl cyclic AMP (Kaukel and Hilz, 1972), and for this
reason must be used as a control in studies involving the use of
this cyclic nucleotide, is a good example. Striking effects of
butyric acid on neuroblastoma cells in culture had been reported
previously, including inhibition of cell division (Prasad and Hsie,
1971) and induction of tyrosine hydroxylase (Waymire et al., 1972)
and acetylcholinesterase (Prasad and Vernadakis, 1972) activity;
sodium butyrate did not stimulate neurite formation in these studies.
However, an examination of the effects of a wide range of concentrations of sodium butyrate (Glazer and Schneider, 1975; Schneider,
1976) revealed that neuroblastoma cells developed neurite-like
processes in concentrations of sodium butyrate between 10^{-6} and 3
x 10^{-4}M, with the maximum effect at 10^{-5}M. Process formation was
decreased at higher concentrations, with no effect at 5 x 10^{-4}M.
It can be concluded that sodium butyrate is fully capable of
stimulating process formation, but as the concentration is increased
an additional effect is produced which counteracts neurite formation.
It is interesting that the higher concentrations are required for
inhibition of cell division and induction of acetylcholinesterase
activity.

B. Development of resistant clones

     Various neuroblastoma lines have been reported to develop
resistance to the effects of 6-thioguanine (Wood et al., 1973) and
6-mercaptopurine (Baskin and Rosenberg, 1975) and to the growth
inhibitory effects of prostaglandin E_1 (Rehnberg and Schneider,
unpublished observations) and sodium butyrate (Schneider, 1976).
Clearly, development of resistant clones must be considered a real
possibility when using chemical agents or altered environmental
conditions to abolish cell division. Concentrations of the agents
being used for this purpose should be at sufficiently high levels
to reduce development of the resistant clones, but at the same
time less than those which produce toxic effects.

IV. Age-related changes in neuroblastoma cells in culture

     A wide variety of biochemical, functional and morphological
parameters have been used to assess the effects of aging in cultures
of dividing human diploid fibroblasts. Some of these parameters
may reflect to some degree analogous events in vivo, such as lipofuscin formation and alterations in various enzyme levels. Age-related
changes in several cell characteristics also occur in neuroblastoma
cells which are maintained in a nondividing state. As examples,
data will be presented in this section on cell viability, lipofuscin
formation, lysosomal enzyme levels, acetylcholinesterase activity,
cell size distribution and latency for cell division upon reseeding.

A. <u>Cell number and viability</u>

Although there are numerous agents and conditions which will
reduce growth of cells in culture, our initial studies utilized
maintenance of cells at confluent density or treatment with
papaverine. More recently we have investigated the use of low pH
to reduce cell division for relatively long periods of time. Table
2 compares cell growth for T59 neuroblastoma cells which were
allowed a) to remain at confluent density, b) were treated with
10^{-6}M papaverine and c) were exposed to pH 6.6-6.8 for varying
lengths of time. Untreated cells reach a value for cell number
around 8 to 9 x 10^6, whereas papaverine-treated cultures in low
pH attain only approximately one-third to one-half that amount.
Cell viability remains high in these long-term nondividing cultures,
then decreases to around 40 percent by day 25; average percent
viability values for a large number of cultures allowed to remain
at confluency are given in Table 3. These values are similar to
previously published data on neuroblastoma cell viability over long
periods of culture (Nandy and Schneider, 1976). Treatment with
papaverine or exposure to low pH did not significantly change viability
values at the various time periods.

These experiments indicate that populations of nondividing cells
can be obtained which are sufficiently viable for biochemical and
physiological measurements, even though it appears that cell viability
can decrease significantly after 20 days in culture. Conditions
which could increase percent cell viability or separate viable from
nonviable cells would extend the period of time for which nondividing
neuroblastoma cells could be used for studies of age-related alterations, and would be quite useful in <u>in vitro</u> aging studies. One
procedure which might prove useful for separating viable from nonviable cells is by harvesting and reseeding. Presumably only viable
cells will reattach to the flask surface, and a medium change at
the appropriate time after reseeding would remove nonviable unattached
cells. An experiment to test this procedure was carried out with
T59 neuroblastoma cells harvested after 20 days in culture at confluent
density; medium had been changed every day. Cell viability on the
day of harvest was 43%. The cells (0.15 x 10^6) were reseeded in 5 ml
of medium and subsequently harvested for measurement of viability over
the next 6 days. The viability values for the cells which attached
after reseeding were 90% 24 hr. later, 88% 48 hr. later, 83% 96 hr.
later and 90% 144 hr. later. These data indicate that the nonviable
cells did not reattach and were lost at the first medium change.
However, it should be pointed out that the reattachment efficiency
of the viable cells of an aged culture may not be as great as for
younger cultures, and consequently some viable cells might be lost
due to lack of reattachment. Nevertheless, those cells which do
attach will represent viable cells which have been maintained in a
nondividing state for a known period of time.

Table 2.   Growth of T59 neuroblastoma cells.

	DAYS IN CULTURE			
	5	10	15	20
UNTREATED	3.3	6.7	7.8	9.2
PAPAVERINE	1.9	2.7	3.6	3.8
pH 6.6-6.8	2.4	2.5	2.4	---

Values are presented as million cells and represent the averages of duplicate flasks. On day zero .075 x 10^6 cells were seeded in 5 ml of medium in T25 Falcon plastic tissue culture flasks under the conditions described in Table 1.   Treatment with 10^{-5}M papaverine was initiated 24 hr. after seeding; exposure of cells to low pH began 5 days after seeding.   Medium was changed every 24 hrs.

B.   Lipofuscin pigment formation

Aging in animals is accompanied by increases in the amount of cytoplasmic lipofuscin, a dense pigment identifiable by its characteristic yellow autofluorescence and by its histochemical staining properties. Lipofuscin has been shown to accumulate in several human tissues (Toth, 1968). Dividing and nondividing cells in tissue culture also accumulate increasing amounts of lipofuscin when they are maintained in culture for prolonged periods of time; pigment accumulation has been demonstrated in WI-38 fibroblasts (Deamer and Gonzales, 1974), human glial cells (Brunk et al., 1973), and mouse neuroblastoma cells (Nandy and Schneider, 1976).   The pigment which develops in vitro appears to be similar to that found in nerve cells in vivo when examined by fluorescence, histochemical and electron microscopic techniques. Confluent neuroblastoma cell cultures accumulate significant amounts of pigment over periods of a few weeks, and the amount of pigment can be increased considerably by inhibiting cell division further with drugs or by environmental conditions.   The data in Table 4 show the percent of cells which contain detectable pigment in young and older cultures under different conditions. Acid phosphatase-positive dense clumps of pigment were used as an indicator of lipofuscin since previous work showed a good correlation between acid phosphatase staining, yellow autofluorescence and the acid-Schiff staining procedure (Nandy and

Table 3. Viability for long-term T59 neuroblastoma cultures.

	DAY INTERVALS				
	1-5	6-10	11-15	16-20	21-25
UNTREATED	89.5 ±1.1 (57)	90.7 ±1.2 (32)	83.6 ±2.3 (13)	67.3 ±9.7 (4)	42.7 ±14.0 (3)
CENTROPHENOXINE 10-4M	85.8 ±1.3 (5)	83.1 ±6.2 (7)	82.1 ±4.4 (8)	71.4 ±5.8 (5)	43.7 ±22.0 (3)

Values are presented as million cells with ±SE and with the number of observations in parantheses. Centrophenoxine treatment was initiated 2 days after initial seeding; medium was changed every 24 hr. Culture conditions were as described in Table 1.

Table 4.   Effects of culture conditions and aging on acid phosphatase-positive pigment content in neuroblastoma cells.

	DAYS IN CULTURE		
	8	13–15	17
UNTREATED	3±1	32±4	59±2
PAPAVERINE	40±9	71±9	79±21
pH 6.6–6.8	21±5	61±3	49±5

Cells were grown on glass coverslips.   Change to low pH or treatment with 10^{-5}M papaverine was initiated 3 days after initial seeding.   Each value (percent of cells with pigment) represents the average of 20 counts on each of 2 coverslips.   There were no differences in cell viabilities between untreated and treated cells.   Acid phosphatase was detected histochemically by the naphthol AS-BI phosphate procedure of Burstone (1958).

Schneider, 1976).   Each of these procedures showed a gradual accumulation of pigment with time in culture and an increase in pigment after treatment with papaverine or prostaglandin E_1 or in serum-free medium, all of which are conditions that reduce cell division.   The more recent results presented in Table 4 are in agreement with the previously published data showing that papaverine enhances pigment content, and also shows that low pH increases pigment above that for untreated cells of the same age.

The biochemical events involved in lipofuscin formation are at present unknown.   The relative ease of working with cells in culture and the comparative short time span of pigment formation in vitro suggest that dynamics of lipofuscin formation, fate, and effect on cell function could be profitably studied with cell culture systems. Furthermore, the effects of various chemical agents and conditions on lipofuscin formation can also be examined with relative ease in these in vitro systems (See section below on centrophenoxine).

C.   Lysosomal Enzyme Levels

It has been suggested that lysosomes may play a role in lipofuscin pigment formation, a topic which has received considerable attention (Toth, 1968; Daems et al., 1969 and Siakotos and Armstrong, 1975).   Furthermore, cells in culture show age-related increases

Table 5. Lysosomal Enzyme Activity in T59 Mouse Neuroblastoma
          Cells in Culture.

DAYS IN CULTURE	ACTIVITY		
	Acid Phosphatase	β-Glucuronidase	N-Acetyl-β-D-glucos-aminidase
5-8	15.1±3.1	3.7±1.7	5.8±.7
21-32	26.1±3.3	4.1± .4	13.8±1.8

Cells were grown in culture as described in Table 1, and were
seeded in 5 ml of medium at 0.15 x 10^6. Enzyme activity is presented
as μmoles of substrate produced/hr/10^6 cells. Acid phosphatase and
β-glucuronidase activities were measured in 0.1% Triton-X100 extracts
of the cells by the procedure of Gianetto and DeDuve (1955);
N-acetyl-β-D-glucosaminidase was measured by the same procedure as
for acid phosphatase with a final concentration of p-nitrophenyl-N-
acetyl-β-D-glucosaminide of .5 mg/ml.

in lysosomal enzymes, as shown by electron microscopy (Robbins et al.,
1970 and Lipetz and Cristofalo, 1972) and by biochemical findings
(Cristofalo, 1970).

Analysis of cultured mouse neuroblastoma cells revealed that
each of three lysosomal enzyme assayed (acid phosphatase, β-glucuronidase and N-acetyl-β-D-glucosaminidase) increased with aging in
culture (Table 5). The increases for acid phosphatase and N-acetyl-
β-D-glucosaminidase were greater than that for β-glucuronidase.
Very little β-glucuronidase or acid phosphatase activities were found
in the media from either young or old cells. Acid phosphatase
activity accumulated in the medium over a 24 hr. period was 0.9±0.2
units for 6-10 day-old (n=3) and 0.9±0.2 for 11-15 day-old (n=6)
cells; the corresponding values for β-glucuronidase activity were
.3±.03 (n=3) and .4±.03 (n=6). N-Acetyl-β-D-glucosaminidase activity,
on the other hand, was relatively high compared to the N-acetyl-β-D-
glucosaminidase activity in the cells. Three times more N-acetyl-β-
D-glucosaminidase activity than was in the cells was released into
the medium in 24 hr. These preliminary findings indicate that nondividing neuroblastoma cells are similar to dividing diploid cells
in that there is an age-related increase in lysosomal enzyme activity.
Further work is necessary before it will be possible to establish
whether or not the increases in lysosomal enzyme activity is
responsible for certain aspects of cellular aging or, on the other

hand, is only one of the many results of cell aging. The relationship between lysosomal dynamics and lipofuscin pigment can also be
investigated in the in vitro system, and should provide valuable
information in this area.

D. Changes in other enzymes

The enzyme acetylcholinesterase is found in all lines of mouse
neuroblastoma cells, and can be elevated under a variety of conditions, many of which also reduce cell division (Prasad, 1975). The
increases in enzyme activity is reduced by the protein synthesis
inhibitor cycloheximide (Schneider, 1976 and Lanks et al., 1974).
Lanks et al. (1974) have shown that the increase in acetylcholinesterase activity which occurs upon inhibition of cell division in
serum-free medium is accounted for by a higher rate of enzyme
synthesis. These findings are consistent with true enzyme induction.

In order to measure the ability of aging neuroblastoma cells to
maintain the elevated rate of acetylcholinesterase activity associated
with the induced steady state level, enzyme activity was measured
in cells at confluent density for up to 4 weeks in culture. Enzyme
activity (measured by the procedure of Ellman, et al., 1961) increased
from a low level of 2 nmoles of product formed/min/mg protein five
days after seeding, when the cells were still in log growth, to 23
nmoles/min/mg protein five days later, at which time confluent density
had been reached. The increase in enzyme activity continued until
day 19 at which time 43 units of activity was reached, but thereafter
decreased to 24 units by day 24 and 14 units by day 30. The fall of
in enzyme activity was greater than the drop in cell viability, which
in this experiment decreased from 95% at day five to 70% at day 20
and remained at this level to day 30. It would appear from these
results that the cells are unable to maintain for a prolonged period
of time the elevated rate of acetylcholinesterase synthesis normally
associated with decreased cell division. On the other hand, lactate
dehydrogenase and glucose-6-phosphate dehydrogenase activities
remained relatively constant over the entire time interval, indicating that the decrease in acetylcholinesterase activity did not merely
reflect an overall decrease in protein synthesis. Thus, it may be
that the ability to maintain an induced level of enzyme synthesis
decreases with age in nondividing neuroblastoma cells.

E. Cell Size Changes

One of the characteristics of aging cells in culture is a gradual
shift to a larger mean volume (Cristofalo, 1970 and Simons, 1967).
This shift in size is compatible with an increase in the percentage
of nondividing cells in the late passage cultures. Bowman et al.
(1975) conclude that cell aging in culture may involve a progressive
loss of DNA synthesis capability, which in turn, lead to other

Table 6. Effect of culture age on T59 neuroblastoma cell size distribution.

CULTURE AGE	PERCENT OF CELL IN EACH SIZE CLASS									
	.8-2	.2-3	3-4	4-5	5-6	6-7	7-8	8-9	9-10	19-∞
7 days	11 ±3	21 ±2	23 ±4	15 ±2	9 ±1	6 ±1	4 ±.4	2 ±1	2 ±.3	7 ±1
23-24 days	17 ±1	11 ±3	11 ±2	11 ±1	9 ±.3	7 ±.4	6 ±1	4 ±1	3 ±1	10 ±2

Culture age is the number of days after initial plating. Culture conditions were as described in Table 1. Size classes are expressed as arbitrary units: 1 unit equals approximately 5.7μ in diameter. Values are given as mean ±standard error; n=4 in each case. Overall recovery for cells counted was 100% for the 7-day old cultures and 89% for the 23-24 day old cultures.

age-related changes, including an increase in cell size.

Since aging post mitotic neuroblastoma cells are in a non-dividing state, cell size distribution was examined for different periods of time in culture. Electronic analysis of cell size with a Particle Data Inc. cell sizer showed that relatively young cultures gave a sharp peak in cell size at the 3-4 unit size range (Table 6). In contrast, this peak was lost in 23-24 day-old cultures, with a greater spread of cell size over the full range of sizes measured. The ratio of cells in the 5-6 unit range or less to those above the 5-6 range is 3.8 for the young cultures and 1.8 for the older cultures, reflecting a greater cell size spread in the latter case. It appears from these preliminary experiments that nondividing neuroblastoma cells undergo cell size changes which are comparable to those reported for nondividing fibroblast cultures. Further work on DNA, RNA and protein synthesis is needed in order to gain an understanding of the full significance of the change.

F. Latency for Cell Division Upon Reseeding

In addition to the limited in vitro life span of diploid cells cultured from mammalian species, it is also well known that the age of the donor affects the behavior of the cells explanted. Cell senescence in culture occurs earlier in cells from older donors, and there is a greater period of time between initial explant and the onset of cell division than in cells from younger donors (see Soukupova et al., 1970). In view of this phenomenon, we examined the latency in onset of cell growth after reseeding neuroblastoma cells from cultures of different ages. Replating cultures under standard conditions showed that there was a progressive increase with age in the time between replating and the onset of cell division. Table 7 shows that the average generation time over the first 4 days in culture increased progressively from 22±2 hr. for 5 day old cultures to 147±86 hr. for 20-30 day old cultures. However, all cultures eventually grew to the same confluent density. The greater average generation times for the older cultures reflected initial delays before growth started. Cell viabilities were between 45 and 60% for the 15 through 30 day old cultures.

It is possible that the delay in growth observed in the older cultures reflects age-related changes in the ability to initiate mitosis or progress through the cell cycle. Perhaps age-dependent changes occur which make more difficult the transition from the G_1 stage of the cell cycle to the S phase, and that a certain amount of time is required for synthesis of cellular components necessary for this transition. On the other hand, it is possible that a sub-population of the older cells is permanently incapable of cell division, and that the remainder of the cell population, possibly only a small portion, must undergo a sufficient number of division in order to bring the culture into apparent log growth based on the

Table 7.   Generation times for neuroblastoma cells upon reseeding.

AGE OF CULTURE (days)	GENERATION TIME (HRS) (over initial 4 days)
5	22±2 (8)
7-10	28±2 (6)
15-19	44±12(5)
20-30	147±86(5)

T59 neuroblastoma cells from cultures of different ages were harvested with .25% Viokase and reseeded at a concentration of 0.075×10^6 cells in 5 ml of medium in 25 cm^2 Falcon plastic tissue culture flasks. Generation times are given as means ±SE for the initial 4 days after reseeding; the number of separate experiments at each age is shown in the parantheses.

total number of cells seeded. Studies with autoradiographic analysis of ^{3}H-thymidine incorporation will be useful in differentiating between these possibilities.

V.   Effects of centrophenoxine on age-related changes in neuroblastoma cells

Centrophenoxine, an ester of dimethylaminoethanol and p-chloro-phenoxyacetic acid, has been reported to cause improvement of certain symptoms of senile dementia (Destrem, 1961 and Thuillier et al., 1959). The drug has also been shown to improve learning and memory in twelve-month old mice, compared to the corresponding controls (Nandy, unpublished observations).

The mechanism by which centrophenoxine acts is not known, due in part to the difficulties of working with the in vivo model systems available for investigating the long-term actions of agents which may influence aging or lipofuscin deposition. Drug metabolism and distribution, assessment of drug concentration at the sites of action and the prolonged time required for age-related cellular changes in vivo contribute to these difficulties. The use of cell culture systems for studying effects of chemicals on cellular aging could circumvent some of these difficulties. The results presented in this section indicate that centrophenoxine does in fact alter some of the age-related changes in neuroblastoma cells, and that this cell culture model may provide a profitable system for further pharmacological analysis of the mechanism of action of this and other agents.

A.   Cell number and viability

Table 3 shows that cell viabilities in long-term cutlures treated with 10^{-4}M centrophenoxine were similar to those for cells in regular medium.   Short-term toxicity studies, up to 5 days, showed that even in high concentrations (3 x 10^{-3}M) centrophenoxine did not reduce cell viability.

Centrophenxoine has little effect on cell growth, and in the concentrations used in this study (10^{-4} and 3 x 10^{-4}M) did not alter cell number in the long-term cultures.   For example, cell numbers in 25 cm^2 Flacon tissue culture flasks for cells 11-15 day old cultures in regular medium was 14.9±1.9 x 10^6, and the corresponding value for cells treated with 10^{-4}M centrophenoxine from the second day of culture was 14.3±1.8 x 10^6.   Thus, it can be inferred that centrophenoxine-induced alterations in other cell parameters are not merely secondary to effects on cell division or on cell viability.

B.   Lipofuscin

Since centrophenoxine causes a reduction in lipofuscin pigment in vivo (Nandy and Bourne, 1966), we tested its ability to cause a similar reduction of pigment in neuroblastoma cells in culture (Nandy and Schneider, 1976).   Treatment of cells with 10^{-4}M or 3 x 10^{-4}M centrophenoxine resulted in a marked reduction in the amount of lipofuscin in cells which had been treated with 1.1 x 10^{-5}M papaverine for 16 days.   The reduction of pigment with centrophenoxine was evident from analysis of the cells by autofluorescence and by periodic acid-Schiff and acid phosphatase staining.   Reseeding (at a lower density) cells which have been allowed to accumulate pigment results in cell division and a concomitant decrease in pigment content. This decrease in pigment is apparently due to dilution of pigment upon mitotic division.   However, the reduction in pigment in the presence of centrophenoxine is not associated with altered rates of cell division or with significant alterations in cell viability. It may be that the ability of centrophenoxine to reduce lipofuscin content of neuroblastoma cells in vitro is related to its analogous effect in vivo.   If this is true, the neuroblastoma culture system should provide an excellent model in which to examine the mechanism by which this agent causes lipofuscin reduction.

C.   Lysosomal enzyme levels

Due to the suggested involvement of lysosomes in lipofuscin formation, and to the ability of centrophenoxine to reduce neuronal lipofuscin content in vivo, the effects of centrophenoxine on

lysosomal enzyme levels in neuroblastoma cells were measured. Acid
phosphatase, β-glucuronidase and N-acetyl-β-D-glucosaminidase were
assayed in cell extracts and in the corresponding media from untreated
T59 cultures and from those which had been treated for 10 to 14 days
with 3 x 10^{-3}M centrophenoxine; the cultures were all 11 to 15 days
old. Centrophenoxine caused a 36-38% increase in the levels of
these enzymes in the cell extracts. The values for untreated cells
were 19.1±2.2 (n=7) for acid phosphatase, 3.9±0.9 (n=7) for N-acetyl-
β-D-glucosaminidase and 1.1±0.2 (n=7) for β-glucuronidase; the
corresponding values for centrophenoxine-treated cells were 26.0±2.9
(n=6), 5.4±0.9 (n=6) and 1.4±0.3 (n=6). The centrophenoxine treatment
did not alter the amount of enzyme activity in media for acid phosphatase or β-glucuronidase, but did cause a 54% increase in N-acetyl-
β-D-glucosaminidase activity. It is of interest that the amount of
N-acetyl-β-D-glucosaminidase in media from cells for a 24 hr. period
is much higher relative to the amount of activity of the other two
enzymes. The amount of enzyme activity per 10^6 cells in media in
which 11-15 day-old untreated T59 cells had been incubated for 24
hrs. was only 0.9±0.2 (n=6) and 0.4±0.03 (n=6) for acid phosphatase
and β-glucuronidase, respectively, but was 14.9±3.6 (n=6) for N-
acetyl-β-D-glucosaminidase.

   D.   Acetylcholinesterase activity

   Centrophenoxine (10^{-3}M or 3 x 10^{-3}M) had no effect on
acetylcholinesterase activity in T59 cells which were treated up to
4 days with the agent. However, it did cause an elevation and a
prolongation of the increase in acetylcholinesterase activity
resulting from attainment of confluent density (See Section IV D).
For example, enzyme activity in 19 day old untreated cells was 43
units/mg protein, whereas for 10^{-3}M centrophenoxine-treated cells
of the same age, activity was 60. Activity then decreased in untreated cells (24 units/mg protein on day 24), but remained at 58 for
centrophenoxine-treated cells. However, even in the treated cells
the activity eventually decreased, reaching 24 by day 30.

   E.   Cell size

   Treatment of neuroblastoma cells with centrophenoxine (10^{-4} -
3 x 10^{-3}M) had no significant effect on the age-related shift to a
larger mean cell size. In contrast, a number of other agents, such
as sodium butyrate and prostaglandin E_1, cause pronounced alterations
in cell size distribution. It appears from these experiments that
cell size changes are not mediated by mechanisms which are responsible
for the other centrophenoxine-responsive changes associated with
aging of the cells in culture. It is likely that the shift to larger
cells reflects, at least in part, inhibition of cell division with
resultant unbalanced growth.

F.   Summary

It appears from the results presented in this section that
centrophenoxine can modify some of the age-related changes which
have been shown to occur in nondividing neuroblastoma cells in
culture. The drug causes the cells to resemble younger cells in
those parameters which are affected, which include reduction of
lipofuscin pigment content and maintainence of induced acetylcholinesterase levels.

It is also interesting that centrophenoxine produced an elevation
in lysosomal enzymes, at the same time causing a reduction in
lipofuscin pigment. Although the mode of lipofuscin formation is
not known with certainty, it may be that lysosomes at some stage of
their life cycle are precursors to lipofuscin pigment. If centrophenoxine prevents lysosomes from participating in pigment formation,
an accumulation of lysosomes and a diminution of pigment might result.
This explanation, of course, implies that neuroblastoma lipofuscin
has a lower content of these three lysosomal enzymes than do neuroblastoma lysosomes.

Further work is needed to shed light on the mechanism whereby
centrophenoxine alters pigment formation and reverses some of the
age-related changes in this particular system. However, it is felt
that this model offers a cell system in which this drug, as well as
others, can be studied more easily than in available in vivo systems.

Acknowledgements: The authors express their appreciation to
Miss Susan Dexter for excellent technical assistance and to Mrs.
Terry Laffey for assistance in the preparation of this manuscript.
This work was supported in part by USPHS grant NS11365 and by funds
provided by the Veterans Administration.

REFERENCES

Amano, T., Richelson, E. and Nirenberg, M. Neurotransmitter synthesis
    by neuroblastoma clones. Proc. Nat. Acad. Sci. U.S.A. 69:258-263,
    1972.

Anagnoste, B., Freedman, L.S., Goldstein, M., Broome, J. and Fuxe, K.
    Dopamine-β-hydroxylase activity in mouse neuroblastoma tumors
    and in cell cultures. Proc. Nat. Acad. Sci. U.S.A. 69:1883-1886,
    1972.

Augusti-Tocco, G. and Sato, G. Establishment of functional clonal
    lines of neurons from mouse neuroblastoma. Proc. Nat. Acad. Sci.
    U.S.A. 64:311-315, 1969.

Baskin, F. and Rosenberg, R.N. Decreased 6-mercaptopurine retention by two resistant variants of mouse neuroblastoma with normal hypoxanthine-guanine-phosphoribosyltransferase activities. J. Pharmacol. Exp. Ther. 193:293-300, 1975.

Bear, M.P. and Schneider, F.H. The effect of media pH on the rate of growth, neurite formation and acetylcholinesterase activity in mouse neuroblastoma cells in culture. J. Cellular Physiol., In press, 1976.

Bowman, P.D., Meek, R.L. and Daniel, C.W. Aging of human fibroblasts in vitro. Correlations between DNA synthesis ability and cell size. Exp. Cell Res. 93:184-190, 1975.

Breakefield, X.O. Neurotransmitter metabolism in murine neuroblastoma cells. Life Sci. 18:267-278, 1976.

Brunk, U., Ericsson, J.L.E., Ponter, J. and Westermark, B. Residual bodies and "aging" in cultured human glial cells. Exp. Cell Res. 79:1-14, 1973.

Burstone, M.S. Histochemical demonstration of acid phosphatases with napthol. J. Nat. Cancer Inst. 21:523-539, 1958.

Cristofalo, V.J. Metabolic aspects of aging in diploid human cells. In: Aging in Cell and Tissue, (Eds. E. Holeckova and V.J. Cristofalo), Plenum Press, New York, pp. 83-119, 1970.

Daems, W.T., Wisse, E. and Brederoo, P. Electron microscopy of the vacuolar apparatus in lysosomes. In: Biology and Pathology, Vol. 1, (Eds. J.T.D. Ingle and H.B. Fell), Am. Elsevier Pub. Co., New York, pp. 97-103, 1969.

Deamer, D.W. and Gonzales, J. Autofluorescent structures in cultured WI-38 cells. Arch. Biochem. Biophys. 165:421-426, 1974.

Destrem, H. Essai clinique de la centrophenoxine en geriatrie (52 cas). Presse Med. 69:1999-2001, 1961.

Dunham, L.J. and Stewart, H.L. A survey of transplantable and transmissible tumors. J. of the Nat. Cancer Inst. 13:1299-1377, 1953.

Ellman, G.L., Courtney, K.D., Andres, V. and Featherstone, R.M. A new and rapid colorimetric determination of acetylcholinesterase activity. Biochem. Pharmacol. 1:88-95, 1961.

Furmanski, P., Silverman, D.J. and Lubin, M. Expression of differentiated functions in mouse neuroblastoma mediated by dibutyryl-cyclic adenosine monophosphate. Nature 233:413-415, 1971.

Gianetto, R. and DeDuve, C. Tissue fractionation studies: comparative study of binding of acid phosphatase, β-glucuronidase and cathepsin by rat liver particles. Biochemical Journal 59:433-438, 1955.

Glazer, R.I. and Schneider, F.H. Effects of adenosine 3':5'-Monophosphate and related agents on ribonucleic acid synthesis and morphological differentiation in mouse neuroblastoma cells in culture. J. Biol. Chem. 250:2745-2749, 1975.

Harris, A.J. and Dennis, M.J. Acetylcholine sensitivity and distribution on mouse neuroblastoma cells. Science 167:1253-1255, 1970.

Hay, R.J. Cell strain senescence in vitro: Cell culture anomaly or an expression of a fundamental inability of normal cells to survive and proliferate. In: Aging in Cell and Tissue Culture, pp. 7-24, 1970.

Hayflick, L. Cytogerontology. In: Theoretical Aspect of Aging, (Ed. M. Rockstein), Academic Press, New York, pp. 83-103, 1974.

Hinkley, R.E. and Telser, A.G. The effects of halothane on cultured mouse neuroblastoma cells. I. Inhibition of morphological differentiation. J. Cell Biol. 63:531-540, 1974.

Kates, J.R., Winterton, R. and Schlessinger, K. Induction of acetylcholinesterase activity in mouse neuroblastoma tissue culture cells. Nature 229:345-347, 1971.

Kaukel, E. and Hilz, H. Permeation of dibutyryl-cAMP into HeLa cells and its conversion to monobutyryl cAMP. Biochem. Biophys. Res. Commun. 46:1011-1018, 1972.

Lanks, K.W., Dorwin, J.M. and Papirmeister, B. Increased rate of acetylcholinesterase synthesis in differentiating neuroblastoma cells. J. Cell Biol. 63:824-830, 1974.

Lipetz, J. and Cristofalo, V.J. Ultrastructural changes accompanying the aging of human diploid cells in culture. J. Ultrastruct. Res. 39:43-56, 1972.

Littlefield, J.W. Variation, Senescence and Neoplasia. Harvard University Press, Cambridge, MA., 1976.

Nandy, K. and Bourne, G.H. Effect of centrophenoxine on the lipofuscin pigment in the neurons of senile guinea pigs. Nature (Lond.) 210: 313-314, 1966.

Nandy, K. and Schneider, F.H. Lipofuscin pigment formation in neuro-
    blastoma cells in culture. In: Neurobiology of Aging, (Eds.
    R. D. Terry and S. Gershon), Raven Press, New York, pp. 245-264,
    1976.

Nelson, P.G., Peacock, J.H. and Amano, T. Responses of neuroblastoma
    cells to iontophoretically applied acetylcholine. J. Cell
    Physiol. 77:353-362, 1971.

Orgel, L.E. Ageing of clones of mammalian cells. Nature 243:441-445,
    1973.

Peacock, J.H., McMorris, F.A. and Nelson, P.G. Electrical excit-
    ability and chemosensitivity of mouse neuroblastoma X mouse on
    human fibroblast hybrids. Expl. Cell Res. 79:199-212, 1973.

Prasad, K.N. Differentiation of neuroblastoma cells in culture.
    Biol. Rev. 50:129-165, 1975.

Prasad, K.N. and Hsie, A.W. Morphological differentiation of mouse
    neuroblastoma cells induced in vitro by dibutyryl adenosine 3':5'-
    cyclic monophosphate. Nature New Biology 233:141-142, 1971.

Prasad, K.N. and Vernadakis, A. Morphological and biochemical study
    in x-ray and dibutyryl cyclic AMP-induced differentiated neuro-
    blastoma cells. Exp. Cell Res. 70:27-32, 1972.

Robbins, E., Levine, E.M. and Eagle, H. Morphologic changes
    accompanying senescence of cultured human diploid cells. J.
    Expl. Med. 131:1211-1222, 1970.

Schneider, F.H. Effects of sodium butyrate on mouse neuroblastoma
    cells in culture. Biochem. Pharmacol. 25:2309-2317, 1976.

Schubert, D., Humphreys, S., Baroni, C. and Cohn, M. In vitro
    differentiation of a mouse neuroblastoma. Proc. Natl. Acad. Sci.
    U.S.A. 64:316-323, 1969.

Siakotos, A.N. and Armstrong, D. Age pigment, a biochemical indicator
    of intracellular aging. In: Neurobiology of Aging, (Eds. J. M.
    Ordy and K.R. Brizzee), Plenum Press, New York, pp. 369-399, 1975.

Simantov, R. and Sachs, L. Regulation of acetylcholine receptors in
    relation to acetylcholinesterase in neuroblastoma cells. Proc.
    Natl. Acad. Sci. U.S.A. 70:2902-2905, 1973.

Simons, J.W.I.M. The use of frequency distribution of cell diameters
    to characterize cell populations in tissue cultures. Exp. Cell
    Res. 45:336-350, 1967.

Soukapova, M., Holeckova, E. and Hnevkovsky, P. Changes of the
    latent period of explanted tissues during ontogenesis of aging.
    In: Cell and Tissue Culture, (Eds. E. Holeckova and V. J.
    Cristofalo), Plenum Press, New York, pp. 41-56, 1970.

Thuillier, G., Rumpf, P. and Thuillier, J. Preparation et. etude
    pharmacologique preliminaire des esters dimethylaminoethyliques
    de divers acides agissant comme regulateurs de croissance des
    vegetaux. Compt. Rend. Heb. Sean. L'Acad. Sci. Paris 249:2081-
    2083, 1959.

Toth, S.E. The origin of lipofuscin age pigments. Exp. Gerontol.
    3:19-30, 1968.

Varon, S. In vitro approaches to the study of neural tissue aging.
    In: Survey Report on the Aging Nervous System, (Ed. G.J. Maletta),
    U.S. Government Printing Office, Washington, D.C., pp. 59-76,
    1975.

Waymire, J.C., Weiner, N. and Prasad, K.N. Regulation of tyrosine
    hydroxylase activity in cultured mouse neuroblastoma cells:
    Elevation induced by analogs of adenosine 3':5'-cyclic mono-
    phosphate. Proc. Nat. Acad. Sci. U.S.A. 69:2241-2245, 1972.

Wood, A.W., Becker, M.A., Minna, J.D. and Seegmiller, J.E. Purine
    metabolism in normal and thioguanine resistant neuroblastoma.
    Proc. Nat. Acad. Sci. U.S.A. 70:3880-3883, 1973.

II.
Neuropathological and Clinical Aspects

IMMUNE REACTIONS IN AGING BRAIN AND SENILE DEMENTIA

Kalidas Nandy

Geriatric Research, Educational and Clinical Center
Veterans Administration Hospital
Bedford, MA. 01730

The immune system which provides specific defense mechanisms in our body may prove destructive in senescence. Immunologic competence is a growth-related process and may undergo deteriorative changes during aging. Such a self-destructive immunological reaction, often referred to as an autoimmune phenomenon, may give rise to pathological changes and reduction of life expectancy. There is considerable evidence in the literature to indicate that autoimmune reactions occur with increased frequency in the aged (Comfort, 1963). Although controversy exists on the processes underlying these changes, it is generally believed to result from the emergence of new antigenic stimuli or from the loss of acquired immunologic tolerance associated with aging. The autoimmune theory was first proposed by Burnet (1959). He described these changes as being due to the formation of 'forbidden clones of cells' arising from the derranged stem cells located in the reticulo-endothelial system, lymph nodes, spleen or bone marrow. Burch (1968), the leading proponent of the autoimmune theory of aging, proposed that several factors acting throughout life may significantly alter the process of acquired immunologic tolerance resulting in the increase of forbidden clones and incidence of auto-immune disorders. Walford (1962, 1967 and 1970), on the other hand, hypothesized that aging may be due to long-term low-grade histo-incompatability reactions among the body's population of cells resulting in cell death. The possible deterioration of the immune system during aging in mammals has been studied by Makinodan (1976) who suggested that this might be due to either intrinsic changes in T and B cells or their interaction, thus making them less efficient.

Aging is associated with a number of changes in the mammalian brain such as neuronal loss, lipofuscin pigment formation, loss of

dendritic spines, and formation of amyloid lesions and senile plaques.
Among these changes, the loss of nerve cells is probably the most
consistent one in the mammalian brain. This change is quite marked
in the brain of patients with senile and presenile dementia. This
is also important from the physiological points of view as the
neurons are post-mitotic and are not replaced by the division of the
remaining cells. The number of Purkinje cells in the human cerebellum
at different ages was studied by Ellis (1920) who noted a consistent
decrease of these cells with age in subjects dying of causes which
are not expected to affect the brain. Brody (1955) also demonstrated
a similar reduction in the number of neurons in human cerebral cortex
ranging from newborn to 95 years of age. The greatest loss was in
the superior temporal gyrus, area striata and hippocampus. In
contrast with normal aging, this cell loss in the brain of dementia
patients is not continuous over the whole cortex. An analysis of
four areas of the cerebral cortex, from pia to white matter, in
presenile dementia, demonstrated a neuron loss of 57 percent in all
areas, the superficial layers of the cortex being less affected
than the deeper ones (Colon, 1973). The absolute number of neurons
and thickness of the cortex were also studied in different areas
of cortex of mentally healthy subjects of different ages and in
patients with senile and vascular dementia, Alzheimer's or Pick's
disease (Shafer, 1972). According to this study, the absolute
number of neurons in mentally healthy old persons may be reduced by
20 percent, while that in senile dementia may be reduced by 35-38
percent. Although the loss of neurons appears to be an important
change in the brain of aging mammals, its underlying physio-pathology
or precise significance is not clearly understood.

        The possible role of immunological reactions in neuronal
degeneration in aging has been investigated in our laboratories.
Female C57 BL/6 mice of different ages were kept in constant
temperature and humidity controlled environmental chamber. Fluorescein
isothiocyanate (FITC) labeled rabbit anti-mouse gamma-globulin
(Cappel Laboratories, PA.), were used to demonstrate antigen-antibody
reaction in mouse brain. An intravascular perfusion with phosphate
buffered saline (PBS) was used to remove all traces of gamma-globulin
in the blood vessels of the brain. Frozen sections of both young
and old mice were treated with sera from mice of different ages
prior to incubation with FITC-labeled antimouse gamma-globulin. A
positive reaction as demonstrated by a bright greenish fluorescence
was mostly located on the cell wall, cytoplasm or the nucleus.
Specific fluorescence was observed in the neurons of both young and
old mice when the brain sections were treated with sera from old
mice but none when sera from young mice were used. Protein fractions
of old mouse serum (albumin, β-globulin and gamma-globulin) were used
in place of sera and only the gamma-globulin fraction gave the
positive reactions in the neurons. Control tests for specificity
of the reaction were carried out by absorption of the antimouse

gamma-globulin with normal mouse serum prior to incubation and also by treating mouse brain sections with FITC-labeled normal rabbit globulin. It appears, therefore, that gamma-globulin binding fractions (most likely an antibody) are present in the sera of old mice and not of young and these are gamma-globulin in nature (Threatt et al., 1971).

An attempt has also been made to determine the age at which brain-reactive antibodies (BRA) in sera first appears in C57 BL/6 mice. Sera in different dilutions from mice of different ages were studied using frozen brain sections by indirect immunofluorescence method. It was noted that dilution at which specific fluorescence was completely eliminated increased progressively with the age of the serum donor starting from the age of 6-15 months. There was also a progressive increase in the percentage of cells in the cerebral cortex showing a positive reaction when undiluted serum from mice of increasing age was used. It appeared in this study that the age of onset of BRA in sera probably is between 6-15 months of age and thereafter increased progressively as a function of age (Nandy, 1972a).

A study has also been carried out to determine whether the antigen responsible for the induction of antineuron antibodies is endogenous or exogenous. Young (2 months) and relatively old (12 months) germ-free female mice (Charles River Laboratories) and a similar number of control mice of same age, sex were used. The animals were sacrificed and brain-sections from each mouse were pretreated with their own serum prior to incubation with FITC-labeled antimouse rabbit gamma-globulin. There was no significant difference in the number of germ-free and control old mice showing positive sera. Sera from all young mice, both germ-free and control, were negative. Although it is possible that these germ-free mice were exposed to viruses and the antibodies thus formed cross-reacted with brain antigen, the study indicates that development of the brain-reactive antibodies in the sera of these mice is probably due to stimulation of the animals' immune system by an autogenous antigen (Nandy, 1972b).

The specificity of BRA to neuronal antigen has also been investigated. Sera of old mice (18-30 months) were first tested for the presence of BRA by the immunofluorescence method and the positive sera were incubated separately with the homogenates made from a number of organs (liver, kidney, myocardium, skeletal muscle, testes, pancreas, adrenal) for possible absorption of the antibodies by the tissues. The sera mixed with the organ homogenates were then centrifuged and the clear supernatant was then applied to brain sections prior to incubation with FITC-labeled antimouse gamma-globulin. It was interesting to note that BRA were to a very slight degree absorbed by liver, kidney, adrenal, testes and pancreas and not at all by skeletal and heart muscles. When sections of each of the organs

were also treated with positive sera, a positive reaction was noted
in occasional epithelial cells in most organs but not in heart
and skeletal muscle cells. The study indicated that the antibodies
against brain antigen are specific to neuronal antigen (Nandy, 1975a).

Since the old mice with high titers of BRA were healthy before
sacrifice and since death of a large number of neurons was not
noted in the brain at any time, the possible role of blood-brain
barrier (BBB) in separating the circulating antibodies from the
brain antigen in old mice was explored. Sera from old mice were
injected directly into one cerebral hemisphere (intracerebral
injection) in both young and old mice and antigen-antibody reaction
was noted in a large number of neurons around the area of injection
in both groups. No such reaction was noted on the contralateral
side or when the sera from young mice were injected. Damage to
BBB by mechanical injury to the cerebrum of one side in old mice
demonstrated similar reaction around the injured area. No reaction
was noted in the neurons of young mice after similar damage to BBB
(Threatt et al., 1971).

Serial sections of the brains of old mice were examined at
variable intervals following damage to this BBB by histological,
histochemical and electron microscopic methods. Evidence of
morphological damage was noted in 20-50 percent of the cells showing
antigen-antibody reaction by immunofluorescence method within 48
hours (Nandy, 1972c).

The possible migration of gamma-globulin across BBB was studied
in 2-3 month old C57 BL/6 female mice using ^{125}I-labeled gamma-
globulin. 10μc of ^{125}I-gamma-globulin (0.3 mg of gamma-globulin
in 0.1 ml of solution) was injected into the peritoneal cavity of
mice and a sample of blood (0.5-1.0 ml) was drawn from the heart
of each animal under nembutal anesthesia prior to sacrifice. At
least three animals were sacrificed at different time intervals
(6, 12, 18, 24, 36, 48, 72, 96, 120 hours) after the administration
of the isotope. The animals were thoroughly perfused by injecting
20 ml of PBS (pH 7.1) into the left ventricle and draining out through
cut right atrium. The ventricles of the brain were also perfused
with the same fluid by injecting the fluid into the two lateral
ventricles and draining it out through the cut brainstem. The
parts of brain (brainstem cerebrum and cerebellum), liver, kidney,
adrenal, heart, quadriceps femoris muscle, spleen, thyroid were
dissected out and weighed. The samples of blood (0.1 ml), pieces
of various organs and different parts of the brain (10 mg each)
from each animal were placed in the glass tubes for gamma-counting
and were stored at -60°C till ready for use. All samples, the
total dose of isotope in a tube, an empty tube (for background count),
and also samples of blood and organs from two uninjected mice
(control) were counted in a gamma-counter (Biogamma II, Beckman)

for ten minutes or 10,000 counts. The background count was sub-
tracted from all other counts before analysis of the data.

A high level of radioactivity was observed in the samples of
blood and various organs within 6 hours and the activity declined
rather rapidly by 120 hours. The activity of the isotope in the
brain increased slowly from 6 hours to 24 hours and thereafter slowly
declined by 120 hours. While a low level of radioactivity was noted
consistently in the brain tissue in all the animals, the hypothalamus
showed a relatively higher concentration of the isotope than the
samples of cerebrum and cerebellum. An electrophoretic study on
the extracted gamma-globulin from blood samples and cerebral cortex
was carried out on samples of blood and brain of two mice and it
was noted that 90 percent of the activity migrated at the same speed
as the gamma-globulin peak of the simultaneously tested original
radio-globulin. It was, therefore, assumed that the radioactivity
counted in the tissues is still bound to the gamma-globulin and not
free or even bound to some other compound. It appears from this
study that blood-brain barrier largely prevents the migration of
gamma-globulin to the neural tissue from the circulating blood and
only a small quantity is allowed to reach the brain tissue (Nandy,
1975b). The results of the various experiments on the role of
BRA in neuronal degeneration in aging are summerized in Table 1.

There has been considerable speculation on the underlying
etiology of neuronal degeneration in the aging mammalian brain.
The studies in our laboratory indicated that antineuron antibodies
formed in the sera of aging mice appeared to play an important
role in the age-related loss of nerve cells. Ingram et al. (1974)
studied the age-related frequency of gamma-globulin fraction of
human sera which binds with neurons in sections of human brain
tissue. This fraction, presumably a humoral antibody, was found to
bind to cytoplasmic constituents of neurons with increased frequency
and intensity with advancing age.

Autoantibodies against CNS structures in man have been reported
by a number of investigators in different pathological conditions.
The incidence of antibodies to neuronal structures have been reported
in cases of multiple sclerosis and lupus erythematosus (Diederichsen
and Pyndt, 1968), and in schizophrenia (Heath and Krupp, 1967) using
fluorescent antibody techniques. When sera and immunoglobulins from
apparently healthy men and rhesus monkeys were tested against nerve
cells and myelin proteins of brains of the same species, an increasing
number yielded positive results with advancing age (Felsenfeld and
Wolf, 1972; Eddington and Dalessio, 1970). Husby et al. (1976)
demonstrated that 46 percent of the children with reheumatic chorea
showed IgG antibody reacting with neuronal cytoplasm of human caudate
and subthalamic nuclei. The presence of these antineuron antibodies
appeared to correlate with the severity and duration of the clinical

Table 1.   Results of various experiments on the brain-reactive anti-
           bodies in mouse sera done in our laboratories.

No.	Experiments	Nature of Fluorescein Staining of Neurons
I	Sections of brain of old mice + anti-mouse gamma-globulin	Positive (in a few cells only)
II	Brain sections of old mice + serum of old mouse + anti-mouse gamma-globulin	Positive
III	Brain sections of young mice + serum of old mouse + anti-mouse gamma-globulin	Positive
IV	Brain sections of old mice + serum of young mice + anti-mouse gamma-globulin	Negative
V	Brain sections of young mice + serum of young mice + anti-mouse gamma-globulin	Negative
VI	Brain sections + gamma-globulin from old mice + anti-mouse gamma-globulin	Positive
VII	Serum of old mouse injected into the cerebral hemisphere of old mouse and brain sections treated with anti-mouse gamma-globulin	Positive
VIII	Contralateral hemisphere injected with normal saline	Negative
IX	Serum of old mouse injected into the cerebral hemisphere of young mouse + brain section treated with anti-mouse gamma-globulin	Positive
X	Serum of young mouse injected into the cerebral hemisphere of old mouse + brain sections treated with anti-mouse gamma-globulin	Negative

Table 1.   Results of various experiments on the brain-reactive anti-
           bodies in mouse sera done in our laboratories (Cont'd).

No.	Experiments	Nature of Fluorescein Staining in Neurons
XI	Blood-brain barrier damaged in old mice and brain sections treated with anti-mouse gamma-globulin	Positive
XII	Contralateral hemisphere	Negative
XIII	Blood-brain barrier damaged in young mice and brain section treated with anti-mouse gamma-globulin	Negative
XIV	Sera from germ-free (11-12 mos.) + brain sections + anti-mouse gamma-globulin	Positive in 50% mice
XV	Similar study with control mice (11-12 mos.)	Same
XVI	Specificity of BRA by absorption with various tissues	Specific to brain tissues
XVII	Permeability gamma-globulin across BBB	Slow entry and slow exit

attacks and cross-reacted with Group A streptococcal membranes.
Antibodies against CNS structures were also observed in patients
with cerebro-vascular accidents and the extent of the damage was
correlated with the severity of the ischaemia of the cerebral structures involved (Motycka and Jezkova, 1975).   Antibodies and lymphocytes specifically reacted with nicotinic acetylcholine receptors in
90% of patients with another autoimmune disease, myasthenia gravis
(Lennon, 1976).

     Filppi et al. (1976) studied the effects of mouse anti-brain
antibodies produced in rabbit on the mouse bone-marrow and observed
a reduction of the bone-marrow colony-forming units or hemopoetic
stem cells.   The intraventricular and suboccipital innoculation of
normal recipient rabbits with serum from donor rabbit immunized with

brain homogenates induced transient neurological symptomatology and
reversible EEG changes (Simon and Simon, 1975). On the other hand,
Rapport and Karpiak (1976) studied the effects of antibodies against
whole brain and specific brain fractions on the EEG and a number of
behavioral tests such as conditioned alternations, spontaneous
alternation, a visual discrimination task, DRL behavior, maze
behavior, and passive avoidance. The authors noted the antiserum
against the synaptic membrane fraction to be most effective in
altering EEG pattern and interferring in the retention or acquisition
of all behavioral tasks except visual discrimination.

The possible cytotoxic effects of BRA on the brain tissue was
observed in our study following the damage to the blood-brain barrier
in old mice. A large number of neurons around the area of damage
showed antigen-antibody reaction and evidences of morphological
damage indicated by severe chromatolysis, disruption of cell membrane
under electron microscopy and greatly increased acid phosphatase
activity by histochemical methods (Nandy, 1972c). The precise
mechanism of action of these antibodies in neuronal degeneration in
aging is not clear at this time. The antibody in the presence of
complement could exert a cytotoxic effect upon the neuron. On the
other hand, the reaction of antibody even in minute amounts might
attract the microglia toward the neurons leading to their destruction.
It may be pointed out that microglia were found clustered around the
neurons in the brain of old mice without morphological signs of
degeneration (Nandy, 1972c). While studying the cytotoxic effect of
immune gamma-globulin and complement on Krebs ascites tumor cells,
Green et al. (1959) noted severe damage to the structure of the
cellular membranes, cytoplasmic matrix, mitochondria and endoplasmic
reticulum. Goldberg and Green (1959) studied the problem biochemically and observed a marked loss of free amino acids, RNA and
90 percent of intracellular potassium from cells treated with antibody and complement.

The possible mode of origin of anti-neuron antibodies is also
a matter of considerable speculation. The antigen responsible for
the production of these antibodies could be endogenous or exogenous
in origin. It is possible that autostimulation of the immune system
by the altered brain tissue of the affected mice could take place
during aging. Another possibility is that such antibodies may arise
by stimulation of the immune system of the mouse by microbial agents.
In our studies using sera from germ-free mice by fluorescence methods
did not reveal any significant difference in the serum antibody content
in the two groups. The other possibility might be the dysfunction
of the immunocompetent cells associated with aging. Makinodan (1976)
reported that the decline in immune function may occur in normal
individuals following sexual maturity and this age-related decline
may be associated with increased frequency of autoimmune disorders.
Both cellular and humoral immunity may be affected in this process

(Price and Makinodan, 1975). Makinodan (1976) suggested that this decline might be due primarily to changes in T-lymphocytes and to some extent stem cells. Animal studies by Makinodan et al. (1971) have revealed that mice 100 weeks old retain only 10 percent of their humoral response to sheep erythrocytes found in animals 20 weeks old. Weksler and Hutteroth (1974) studied the response of lymphocytes from young and old persons to plant mitogens and allo-genic cells and found a significantly depressed response by the lymphocytes from the old persons. Based on numerous pieces of evidence, Burnet (1970) and Walford (1969) suggested that the age-related immunologic incompetence may be causally related to the aging process itself. The precise role of the altered immunologic competence in aging in the formation of brain-reactive antibodies requires further investigation.

Another conspicuous change in the brain of patients with senile dementia is the formation of senile or neuritic plaques. These have been demonstrated by both histochemical (Divry, 1952; Ishii, 1958; Margolis, 1959) and electron microscopic methods (Terry et al., 1964; Kidd, 1964; Krigman, 1965; Suzuki, 1967; Wisniewski and Terry, 1975). Microscopically, the plaques consist of an amyloid core surrounded by degenerating fibers and reactive cells. Amyloid lesions are also found in the brain of aging mammals (Walford and Hildeman, 1964; Schwartz, 1970). Glenner et al. (1970, 1972) demonstrated a marked similarity between certain amyloid protein and the light and heavy chains of immunoglobulin and suggested that these amyloid proteins are antigen-antibody complexes catabolized by phagocytes and degraded by lysosomes. Another investigator claimed that amyloid is a direct toxic cause of neuritic degeneration and senile plaque formation (Schwartz, 1970). Amyloid fibrils have also been demonstrated in senile plaques of the brain of patients with senile dementia and Alzheimer's disease (Ishii and Haga, 1976) using immunoperoxidase technique. Furthermore, Kalter and Kelly (1975) demonstrated a lower level of albumin and higher levels of certain immunoglobulins in 16 patients of Alzheimer's disease than in a control group of institutionalized patients. The study indicated a greater involve-ment in the humoral than the cell-mediated immune mechanism.

More recently, evidences have been offered in favor of possible infectious etiology of senile dementia. Neuritic plaques containing amyloid have been demonstrated in the brains of mice infected with certain strains of scrapie agents using silver impregnation and electron microscopic methods (Fraser and Dickinson, 1973; Fraser and Bruce, 1973; Wisniewski, 1975). Although the involvement of antigen-antibody complex in senile plaques has been suggested, no specific humoral antibody has been identified to scrapie agents. Further support for the infectious etiology of senile dementia is found in the successful transmission of Creutzfeld-Jakob disease from both affected human and Chipmanzee brain to stumptail Macaques

Table 2.   References listed in the text are classified according to
           subject

Subjects	References
1. Autoimmunity	Burch, 1968; Burnet, 1959, 1970; Comfort, 1963; Walford, 1962, 1967, 1969, 1970; Walford and Hildeman, 1964.
2. Immune dysfunction in aging	Makinodan, 1976; Makinodan et al., 1971; Price and Makinodan, 1975; Walford, 1967; Weksler and Hutteroth, 1974.
3. Cell loss: in aging	Brody, 1955; Ellis, 1920.
: in dementia	Colon, 1973; Shafer, 1972.
4. Brain-reactive antibodies	
: in aging	Ingram et al., 1974; Nandy, 1972a, 1972b, 1972c, 1975a, 1975b; Threatt et al., 1971.
: in senile dementia	Diederichsen and Pyndt, 1968; Felsenfeld and Wolf, 1972; Heath and Krupp, 1967; Hushby et al., 1976; Kalter and Kelly, 1975.
: in cerebro-vascular stroke	Motycka and Jezkova, 1975.
: in antimyelin antibody	Eddington and Dalessio, 1970.
: in experimental allergic encephalomyelitis and multiple sclerosis	Field et al., 1963.
: in cytotoxic effects	Goldberg and Green, 1959; Green et al., 1959; Nandy, 1972c; Rapport and Karpiak, 1976; Simon and Simon, 1975.
5. Autoantibodies in myasthenia gravis	Lennon, 1976.

Table 2.   References listed in the text are classified according to
           subject (Cont'd)

Subjects	References
6. Amyloid in CNS	Glenner et al., 1970, 1972; Harada et al., 1971; Schwartz, 1970; Wagner, 1955; Walford and Hildeman, 1964.
7. Senile plaques in CNS	Bruce and Fraser, 1975; Divry, 1952; Fraser and Bruce, 1973; Fraser and Dickinson, 1973; Ishii, 1958; Ishii and Haga, 1976; Kidd, 1964; Krigman, 1965; Margolis, 1959; Suzuki and Terry, 1967; Terry et al., 1964; Wisniewski and Terry, 1975.
8. Infectious etiology of senile dementia	Bruce and Fraser, 1975; Espana et al., 1975; Fraser and Bruce, 1973; Fraser and Dickinson, 1973; Grunnet, 1975; Wisniewski, 1975.

(Espana et al., 1975). Grunnet (1975) reported the appearance of
nuclear body types in Creutzfeldt-Jakob disease, a known slow virus
disease and Alzheimer's disease, the presenile dementia of unknown
etiology, and suggested a possible viral etiology of Alzheimer's
disease as well.

There is evidence in the literature on the possible involvement
of immune disorders in the production of certain changes in the brain
of aging mammals as well as patients with senile dementia. The
formation of amyloid and senile plaques and brain-reactive antibodies
offer more direct evidences on the involvement of immune system.
Although there are evidences for viral etiology of Creutzfeldt-Jakob
disease, a similar etiology for age-related changes in the brain and
of Alzheimer's disease is highly speculative. The results of the
recent investigations on the role of immune disturbance in the
pathogenesis of aging changes and in senile dementia are rather
encouraging and hold much future promise (Table 2).

SUMMARY

Immune dysfunction has been implicated as an important factor

in the production of changes in the brain related to aging and
senile dementia such as neuronal loss, amyloid changes, and senile
plaques. Antibodies specific against neuronal tissues have been
demonstrated in the sera of old mice and not of young. These
antibodies begin to form at 6-12 months of age and thereafter
increase progressively as a function of age. The blood-brain
barrier appears to play an important role in separating the
circulating antibodies from the brain antigen and a damage to the
barrier resulted in antigen-antibody reaction and morphological
damage in the cells around the area of damage. There are also
evidences in the literature to indicate that antineuron antibodies
are found in certain pathological conditions in human and that such
antibodies may have some cytotoxic effects as well. The precise role
of immunological dysfunction in the genesis of changes in the brain
relating to aging and dementia is not clear at this stage and requires
further investigation.

REFERENCES

Brody, H. Organization of the cerebral cortex. III. A study of
    aging in the human cerebral cortex. J. Comp. Neurol. 102:511-
    556, 1955.

Bruce, M.E. and Fraser, H. Amyloid plaque in brain of mice infected
    with scrapie morphological variation and staining properties.
    Neuropathol. Appl. Neurobiol. 1:189-192, 1975.

Burch, P.R.J. An inquiry concerning growth, disease and aging.
    Oliver and Boyd, Ltd., Edinburgh, 1968.

Burnet, F.M. Auto-immune disease. II. Pathology of the immune response.
    Brit. Med. Journal 2:720-725, 1959.

Burnet, F.M. An immunological aspect of aging. Lancet 2:358-360,
    1970.

Colon, E.J. The cerebral cortex in presenile dementia. Acta Neuro-
    path. (Berl) 23:281-290, 1973.

Comfort, A. Mutation, autoimmunity and aging. Lancet 2:138-140, 1963.

Diederichsen, H. and Pyndt, I.C. Antibodies against neuron in a
    patient with systemic lupus erythematosis, cerebral palsy and
    epilepsy. Brain 93:407-412, 1968.

Divry, P. La pathochimie generale et cellular des processus senile
    et preseniles. In: Proc. First International Congress,
    Neuropath., Rome, 2:313, 1952.

Eddington, T.S. and Dalessio, D.J. The assessment of immunofluor-
    escence methods of humoral and antimyelin antibodies in man.
    J. Immunol. 105:248-255, 1970.

Ellis, R.S. Norms for some structural changes in the human cerebellum
    from birth to age. J. Comp. Neurol. 32:1-33, 1920-1921.

Espana, C., Gajdusek, C., Gibbs, C.J., Osburn, B.J., Gribble, D.H.
    and Cardinet, G.H. Transmission of Creutzfeldt-Jakob disease
    to the stumptail Macaque. Proc. Soc. Exp. Biol. Med. 149:723-
    724, 1975.

Field, E.J., Caspary, E.A. and Ball, E.J. Some biological properties
    of a highly active encephalitogenic factor isolated from human
    brain. Lancet 2:11, 1963.

Filppi, J.A., Rheins, M.S. and Nyerges, C.A. Antigenic cross-re-
    activity among rodent brain tissues and stem cells. Transplant-
    ation 21:124-128, 1976.

Fraser, H. and Bruce, M.E. Argyrophilic plaques in mice inoculated
    with scrapie from particular sources. Lancet 1:617-618, 1973.

Fraser, H. and Dickinson, A.G. Scrapie in mice. Agent strain
    differences in the distribution and intensity of grey matter
    vacuolation. J. Comp. Pathol. 83:29-40, 1973.

Glenner, G.G., Ein, D. and Terry, R.D. The immunoglobulin origin
    of amyloid. Am. J. Med. 52:141-147, 1972.

Glenner, G.G., Harbough, J., Ohms, J.I., Harada, M. and Cuatrecasas,
    P. Amyloid protein: the amino-terminal variable fragment of
    immunoglobulin light chain. Biochem. Biophys. Res. Commun.
    41:1287-1289, 1970.

Goldberg, B. and Green, H. Cytotoxic action of immune gamma-globulin
    and complement on Krebs ascites tumor cells. J. Exp. Med. 109:
    505-510, 1959.

Green, H., Fleischer, R.A., Barrow, P. and Goldberg, B. The cytotoxic
    action of immune gamma-globulin and complement of Krebs ascites
    tumor cells. J. Exp. Med. 109:511-521, 1959.

Grunnet, M.L. Nuclear bodies in Creutzfeldt-Jakob and Alzheimer's
    disease. Neurology, Minn. 25(1):1091-1093, 1975.

Heath, R.G. and Krupp, I.M. Schizophrenia as an immunologic disorder.
    Arch. Gen. Psychiat. 16:1-9, 1967.

Husby, G., Rijn, I.V.E., Zabriskia, J.B., Abdin, Z.H. and Williams,
    R.C. Antibodies reacting with cytoplasm of subthalamic and
    caudate nuclei neurons in chorea and acute rheumatic fever.
    J. Exp. Med. 144:1094-1110, 1976.

Ingram, C.R., Phegan, K.J. and Blumenthal, H.T. Significance of an
    aging-linked neuron binding gamma-globulin fraction of human
    sera. J. Geront. 29:20-27, 1974.

Ishii, T. Histochemistry of the senile changes of the brain of
    senile dementia. Psychiat. Neurol. Jap. 60:768-781, 1958.

Ishii, T. and Haga, S. Immuno-electron microscopic localization of
    immunoglobulins in amyloid fibrils of senile plaques. Acta
    Neuropath. (Berl) 36:243-249, 1976.

Kalter, S. and Kelly, S. Alzheimer's disease. Evaluation of
    immunologic indices. N.Y. State J. Med. pp. 1222-1225, July,
    1975.

Kidd, M. Alzheimer's disease. An electron microscopic study. Brain
    87:303-320, 1964.

Krigman, M.E., Feldman, R.G. and Bensch, K. Alzheimer's presenile
    dementia. A histochemical and electron microscopic study. Lab.
    Invest. 14:381-396, 1965.

Lennon, V.A. Immunology of the acetylcholine receptors. Immunol.
    Commun. 5(4):323-344, 1976.

Makinodan, T. Immunobiology of aging. J. Am. Ger. Soc. 24:249-252,
    1976.

Makinodan, T., Perkins, E.H. and Chen, M.G. Immunologic activity in
    the aged. Adv. Gerontol. Res. 3:171, 1971.

Margolis, F. Senile cerebral disease: A critical survey of traditional
    concepts based upon observation with newer technique. Lab.
    Invest. 8:335, 1959.

Motycka, A. and Jezkova, Z. Autoantibodies and brain ischaemia
    topography. Cas. Lek. Ces. 114:1455-1457, 1975.

Nandy, K. Brain-reactive antibodies in mouse serum as a function of
    age. J. Geront. 27:173-177, 1972a.

Nandy, K. Neuronal degeneration in aging and after experimental
    injury. Exp. Geront. 7:303-311, 1972b.

Nandy, K. Brain-reactive antibodies in serum of germ-free mice.
    Mech. Age. Dev. 1:133-138, 1972c.

Nandy, K. Significance of brain-reactive antibodies in serum of aged
    mice. J. Geront. 30:412-416, 1975a.

Nandy, K., Fritz, R.B. and Threatt, J. Specificity of brain-reactive
    antibodies in serum in old mice. J. Geront. 30:269-274, 1975b.

Price, G.B. and Makinodan, T. Immunologic deficiencies in senescence.
    I. Characterization of intrinsic deficiencies. II. Characterization
    of extrinsic deficiencies. J. Immunol. 108:403-413, 1975.

Rapport, M.M. and Karpiak, S.E. Discriminative effects of antisera
    to brain constituents on behavior and EEG activity in the rat.
    Res. Commun. in Psych. Psychiat. and Behavior 1:115-124, 1976.

Shafer, V.P. Absolute number of neurons and thickness of the cere-
    bral cortex during aging, senile and vascular dementia, and
    Pick's and Alzheimer's diseases. Zhurnal Nevropatologii i
    Psikkiatrii imeni S.S. Korsakova 72:1024-1029, 1972.

Simon, J. and Simon, O. Effect of passive transfer of anti-brain
    antibodies to a normal recipient. Exp. Neurol. 47:523-534, 1975.

Suzuki, K. and Terry, R.D. Fine structural localization of acid
    phosphatase in senile plaques in Alzheimer's presenile dementia.
    Acta Neuropath. (Berl) 8:276-284, 1967.

Terry, R.D., Gonatas, N.K., Weiss, M. Ultrastructure of senile
    plaques in Alzhimer's presenile dementia. Amer. J. Path. 44:
    269-281, 1964.

Threatt, J., Nandy, K. and Fritz, R. Brain-reactive antibodies in
    serum of old mice demonstrated by immunofluorescence. J. Geront.
    26:316-323, 1971.

Walford, R.L. Autoimmunty and aging. J. Geront. 17:281-285, 1962.

Walford, R.L. General immunology of aging. In: Advances in
    Gerontological Research, (Ed. B. L. Strehler), Vol. 2, Academic
    Press, New York, pp. 159-204, 1967.

Walford, R.L. Immunologische aspekte des alterns. Klin. Wschr. 47:
    599-605, 1969.

Walford, R.L. Immunologic theory of aging. Williams and Wilkins, Co.,
    Baltimore, 1970.

Walford, R.L. and Hildemann, W.H. Chronic and subacute parabiotic
     reactions in the syrian hamster: Significance with regard to
     transplantation immunology, experimental amyloidosis and an
     immunologic theory of aging. Transplantation 2:87–115, 1964.

Weksler, M. and Hutteroth, T.H. Impaired lymphocyte function in
     aged human. J. Clin. Invest. 53:99–104, 1974.

Wisniewski, H. Infectious etiology of neuritic (senile) plaques
     in mice. Science 190:1108–1110, 1975.

REVERSIBLE MODIFICATION OF BLOOD-BRAIN BARRIER PERMEABILITY TO

PROTEINS

Stanley I. Rapoport

Laboratory of Neurophysiology
National Institute of Mental Health
Bethesda, MD. 20014

SITES AND DEFECTS OF BLOOD-BRAIN BARRIER

Entry of proteins into the central nervous system (CNS) is severely restricted by the blood-brain barrier (BBB), which is interposed between brain and cerebrospinal fluid (CSF) on the one hand, and blood on the other. The BBB has been demonstrated at three separate sites: the cerebrovascular endothelium, the epithelium of the choroid plexus, and the arachnoid membrane that separates the subdural from the subarachnoid space (reviewed by Rapoport, 1976). Each of these sites restricts protein and ion exchange because it contains a continuous layer of cells connected by tight junctions, or close intercellular adhesions. These make the cell layer have the approximate permeability properties of an extended cell membrane and limit passive protein and ion diffusion into the brain (Fig. 1). In addition, cerebrovascular endothelial cells have very little vesicular transport activity as compared to peripheral vascular endothelia, further limiting transport of protein across cerebral blood vessels (Reese and Karnovsky, 1967; Crone, 1965).

Peripheral nerves have a barrier which, is an extension of the central barrier, at the perineurium (corresponding to the arachnoid membrane) and at the continuous layer of vascular endothelium of the endoneurium (Olsson and Reese, 1971). At peripheral nerve terminals, however, this barrier is defective and allows occasional entry and retrograde axonal transport of protein toxins and some viruses into the CNS. Peripheral barrier defects also exist at the olfactory mucosa, sensory ganglia and lamina cribrosa of the optic nerve. In the CNS, there are additional special, nonbarrier regions which function in the neuroendocrine system and which have permeable

197

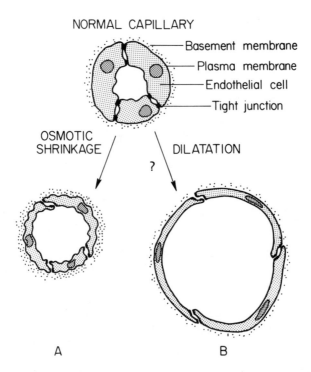

Fig. 1. <u>Schematic models for barrier opening</u>. A. When endothelial cells shrink in a hypertonic environment, their membranes pull on and widen tight junctions. B. Increased intraluminal pressure dilates capillaries and stretches endothelial cells and junctions. Another possibility is that vesicular transport is stimulated.

capillaries with a fenestrated, porous endothelial lining. These regions include the pineal body, posterior lobe of the pituitary, median eminence and wall of the optic recess (reviewed by Rapoport, 1976).

PROTEIN CONCENTRATIONS IN BRAIN AND CSF

Normal protein concentrations in CSF and brain are very low as compared to plasma concentrations, attesting to the overall effectiveness of the BBB to protein. Although electron microscopy demonstrates that some few brain arterioles support vesicular transport of horseradish peroxidase protein into brain (Westergaard and

Brightman, 1973), net protein transport is quantitatively infinitesimal. The brain/plasma ratio of ^{125}I-γ-globulin in experimental animals is about 2% and is due mainly to the cerebrovascular compartment (Sokoloff, 1961; Nandy, 1975). If blood is first washed from the brain by perfusing saline through the left ventricle of the heart, the brain/serum ratio of neutralizing IgG to measles virus is only 0.15%, a quantity ascribable to retention in brain of 10% of blood that was not washed out by perfusion, Table 1, (Hicks et al., 1975, 1977; Rapoport and Fredericks, unpublished).

Protein concentrations in CSF also are below 1% of serum concentrations. For example, the CSF/serum ratio of IgG is 0.13% and that of IgA is 0.075% (Felgenhauer, 1974). Many proteins in CSF are derived under normal conditions solely from blood, and enter CSF mainly via the choroid plexus and not through the cerebral vasculature. Their rates of entry into CSF are proportional to the rate of CSF secretion (Hochwald and Wallenstein, 1967), and they cross choroidal epithelium by ultrafiltration between epithelial cells and by transcellular vesicular transport (Klatzo et al., 1965; Felgenhauer, 1971; Rapoport, unpublished observation). Gamma-globulin equilibrates between CSF and blood in 4 days in man, as compared to 3 days for the smaller albumin molecule; in cats, equilibrium times for these proteins are approximately equal (Frick and Scheid-Seydel, 1958; Hochwald and Wallenstein, 1967; Rapoport, 1976).

Protein may be restricted from brain for several reasons. Because maturation of the peripheral immune system precedes the appearance of at least some brain antigens, the barrier reduces subsequent interaction between brain antigen and the peripheral immune system, including circulating immune agents and lymphocytes participating in cellular immunity (Cohen, 1968; Ruddi et al., 1972; Nandy, 1975; Rapoport, 1976; Gannushkina et al., 1977). In addition, a low concentration of protein in the extracellular brain parenchyma limits osmotically induced filtration of fluid into brain from blood and may prevent brain edema (Rapoport, 1976).

OSMOTIC OPENING OF BLOOD-BRAIN BARRIER

Tight-Junctional Widening

Cerebrovascular endothelial cells, like plant and animal cells, act as osmometers and shrink when placed in a hypertonic solution of a salt or of a lipid insoluble non-electrolyte like mannitol or urea. We demonstrated this by applying hypertonic solutions, of different lipid insoluble and partially lipid soluble substances, including NaCl, sugars, urea and lactamide, to the pial surface of the rabbit

brain, so as to open the barrier at pial vessels to the intravascular
Evans blue-albumin complex (Rapoport, 1970; Rapoport et al., 1972).
We showed that the relation between threshold for barrier opening by
reversibly-acting solutes and solute lipid solubility followed
patterns of osmotic shrinkage of single cells, and that barrier
opening to Evans blue-albumin was reversible within about 30 minutes.
We therefore suggested that osmotic shrinkage of cerebrovascular
endothelial cells mechanically distorted tight junctions and increased
junctional permeability. The mechanism was confirmed with electron
microscopy, where the tight junctions that normally prevent passage
of horseradish peroxidase were shown to become permeable to this
intravascular protein after osmotic barrier opening by hypertonic
urea (Figs. 1A, 2) (Brightman et al., 1973).

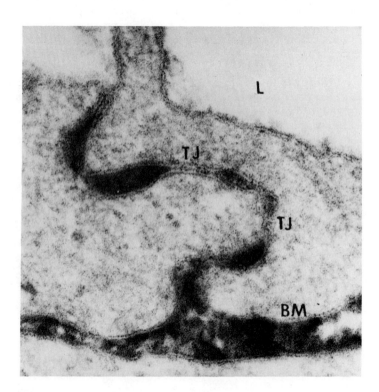

Fig. 2. Opening of tight junctions between endothelial cells to
peroxidase tracer, by intracarotid infusion of 3 M urea in the
rabbit. Peroxidase was given before internal carotid infusion, and
the animal was sacrificed 90 sec later. The peroxidase is washed out
of the capillary lumen (L) during fixation. The tracer is present
along the interface between endothelial cells, in the gaps between
the tight junctions (arrows) and in the basement membrane (BM)
(From Brightman et al., 1973).

We extended these observations by showing that it was possible to reversibly open the blood-brain barrier through tight junctional alteration over large regions of brain (Rapoport and Thompson, 1973; Rapoport, 1976). A hypertonic solution of urea, lactamide or arabinose, when infused for 20 to 30 seconds into the internal carotid artery of the monkey via the lingual artery, increased barrier permeability to intravascular Evans blue-albumin. When care was taken to maintain normal cerebral blood flow and to prevent cerebral hypoxia, osmotic barrier opening was accomplished without gross neurological sequelae, histological evidence of brain damage or altered water, Na or K composition of brain. Studies with tracers injected at different times after osmotic opening by intracarotid infusion also showed that the barrier remained open for up to 4 hours (Rapoport et al., 1972; Rapoport and Thompson, 1973; Studer et al., 1974; Rapoport et al., 1976).

We are now quantifying the extent of osmotic opening to tracers when altering the concentration of osmotic solute, the duration of perfusion, and the method and agent employed. These empirical parameters must be determined before the procedure can be used routinely to increase entry of blood-borne substances into the brain.

Barrier Opening to Albumin and γ-globulin

Sun et al., 1976, infused a 1.8 molal solution of L(+) arabinose (in 0.9% NaCl) into the internal carotid artery (without clamping the external or common carotids) of anesthetized rats at a rate of 7.4 ml/min. Using intravascular ^{125}I-albumin as a barrier tracer, they found that after one hour the ^{125}I content of the perfused hemisphere increased by a factor of more than 3 as compared to that of the unperfused hemisphere. Because the albumin distribution space in normal brain represents the vascular compartment, which composes 2 to 4% of brain weight (Sokoloff, 1961; Studer et al., 1974), osmotic barrier opening can elevate the albumin space to include a large fraction of the brain extracellular space.

We also measured the extent of osmotic barrier opening to γ-globulin, using circulating neutralizing antibody (IgG) to measles virus as the barrier tracer (Hicks et al., 1975, 1976). Therapy of viral infections of the CNS might be aided if the barrier could be opened to circulating immune proteins, and it might be possible also to test the hypothesis that circulating brain reactive protein within the brain can accelerate death of neuronal cells and the aging process (Nandy, 1975).

Rhesus monkeys were immunized against measles virus so as to elevate the serum concentration of measles neutralizing antibody

Table 1. Barrier opening to measles neutralizing antibody (NU) by perfusion with 1.8 to 2.2 molal arabinose solutions in monkeys.

GRADE OF OPENING	TIME AFTER PERFUSION	NO. OF ANIMALS	BRAIN/SERUM ANTIBODY RATIO $(NU/g)/(NU/ml)$	
			Cortex	Striatum
UNPERFUSED HEMISPHERE	1-14 days	18	1.19 ± 0.68[+]	1.56 ± 1.13
PERFUSED - UNPERFUSED HEMISPHERE				
0 - 1+	1-4 days	3	0.9*	0.6
2+	1-4 days	3 of 5	5.6	4.6
	14 days	2	4.1	4.1
3+	1-4 days	6	54.4	29.1
	14 days	2	1.5	0.3

[+]Mean ± S.D.; *Mean

Data are from Hicks et al. (1975, 1976)

to 80,000 neutralizing units (NU)/ml, as determined by a plaque-dilution technique on Vero cell monolayers. The left cerebral hemisphere was perfused with a 1.8 to 2.2 molal solution of L(+) arabinose via the lingual artery for 20 to 30 seconds when the external and common carotid arteries were temporarily clamped. Barrier opening was graded when the animals were killed 1 to 14 days later, according to the intensity and extent of extravasation of intravascular Evans blue-albumin.

About 50% of the animals had Grade 3+ opening (deep blue, extensive staining of the brain), accompanied by neurological sequelae and evidence of brain damage (Table 1). The remainder had Grade 1+ and 2+ staining without gross neurological sequelae.

Staining was restricted to the perfused, left side of the brain, and in this region Grade 2+ barrier opening elevated the brain/serum antibody ratio, (NU/g brain)/(NU/ml serum), by 0.005 above the value in the unperfused, unstained hemisphere in 5 of 7 animals (Table 1). Furthermore, brain antibody remained elevated for 2 weeks, indicating that IgG is lost slowly from brain and can retain its intracerebral, virus-neutralizing capacity for up to 2 weeks. Grade 3+ barrier opening elevated the brain/serum antibody ratio by 0.05 in perfused brains for 1 to 4 days following perfusion.

Absolute concentrations of brain antibody (NU/g) were estimated by multiplying mean ratios by 80,000 NU/ml, the mean serum concentration of antibody in immunized animals. On the basis of in vitro inhibition studies, the antibody in brain after Grade 3+ barrier opening would be more than sufficient to inhibit measles growth without added complement, and the antibody in brain after Grade 2+ opening would just be sufficient (Albrecht et al., unpublished observations). We are now attempting to produce Grade 2+ opening more consistently in our experiments, by adjusting perfusion rates, perfusion duration and concentration and choice of hypertonic solute.

After osmotic opening, CSF/serum antibody ratios, (NU/ml CSF)/(NU/ml serum), were elevated 10-fold for over 4 days. The rise was equal for both Grade 2+ and 3+ opening (Fig. 2). The lack of correlation between increased CSF antibody and grade of opening suggests that the extra CSF antibody came from an extracerebral source, perhaps the choroid plexus.

BLOOD-BRAIN BARRIER PERMEABILITY AND AUTOREGULATION

With aging, degenerative processes like atherosclerosis and chronic hypertension increase barrier permeability by interrupting normal endothelial continuity at cerebral vessels. In addition,

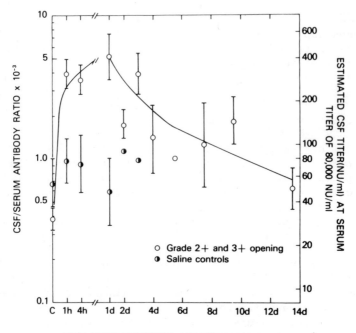

TIME AFTER PERFUSION, HOURS(h) AND DAYS(d)

Fig. 3. CSF/serum antibody ratio following osmotic barrier opening by hypertonic (1.8 – 2.2 molal) arabinose solutions in rhesus monkeys. Geometric means ± S.E.M. are given for the ratio, (NU/ml CSF)/(NU/ml serum). Data for Grade 3+ and 2+ opening are combined. Right hand ordinate gives estimated values of NU/ml CSF for a serum concentration of 80,000 NU/ml. (From Hicks et al., 1976).

the barrier at cerebral venules is made more permeable by neurones undergoing retrograde degeneration, presumably through release of cellular contents (Matthews and Kruger, 1973).

Other pathological conditions also increase vascular permeability, but do not necessarily irreversibly alter cerebrovascular ultra-structure. They include acute hypertension (produced by injection of Aramine or norepinephrine, or by rapid infusion of saline into the internal carotid artery), hypertensive encephalopathy, convulsions, hypercapnia, metabolic and respiratory acidosis with coma, cerebral concussion, intracranial hypertension, and damage due to an ischemic lesion or intracranial tumor (reviewed by Rapoport, 1976). In many of them, autoregulation of cerebral blood flow is lost or changed.

In normal man, cerebral blood flow is constant at systemic

blood pressures of 50 to 150 mm Hg, due to autoregulatory changes in the flow resistance of cerebral arteries and arterioles. At systemic pressures above 150 mm Hg and in response to insults to the brain, autoregulation becomes defective. The elevated systemic blood pressure can be transmitted directly to cerebral capillaries so as to increase blood flow, dilate the vessels, increase capillary and arteriolar luminal pressures and probably increase filtration of water through capillaries so as to produce local edema.

Cerebrovascular permeability is increased as a consequence of these changes, possibly through mechanical distension of inter-endothelial tight junctions as illustrated in Fig. 1B. The model is not unreasonable although ultrastructural evidence for it is lacking. Interendothelial tight junctions are made permeable by osmotic stresses (vide supra), and tight junctions in peripheral cell layers also are made permeable both hydrostatic and osmotic by pressure stresses (Pitelka et al., 1973; Ussing, 1971; Wade et al., 1973). Another possibility, suggested for acute hypertensive and convulsive barrier opening, is that increased barrier permeability is due to increased vesicular transport across arteriolar endothelium rather than increased junctional permeability (Westergaard and Brønsted, 1975; Lorenzo, personal communication).

SUMMARY

The blood-brain barrier to proteins and ions is located at the cerebrovascular endothelium, epithelium of the choroid plexus and arachnoid membrane. Each of these sites contains a continuous layer of cells connected by tight junctions that restrict intercellular diffusion. The vascular endothelium, moreover, supports little if any vesicular transport of proteins. The overall barrier to proteins is so effective that the concentration of γ-globulin (IgG) in brain is less than 0.15% of serum concentration, and the concentration in CSF is 0.13% of the serum concentration. Restricted access of blood-borne protein to the CNS may limit interaction between brain antigen and the peripheral immune system, and also prevent brain edema.

The cerebral vasculature can be made permeable to proteins by infusing hypertonic solutions of urea, lactamide or sugars into the internal carotid artery. Cerebrovascular endothelia shrink osmotically and interendothelial tight junctions widen reversibly so as to allow protein tracers into the brain. Osmotic barrier opening increases the brain concentration of ^{125}I-albumin by a factor of 3 in the rat, and increases the concentration of IgG in both brain and CSF of the monkey. IgG that enters the brain is not completely degraded or excreted even after 4 days.

Blood-brain barrier permeability is altered in a number of degenerative diseases involving the CNS, and also when autoregulation of cerebral blood flow becomes defective. In such conditions, which include acute hypertension, hypercapnia and concussion, the loss of autoregulation results in dilatation and increased intraluminal pressure in cerebral arterioles and capillaries. Cerebrovascular permeability also is increased, either because of widening of interendothelial tight junctions or because of stimulated trans-endothelial vesicular transport, but the exact mechanism remains to be determined.

REFERENCES

Brightman, M.W., Hori, M., Rapoport, S.I., Reese, T.S. and Westergaard, E. Osmotic opening of tight junctions in cerebral endothelium. J. Comp. Neurol. 152:317-326, 1973.

Cohen, S. The immune response in relation to the nervous system. In: Biochemical Aspects of Neurological Disorders, Third Series, (Eds. J. N. Cumings and M. Kremer), Blackwell, Oxford, 1968.

Crone, C. The permeability of brain capillaries to nonelectrolytes. Acta Physiol. Scand. 64:407-417, 1965.

Felgenhauer, K. Protein size and cerebrospinal fluid composition. Klin. Wochenschr. 52:1158-1164, 1974.

Frick, E. and Scheid-Seydel, L. Untersuchungen mit I^{131}-markiertem γ-Globulin zur Frage der Abstammung der Liquoreiweisskörper. Klin. Wochenschr. 36:857-863, 1958.

Gannushkina, I.V., Sukhorukova, L.I. and Baranchikova, M.V. Dependence of traumatic brain edema on immunologic reactivity against tissue antigens. In: Dynamics of Brain Edema, (Eds. H. M. Pappius and W. Feindel), Springer-Verlag, Berlin, 1977.

Hicks, J., Albrecht, P. and Rapoport, S.I. Entry of measles antibody into the central nervous system of Rhesus monkey following osmotic opening of the blood-brain barrier. Abstr. 5th Ann. Meeting Soc. Neurosci., p. 688, 1975.

Hicks, J.T., Albrecht, P. and Rapoport, S.I. Entry of neutralizing antibody to measles into brain and cerebrospinal fluid of immunized monkeys, after osmotic opening of the blood-brain barrier. Exp. Neurol. 53:768-779, 1976.

Hochwald, G.M. and Wallenstein, M.C. Exchange of γ-globulin between
    blood, cerebrospinal fluid and brain in the cat. Exp. Neurol.
    19:115-126, 1967.

Klatzo, I., Wisniewski, H. and Smith, D. E. Observations on pene-
    tration of serum proteins into the central nervous system.
    Progr. Brain Res. 15:73-88, 1965.

Matthews, M.A. and Kruger, L. Electron microscopy of non-neuronal
    cellular changes accompanying neural degeneration in thalamic
    nuclei of the rabbit. I. Reactive hematogeneous and peri-
    vascular elements within the basal lamina. J. Comp. Neurol.
    148:285-312, 1973.

Nandy, K. Significance of brain-reactive antibodies in serum of
    aged mice. J. Gerontol. 30:412-416, 1975.

Olsson, Y. and Reese, T.S. Permeability of vasa nervorum and
    perineurium in mouse sciatic nerve studied by fluorescence and
    electron microscopy. J. Neuropathol. Exp. Neurol. 30:105-119, 1971.

Pitelka, D.R., Hamamoto, S.T., Duafala, J.G. and Nemanic, M.K. Cell
    contacts in the mouse mammary gland. I. Normal gland in post-
    natal development and the secretory cycle. J. Cell Biol. 56:
    797-818, 1973.

Rapoport, S.I. Effect of concentrated solutions on the blood-brain
    barrier. Amer. J. Physiol. 219:270-274, 1970.

Rapoport, S.I. Blood-Brain Barrier in Physiology and Medicine,
    Raven Press, New York, 1976.

Rapoport, S.I., Hori, M. and Klatzo, I. Testing of a hypothesis for
    osmotic opening of the blood-brain barrier. Amer. J. Physiol.
    223:323-331, 1972.

Rapoport, S.I., Matthews, K., Thompson, H.K. and Pettigrew, K.D.
    Absence of brain edema after reversible osmotic opening of the
    blood-brain barrier. Abstracts 6th Ann. Meeting Soc. Neurosci.,
    2:744, 1976.

Rapoport, S.I. and Thompson, H.K. Osmotic opening of the blood-brain
    barrier in the monkey without associated neurological deficits.
    Science 180:971, 1973.

Reese, T.S. and Karnovsky, M.J. Fine structural localization of a
    blood-brain barrier to exogenous peroxidase. J. Cell Biol. 34:
    207-217, 1967.

Ruddy, S., Gigli, I. and Austen, K.F. The complement system of man
    New Eng. J. Med. 287:489-495, 1972.

Sokoloff, L. Local cerebral circulation at rest and during altered
    cerebral activity induced by anesthesia or visual stimulation.
    In: Regional Neurochemistry: Physiology and Pharmacology of the
    Nervous System, (Eds. S.S. Kety and J. Elkes), Pergamon Press,
    Oxford, 1961.

Studer, R.K., Welch, D.M. and Siegel, B.A. Transient alteration of
    the blood-brain barrier: effect of hypertonic solutions ad-
    ministered via carotid artery injection. Exp. Neurol. 44:266-273,
    1974.

Sun, C.L., Chiueh, C.C., Kopin, I.J., Fredericks, W.R. and Rapoport,
    S.I. Entry of ^{3}H-norepinephrine and ^{125}I-albumin from blood
    into brain following osmotic opening of the blood-brain barrier
    in the rat. Abstracts 6th Ann. Meeting Soc. Neurosci. 2:731, 1976.

Ussing, H.H. Introductory remarks. Philosoph. Trans. R. Soc. Lond.
    (Biol.) 262:85-90, 1971.

Wade, J.B., Revel, J.P. and DiScala, V.A. Effect of osmotic gradients
    on intercellular junctions of the toad bladder. Amer. J. Physiol.
    224:407-415, 1973.

Westergaard, E. and Brightman, M.W. Transport of proteins across
    normal cerebral arterioles. J. Comp. Neurol. 152:17-44, 1973.

Westergaard, E. and Brønsted, H.E. The effect of acute hypertension
    on the vesicular transport of proteins in cerebral vessels.
    In: Abstracts Seventh International Congress Neuropathology,
    p. 322, Akademiai Kiado, Budapest, 1974.

NEUROFIBRILLARY PATHOLOGY: AN UPDATE

Khalid Iqbal, Henryk M. Wisniewski, Inge Grundke-Iqbal
and Robert D. Terry

Department of Pathology (Neuropathology Division)
Albert Einstein College of Medicine
Bronx, New York 10461

Neurofibril is the term coined by light microscopists to refer
to the fibrillary structures in the neuron. These neurofibers
correspond to a variety of linear structures as seen with the
electron microscope. The principal fibrils of the normal mature
neuron are the neurotubules and the neurofilaments (Fig. 1).

Neurotubules are the microtubules of the neuron. They are
seen more abundantly in dendrites than in axons. Each measures
20-24nm in diameter, has a lumen of about 15nm, and has short
"sidearms". The function of neurotubules is not yet clearly
understood, but they have been implicated in the movement of cytoplasmic constituents, especially in axoplasmic flow.

Neurofilaments are linear 8-13nm (average, 10nm) fibers, found
sparsely in the cell body, moderately in the dendrites, and most
abundantly in the axon of the neuron. "Sidearms" can also be seen
on neurofilaments. The function of neurofilaments is not yet known.
They may act as a part of the force-generating mechanism in axoplasmic
transport, and as a cytoskeletal element in the preservation of cell
asymmetry.

In several pathological conditions, including Alzheimer presenile-
senile dementia and to a much lesser degree in normal aged humans,
one of the most striking morphological lesions is the presence of
many intraneuronal argentophilic fibrillary tangles (Fig. 2). These
neurofibrillary tangles are composed of bundles of extraordinary
fibers which measure about 22nm in diameter at their widest, periodically reduced to about 10nm at about every 80nm (Terry, 1963; Terry,
Gonatas and Weiss, 1964; Kidd, 1964). Each abnormal fiber is made

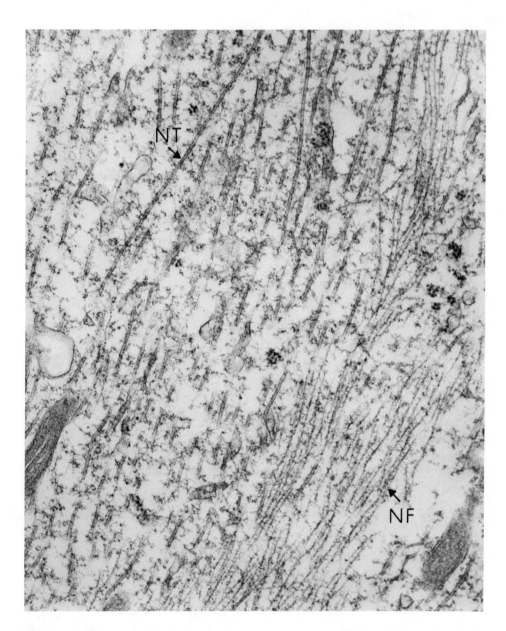

Fig. 1.   An electron micrograph showing normal neurofilaments (NF)
and neurotubules (NT) in a neuronal process; Magnification, X138,500.

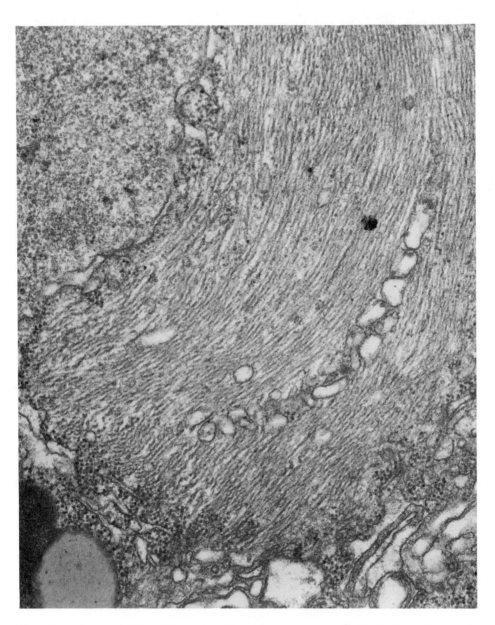

Fig. 2. A neurofibrillary tangle from a case of Alzheimer dementia, showing bundles of paired helical filaments in the neuronal cytoplasm. The neuronal nucleus is at upper left. Magnification, X 53,200.

up of a pair of 10-13nm filaments, apparently lacking in "sidearms", helically wound around each other (Kidd, 1963; Wisniewski, Narang and Terry, 1976). The concentration of these paired helical filaments (PHF) is quantitatively correlated with the degree of psycho-metric deficiency of the patients (Roth, et al., 1966; Blessed et al., 1968; Tomlinson et al., 1970).

The morphological aspects of the neurofibrillary pathology were reviewed by Wisniewski, Terry and Hirano in 1970. Since then neuro-fibrillary degeneration has been reported in certain other disorders. In this paper we shall briefly update the list, and discuss in some detail the chemical studies on neurofibers in normal and in affected neurons.

TYPE AND LOCATION OF NEUROFIBRILLARY CHANGES

The paired helical filaments of the Alzheimer type are also found in great abundance in Guam Parkinsonism dementia complex (Hirano et al., 1968), dementia Pugilistica (Wisniewski et al., 1976), Down syndrome (Olson and Shaw, 1969; Ohara, 1972; Schochet et al., 1973), and postencephalitic Parkinsonism (Hirano, 1970; Wisniewski, Terry and Hirano, 1970), see Table 1. In addition to their presence in small numbers in the normal aged human as mentioned above, the paired helical filaments also have been reported in a single case of Pick disease (Schochet et al., 1968a) and recently by Mandybur et al. (1976) in subacute sclerosing panencephalitis (SSPE).

Not every human disorder characterized by neurofibrillary degeneration contains the paired helical filaments. For instance, in sporadic motor neuron disease (Rewcastle and Ball, 1968; Schochet et al., 1969; Hughes and Jerome, 1971), vincristine neuropathy (Schochet et al., 1968b; Shelanski and Wisniewski, 1969) and infantile neuroaxonal dystrophy (Wisniewski, Terry and Hirano, 1970), there is proliferation of 10nm filaments. In Steele-Richardson-Olszewski syndrome, the abnormal fibers are about 15nm in diameter (Tellez-Nagel and Wisniewski, 1973). Neurofibrillary changes in the human are not only observed in adult and the elderly, but are also observed in children, as in infantile neuroaxonal dystrophy.

The paired helical filaments of the Alzheimer type have not so far been demonstrated in any tissue other than the human brain. The occasional occurrence of somewhat similar structures have recently been reported in the brain of aged Rhesus monkey by Wisniewski, Ghetti and Terry (1973). However, these abnormal fibers seen in animals do not have the same dimensions as those observed in human.

Neurofibrillary pathology has also been demonstrated in animals in several experimentally induced conditions. These are also listed

in Table 1. However, this experimental neurofibrillary proliferation
is always of 10nm filaments, which are morphologically identical
to normal neurofilaments (Fig. 3). The aluminum-induced filamentous
proliferation is apparently specific to the nervous system. In the
case of the mitotic spindle inhibitors similar changes occur not only
in a wide range of cell types but are also reversible. The spindle
inhibitors cause prompt filamentous proliferation in vivo and in
tissue culture. After a few days, these filaments disappear concurrently with an increase in the concentration of normal neurotubules,
and thereafter most of the cells return to a normal state.

Another type of aberrant fibrillar element which has been
observed in small numbers in Alzheimer dementia (Hirano et al., 1968),
Guam Parkinsonism dementia (Hirano et al., 1966) and Pick disease
(Schochet et al., 1968a) in human, and in the Kuru-infected chimpanzee
(Field et al., 1969) and scrapie-infected mice (David-Ferrerira et
al., 1968) are the Hirano bodies; these are filamentous aggregates
frequently juxtoposed to sheet-like material and often resembling
beaded structures. Hirano bodies are sometimes within the neuronal
cell body but are more often in the neurites.

Neurofibrillary pathology also displays certain intracellular
patterns. In some conditions, as shown in Table 1, the neuronal
perikaryon is primarily involved, while in others the cell processes
are more severely affected. The paired helical filaments when
present, are most often seen in the neuronal perikaryon, and in
dendritic endings of the neuritic plaque, and to a lesser extent
in dendrites and synaptic endings outside the plaque area. Furthermore, for the most part the paired helical filaments and 10-15nm
filaments do not occur together in the same disorder. In Pick
disease, although a hyperplasia of the paired helical filaments in
one case (Schochet et al., 1968a), and of 10nm filaments in another
case (Rewcastle and Ball, 1968) have been reported, a combination of
both paired helical filaments, and 10nm filaments has not so far
been observed.

The topographic distribution of neurofibrillary pathology in
each disorder also shows significant consistency. The paired helical
filaments are found predominantly in the cerebral cortex, mesencephalon,
and rostral rhombencephalon. The cerebellum, basal ganglia, lower
rhombencephalon, and spinal cord are rarely affected. The sites of
lesion are generally different in conditions characterized with a
hyperplasia of 10nm filaments. In Steele-Richardson-Olszewski syndrome,
some of the affected areas of the brain are the same as in the group
of disorders where paired helical filaments are observed.

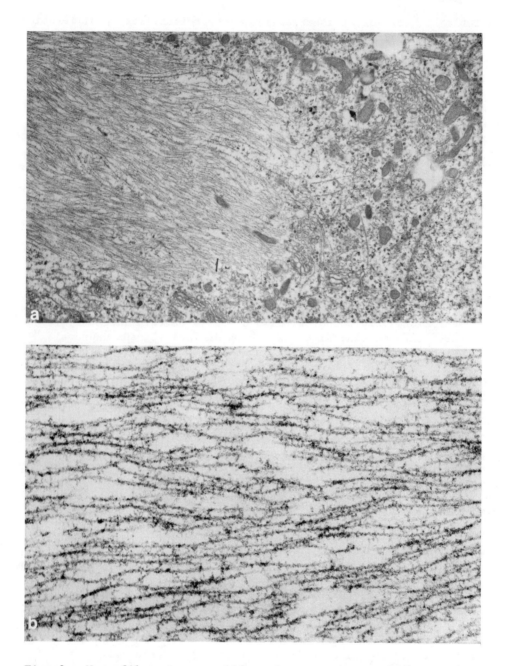

Fig. 3.   Neurofilamentous proliferation seen in a spinal anterior
horn cell of a rabbit treated with aluminum.   The nucleus is at
lower right.   a) Magnification, X 14,500; b) Magnification, X
130,000.

Table 1

Type and Distribution of Neurofibrillary Changes*

Human Conditions	PHF	10nm Filament	Perikaryon Cytoplasm	Neuronal Processes
Alzheimer presenile-senile dementia	+		+++	++
Guam parkinsonism dementia	+		+++	+
Dementia Pugilistica	+		+	++
Down Syndrome	+		++	+
Postencephalitic parkinsonism	+		++	
Subacute sclerosing pan encephalitis (SSPE)	+		+	
Pick disease†	+	+	+++	
Sporadic motor neuron disease		+	+++	
Vincristine neuropathy		+	+++	+
Infantile neuroaxonal dystrophy		+		
Steele-Richardson-Olszewski syndrome		15nm	+	+++
Animal Conditions				
Aged Rhesus monkey	**		+	+
Aluminum encephalopathy		+	+++	+
Spindle inhibitor encephalopathy		+	+++	+
Lathyrogenic encephalopathy (IDPN)		+		+++
Vitamin-E deficiency		+		+++
Copper deficiency		+	+++	
Retrograde and Wallerian degradation		+	+	++

*This is an updated version of that published by Wisniewski, Terry and Hirano, 1970.

†In this disease, the paired helical filaments and the 10nm filaments were observed in two separate cases. See text for details.

**Paired helical filaments with dimensions different from that of Alzheimer dementia.

PROTEIN SUBUNITS OF NORMAL AND ABNORMAL NEUROFIBRILS

Neurotubules

The major constituent from which neurotubules are assembled is tubulin, a dimeric protein with a sedimentation volocity of 6S, and a molecular weight of 108,000 to 130,000 daltons (see review, Olmsted and Borisy, 1973). A characteristic of tubulin is that under optimal conditions each mole of the protein dimer binds one mole of colchicine and two moles of nucleotide. When treated with a reducing agent, the dimeric protein is cleaved into two monomers, the α and the β tubulins, which can be separated by polyacrylamide gel electrophoresis in the presence of denaturants such as sodium dodecyl sulfate, urea, or guanidine hydrochloride. The molecular weights of human brain tubulin monomers are 56,000 daltons for α, and 53,000 daltons for β (Iqbal et al., 1974). These protein subunits are acidic and differ slightly in amino acid composition (Bryan and Wilson, 1971), and tryptic (Iqbal et al., 1976a) and cyanogen bromide (Feit et al, 1971) peptide maps. The neurotubules exist in equilibrium with free tubulin in vitro (Borisy et al., 1974, 1975; Gaskin et al., 1974) and probably in vivo (Inoue and Sato, 1967). They are structurally unstable and can rarely be seen in autopsy tissue. Tubulin is one of the most abundant of brain proteins (Dutton and Barondes, 1969; Shelanski and Taylor, 1970). The presence of tubulin in nerve endings has also been reported (Feit and Barondes, 1970; Blitz and Fine, 1974).

There seem to be no pathologic conditions in which there is a hyperplasia of neurotubules except in the brief and transient state during the recovery phase from treatment with spindle inhibitors (Wisniewski et al., 1968). These drugs cause filamentous proliferation in vivo and in tissue culture followed by disappearance of filaments in a few days with a concurrent increase of neurotubules. Soon after, most of the cells return to a normal state.

Neurofilaments

Neurofilaments have not been studied as extensively as neurotubules. Unlike the latter, the axonal filaments are structurally stable and can be isolated by subcellular fractionation. Neurofilaments and their subunits can be disaggregated in detergents, guanidine hydrochloride and by succinylation (Davison and Taylor, 1960; Schmitt and Samson, 1968). The major neurofilament protein subunit from calf (Shelanski et al., 1971; Davison and Winslow, 1974) and from human (Iqbal et al., 1975) was isolated by making use of the method of DeVries et al. (1972), for the isolation of axons. The major protein subunit of human and calf neurofilament has a molecular weight of 50,000 ± 2000 daltons (Iqbal et al., 1974,

1975; Davison and Winslow, 1974; Schook and Norton, 1975).

Colchicine or nucleotide binding activity could not be demonstrated in calf neurofilaments (Shelanski et al., 1971), but we observed
colchicine binding in human neurofilaments (Iqbal et al., 1976a).
However, our neurofilament fraction did contain some membranes as
contaminant. Stadler and Franke (1974) have recently shown nonspecific
binding of colchicine in liver membranes. Furthermore, the colchicine
binding sites in neurotubules are known to be inaccessible until the
tubules are depolymerized. Since nondenaturing conditions for the
depolymerization of neurofilaments are not yet known, it is not
possible to determine colchicine binding on the neurofilament protein
subunit, as has been done on tubulin.

Very little is known about the chemical or biological relationship between the neurofilaments and the neurotubules. The amino acid
composition of the calf neurofilament subunit (Davison and Winslow,
1974) is closely related to that of the calf neurotubule protein
(Lee and Frigon, 1973). We have recently observed that the tryptic
peptide maps of the major neurofilament protein labelled with ^{125}I
are almost identical to the similarly treated β tubulin, both purified
from human brain (Iqbal et al., 1976a). We also found in the human
neurofilament fraction, the presence of protein bands corresponding
to α and β tubulins, and other high molecular weight proteins observed
in purified human brain tubulin. A trace amount of protein band
corresponding to the major neurofilament protein was also seen in
tubulin. We have also raised antisera against the tubulin-free, human
major neurofilament protein subunit purified by SDS-polyacrylamide
gel electrophoresis. This antiserum formed a specific immuno-
precipitation line in Ouchterlony plates against the neurofilament
protein subunit, purified human brain tubulin and paired helical
filament protein (See below). The details of the immunological cross
reactivity will be published elsewhere (Grundke-Iqbal, Iqbal and
Terry, 1977, in preparation). Yen et al. (1976) were unable to
observe immunological cross reactivity between neurofilament and
tubulin with Ouchterlony immunodiffusion test.

The 10nm filaments observed in certain human pathological conditions or those induced in experimental animals, as described
earlier in this paper, have not yet been isolated and characterized.
It is not, therefore, known for certain if they are chemically
identical to normal neurofilaments, although their appearance is
strikingly similar.

Paired Helical Filaments

No chemical studies have been reported on abnormal neurofibrils
seen in human or in animal except those on the paired helical

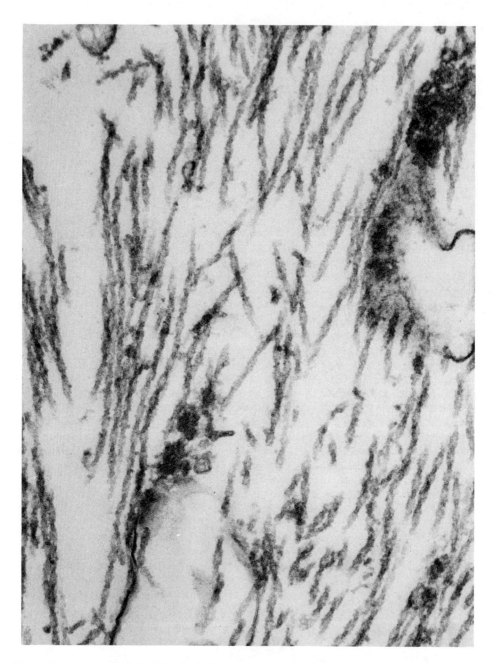

Fig. 4. A paired helical filament enriched fraction prepared from
a case of Alzheimer's dementia; Magnification, X 125,000.

filaments of Alzheimer dementia carried out in our laboratory
(Iqbal et al., 1974, 1975, 1976b, 1976c).

Like neurofilaments, the paired helical filaments are structurally
stable in both fresh and frozen autopsy tissue, and can be isolated
by tissue fractionation. Hippocampus is the area of the brain which
seems to undergo maximal neurofibrillary degeneration. However, the
amount of the paired helical filaments even in the hippocampus is
relatively small, making it difficult to isolate them by direct
subcellular fractionation of whole tissue, especially as to con-
taminating neurofilaments and astrocytic filaments. These difficulties
have been overcome by first isolating neuronal perikarya (Iqbal
and Tellez-Nagel, 1972) from the most severely affected areas of the
demented brains. These isolated perikarya were then subjected to
subcellular fractionation by conventional differential centrifugation
in which a fraction righ in paired helical filaments was sedimented
from the postmitochondrial supernatant (Fig. 4). The contaminants
in this fraction were rough endoplasmic reticulum, lipofuscin and
some mitochondria. This fraction was practically free of neurofilaments, neurotubules and astrocytic filaments as determined by
electron microscopic examination. It may be added here that although
axonal neurofilaments are structurally stable, and are isolated by
subcellular fractionation, this does not seem to be true of those
filaments in the cell body. We have been able to observe neither
neurofilaments with electron microscope nor the major neurofilament
protein subunit with SDS-polyacrylamide gel electrophoresis of
neuronal perikarya isolated from human autopsy tissue. Raine et al.
(1971), and Trapp et al. (1975) were also unable to observe neurofilaments in neuronal perikarya isolated from rat brain.

The paired helical filament and the neuronal fractions from
demented brains revealed a particular protein band on SDS-polyacrylamide gels. This band moved slightly ahead of βtubulin (mol. wt.
53,000) comigrating with the major neurofilament protein (mol. wt.
50,000), both purified from fresh human autopsy tissue. The paired
helical filament protein was observed only in the neuronal perikarya
isolated from areas of the demented brains rich in neurofibrillary
tangles, and was concentrated in the fraction enriched in paired
helical filaments. Similarly processed tissue from the corresponding
areas of the control cases matched for age and hours postmortem, or
from minimally affected areas of the demented brains did not show
the paired helical filament protein. Direct demonstration such as
cytological localization of the paired helical filament protein to
the paired helical filaments, and the reassembly of the paired helical
filaments from the purified paired helical filament protein are still
under investigation.

The two dimensional peptide maps of the tryptic digest of the PHF
protein labelled with ^{125}I are remarkably similar to those of the

Table 2

Similarities and Dissimilarities of Paired Helical Filaments to

Normal Neurofilaments and Neurotubules

Characteristic	Paried Helical Filaments	Neurofilaments	Neurotubules
morphology			
longitudinal section	linear narrowed every 80nm	linear sidearms	linear sidearms
cross-section diameter	22nm to 10nm	10nm	24nm
wall	circular or arciform	circular	circular
stain			
argentophilia	+	+	-?
congophilia	+	+	-?
stability			
autopsy tissue	stable	stable	unstable
long formalin	stable	stable	unstable
direct osmic acid	stable	stable	unstable
glutaraldehyde	stable	stable	stable
colchicine	?, probably stable	stable	unstable

identically treated human neurofilament protein subunit and the
β tubulin, the latter two being almost identical. In contrast,
peptide maps of α tubulin have definite dissimilarities from those
of the rest. The small differences among PHF, neurofilament, and
β tubulin may be due to small amounts of contamination. Alternatively, the small differences in the peptide maps may be real and may
correspond to changes in these proteins such as phosphorylation,
dephosphorylation (Goodman et al., 1970) or addition of sugars
(Barondes, 1968). Such modifications in these proteins may also be
responsible for differences in the electrophoretic mobilities between
β tubulin and the major neurofilament protein, or the PHF protein.

The paired helical filaments also resemble the neurofilaments
in being argentophilic and congophilic, and in their structural
stability characteristics as shown in Table 2.

DISCUSSION

Chemical studies on neurofibers are still in their infancy
except as to neurotubules which have been the target of increasing
attention in the last several years. However, what is clear from
studies described in this paper is that neurotubules, neurofilaments
and paired helical filaments are not only a class of similar
morphological structures but also are chemically very closely related.

Our data suggest that the β protein subunit of neurotubules with
some minor chemical modification may also serve as the principal
protein subunit of neurofilaments as well as of paired helical
filaments. The conditions under which interconversion of neurofibers
might take place are not known. Like neurotubules, the neurofilaments
and the paired helical filaments may be assembled from more than
one protein subunit. Alternatively, if the neurofibers are assembled
from proteins and lipids, the nature of the lipid moieties in the
neurofibers may also determine the assembly of normal and probably
aberrant neurofibers in various morphological structures. Neurofilaments are associated with large amounts of lipids (Schook and
Norton, 1975). Neurotubules have also recently been reported to
require trace amounts of lipids for their assembly (Bryan, 1975).

Very little is known about the function of neurofilaments and
their interaction with neurotubules in the performance of their
function. Since neurofilaments and neurotubules exist in such
close association in the neuron, it is not unreasonable to postulate
that one of the functions of neurofilaments may be the regulation of
the neurotubule function by controlling the assembly of the latter.
As mentioned above, neurotubules are known to exist in equilibrium
with their free protein subunits.

If neurofilaments and paired helical filaments really share a protein subunit with neurotubules as our data suggest, a hyperplasia of the former two neurofibers in pathologic situations may have a deletorius effect on the neuron by disturbing the neurofilament-neurotubule equilibrium. Further characterization of normal and abnormal neurofibers, and studies on the function of normal neurofilaments and neurotubules may lead to a more satisfactory explanation of the pathogenesis of disorders characterized by neurifibrillary degeneration.

SUMMARY

Neurofibrillary changes are of three major types. Paired helical filaments which are about 22nm in width, reduced to about half at about every 80nm from the lesions in Alzheimer presenile/senile dementia, Guam-Parkinsonism dementia, postencephalitic Parkinsonism, adult Down syndrome, dementia pugilistica, subacute sclerosing pan encephalitis (SSPE), and in lesser concentrations in Pick disease, and normal aged humans. Neurofibrillary proliferation of 8-10nm filaments are found in sporadic motor neuron disease, vincristine neuropathy, infantile neuroaxonal dystrophy, and several experimental disorders in animals including encephalomyelopathy caused by aluminum and spindle inhibitors. 15nm fibers are found in the Steele-Richardson-Olszewski syndrome.

The molecular weight of paired helical filament protein subunit and the major neurofilament protein subunit is 50,000 daltons each, as compared to 56,000 daltons for α and 53,000 daltons for β subunits of neurotubule. Two dimensional piptide maps of the paired helical filament protein labelled with ^{125}I are remarkably similar and may be identical to similarly treated major neurofilament protein and β tubulin. The antineurofilament protein antiserum forms specific precipitation line in the Ouchterlony immunodiffusion test with paired helical filament protein, and neurotubule protein. It is postulated that the β subunit of neurotubule with some chemical modification may be shared with the neurofilaments, as well as the paired helical filaments, and that the neuronal degeneration in conditions with neurofibrillary pathology may be related to a disturbance of the neurofilament-neurotubule interaction.

Acknowledgements: We are grateful to Ms. Su Tueh Tsai, Ms. Tanveer Zaidi, Mr. Mohammad Farooq and Ms. Hih-min Wang for their excellent technical assistance. This investigation was supported by grants NS-08180, NS-02255 and NS-03356 from the National Institutes of Health, and by a grant from The Alfred P. Sloan Foundation.

REFERENCES

Barondes, S.H.   Incorporation of Radioactive Glucosamine into
    Macromolecules at Nerve Endings.   J. Neurochem. 15:699–706, 1968.

Blessed, G., Tomlinson, B.E. and Roth, M.   The Association Between
    Quantitative Measures of Dementia and of Senile Change in the
    Cerebral Gray Matter of Elderly Subjects.   Brit. J. Psychiat.
    114:797–811, 1968.

Blitz, A.L. and Fine, R.E.   Muscle-like Contractile Proteins and
    Tubulin in Synaptosomes.   Proceed. Natl. Acad. Sci. USA, 71:
    4472–4476, 1974.

Borisy, G.G., Olmsted, J.B., Marcum, J.M. and Allen, C.   Microtubule
    Assembly in vitro.   Fed. Proc. 33:167–174, 1974.

Borisy, G.G., Marcum, J.M., Olmsted, J.B., Murphy, D.B. and Johnson,
    K.A.   Purification of Tubulin and Associated High Molecular Weight
    Proteins from Porcine Brain and Characterization of Microtubule
    Assembly in vitro.   Ann. N. Y. Acad. Sci. 253:107–132, 1975.

Bryan, J. and Wilson, L.   Are Cytoplasmic Microtubules Heteropolymers?
    Proc. Nat. Acad. Sci. USA, 68:1762–1766, 1971.

Bryan, J.   Preliminary Studies on Affinity Labeling of the Tubulin-
    Colchicine Binding Site.   Ann. N. Y. Acad. Sci. 253:247–259, 1975.

David-Ferreira, J.F., David-Ferreira, K.L., Gibbs, C.J., Jr. and
    Morris, J.A.   Scrapie in Mice: Ultrastructural Observations in
    the Cerebral Cortex.   Proc. Soc. Exper. Biol. Med. 127:313–320,
    1968.

Davison, P.F. and Taylor, E.W.   Physical-Chemical Studies of Proteins
    of Squid Nerve Axoplasm, with Special Reference to the Axon
    Fibrous Protein.   J. Gen. Physiol. 43:801–823, 1960.

Davison, P.F. and Winslow, B.   The Protein Subunit of Calf Brain
    Neurofilament.   J. Neurobiol. 5:119–133, 1974.

Devries, G.H., Norton, W.T. and Raine, C.S.   Axons: Isolation from
    Mammalian Central Nervous System.   Science 175:1370–1372, 1972.

Dutton, G. and Barondes, S.H.   Microtubular Protein: Synthesis and
    Metabolism in Developing Brain.   Science 166:1637–1638, 1969.

Feit, H. and Barondes, S.H.   Colchicine-Binding Activity in Particulate
    Fractions of Mouse Brain.   J. Neurochem. 17:1355–1364, 1970.

Feit, H., Slusarek, L. and Shelanski, M.L. Heterogeneity of Tubulin Subunits. Proc. Nat. Acad. Sci., USA, 68:2028-2031, 1971.

Field, E.J., Mathews, J.D., and Raine, C.S. Electron Microscopic Observations on the Cerebellar Cortex in Kuru. J. Neurol. Sci. 8:209-224, 1969.

Gaskin, F., Cantor, C.R. and Shelanski, M.L. Turbidimetric Studies of the in vitro Assembly and Disassembly of Porcine Neurotubules. J. Mol. Biol. 89:737-758, 1974.

Goodman, D.B.P., Rasmussen, H., DiPells, F. and Guthrow, C.E. Cyclic Adenosine 3:5-monophosphate-stimulated Phosphorylation of Isolated Neurotubule Subunits. Proc. Nat. Acad. Sci., USA, 67:652-659, 1970.

Hirano, A., Malamud, N., Elizan, T.S. and Kurland, L.T. Amyotrophic Lateral Sclerosis and Parkinsonism-Dementia Complex on Guam. Arch. Neurol. 15:35-51, 1966.

Hirano, A., Dembitzer, H.M. and Kurland, L.T. The Fine Structure of Some Intraganglion Alterations. J. Neuropath. & Exper. Neurol. 27:167-182, 1968.

Hirano, A. Neurofibrillary Changes in Conditions Related to Alzheimer's Disease, In: Alzheimer's Disease and Related Conditions, (G.E.W. Wolstenholme and M. O'Connor, Eds.), London, J.&A. Churchill, Ltd. pp. 185-207, 1970.

Hughes, J.T. and Jerome, D. Ultrastructure of Anterior Horn Motor Neurones in the Hirano-Kurland-Sayre Type of Combined Neurological System Degeneration. J. Neurol. Sci. 13:389-399, 1971.

Inoue, S. and Sato, H. Cell Motility by Labile Association of Molecules. J. Gen. Physiol., Suppl. 50:259-292, 1967.

Iqbal, K. and Tellez-Nagel, I. Isolation of Neurons and Glial Cells from Normal and Pathological Human Brains. Brain Res. 45:296-301, 1972.

Iqbal, K., Wisniewski, H.M., Shelanski, M.L., Brostoff, S. Liwinicz, B.H. and Terry, R.D. Protein Changes in Senile Dementia. Brain Res. 77:337-343, 1974.

Iqbal, K., Wisniewski, H.M., Grundke-Iqbal, I., Korthals, J.K. and Terry, R.D. Chemical Pathology of Neurofibrils. Neurofibrillary Tangles of Alzheimer's Presenile-Senile Dementia. J. Histochem. Cytochem. 23:563-569, 1975.

Iqbal, K., Grundke-Iqbal, I., Wisniewski, H.M. and Terry, R.D. On
Neurofilament and Neurotubule Proteins from Human Autopsy Tissue,
In Press, 1976a.

Iqbal, K., Grundke-Iqbal, I., Wisniewski, H.M., Korthals, J.K. and
Terry, R.D. Chemistry of Neurofibrous Proteins in Aging. In:
Neurobiology of Aging, (Eds. S. Gershon and R.D. Terry), Raven
Press, New York, pp. 351-360, 1976b.

Iqbal, K., Grundke-Iqbal, I., Wisniewski, H.M. and Terry, R.D.
Chemical Relationship of the Paired Helical Filaments of
Alzheimer's Dementia to Human Normal Neurofilaments and Neuro-
tubules. Brain Res., In Press, 1976c.

Kidd, M. Paired Helical Filaments in Electron Microscopy of Alzheimer's
Disease. Nature 197:192-193, 1963.

Kidd, M. Alzheimer's Disease-An Electron Microscopical Study. Brain
87:307-320, 1964.

Lee, J.C. and Frigon, R.P. The Chemical Characterization of Calf
Brain Microtubule Protein Subunits. J. Biol. Chem. 248:7253-7262,
1973.

Mandybur, T.I., Nagpaul, A.S., Pappas, Z. and Niklowitz, W.J.
Alzheimer Neurofibrillary Change in Subacute Sclerosing Panencepha-
litic. J. Neuropath. & Exper. Neurol. 35:300, 1976.

Ohara, P.T. Electron Microscopical Study of the Brain in Down's
Syndrome. Brain 95:681-684, 1972.

Olmsted, J.B. and Borisy, G.G. Microtubules. Ann. Rev. Biochem.
42:507-540, 1973.

Olson, M.I. and Shaw, Ch-M. Presenile Dementia and Alzheimer's
Disease in Mongolism. Brain 92:147-156, 1969.

Raine, C.S., Poduslo, S.E. and Norton, W.T. The Ultrastructure of
Purified Preparations of Neurons and Glial Cells. Brain Res.
27:11-24, 1971.

Rewcastle, N.B. and Ball, M.J. Electron Microscopic Structure of the
"Inclusion Bodies" in Pick's Disease. Neurology 18:1205-1213,1968.

Roth, M., Tomlinson, B.E. and Blessed, G. Correlation Between Scores
for Dementia and Counts of Senile Plaques in Cerebral Gray Matter
of Elderly Subjects. Nature 209:109-110, 1966.

Schmitt, F.O. and Samson, F.E., Jr. Neuronal Fibrous Proteins.
Neurosci. Res. Progr. Bull. 6:113-219, 1968.

Schochet, S.S., Jr., Lampart, P.W. and Lindenberg, R.   Fine
     Structure of the Pick and Hirano Bodies in a Case of Pick's
     Disease. Acta Neuropath. 11:330-337, 1968a.

Schochet, S.S., Jr., Lampert, P.W. and Earle, K.M.   Neuronal Changes
     Induced by Intrathecal Vincristine Sulfate. J. Neuropath. &
     Exper. Neurol. 27:645-658, 1968b.

Schochet, S.S., Jr., Hartman, J.M., Ladewig, P.P. and Karle, K.M.
     Intraneuronal Conglomerates in Sporadic Motor Neuron Disease:
     A Light and Electron Microscopic Study. Arch. Neurol. 20:548-553,
     1969.

Schochet, S.S., Jr., Lampert, D.W. and McCormick, W.F.   Neurofibrill-
     ary Tangles in Patients with Down's Syndrome: A Light and Electron
     Microscopic Study. Acta Neuropathol. 23:342-346, 1973.

Schook, W.J. and Norton, W.T.   On the Composition of Axonal Neuro-
     filaments. Transac. Am. Soc. Neurochem. 6:214, 1975.

Shelanski, M.L. and Wisniewski, H.M.   Neurofibrillary Degeneration in-
     duced by Vincristine Therapy. Arch. Neurol. 20:199-206, 1969.

Shelanski, M.L. and Taylor, E.W.   Biochemistry of Neurofilaments and
     Neurotubules. In: Ciba Foundation Symposium on Alzheimer's
     Disease and Related Conditions, (Eds. G.E.W. Wolstenholme and
     M. O'Connor), J.&.A. Churchill, London, pp. 249-266, 1970.

Shelanski, M.L., Albert, S., Devries, G.H. and Norton, W.T.   Isolation
     of Filaments from Brain. Science 174:1242-1245, 1971.

Stadler, J. and Franke, W.W.   Characterization of the Colchicine Bind-
     ing of Membrane Fractions from Rat and Mouse Liver. J. Cell Biol.
     60:297-303, 1974.

Tellez-Nagel, I. and Wisniewski, H.M.   Ultrastructure of Neurofibrill-
     ary Tangles in Steele-Richardson-Olszewski Syndrome. Arch. Neurol.
     29:324-327, 1973.

Terry, R.D.   The Fine Structure of Neurofibrillary Tangles in Alzheimer's
     Disease. J. Neuropath. & Exper. Neurol. 22:629-642, 1963.

Terry, R.D., Gonatas, N.K. and Weiss, M.   Ultrastructural Studies in
     Alzheimer's Presenile Dementia. Am. J. Path. 44:269-297, 1964.

Tomlinson, B.E., Blessed, G. and Roth, M.   Observations on the Brains
     of Demented Old People. J. Neurol. Sci. 11:205-242, 1970.

Trapp, B.D., Dwyer, B. and Bernsohn, J. Light and Electron Microscopic
    Examination of Isolated Neurons, Astrocytes and Oligodendrocytes.
    Neurobiology 5:235-248, 1975.

Wisniewski, H.M., Shelanski, M.L. and Terry, R.D. Effects of Mitotic
    Spindle Inhibitors on Neurotubules and Neurofilaments in Anterior
    Horn Cells. J. Cell. Biol. 38:224-229, 1968.

Wisniewski, H., Terry, R.D. and Hirano, A. Neurofibrillary Pathology.
    J. Neuropath. & Exper. Neurol. 39:163-176, 1970.

Wisniewski, H.M., Ghetti, B. and Terry, R.D. Neuritic (Senile)
    Plaques and Filamentous Changes in Aged Rhesus Monkeys. J.
    Neuropath. & Exper. Neurol. 32:566-584, 1973.

Wisniewski, H.M., Narang, H.K. and Terry, R.D. Neurofibrillary Tangles
    of Paired Helical Filaments. J. Neurol. Sci. 27:173-181, 1976.

Wisniewski, H.M., Narang, H.K., Corsellis, J.A.N. and Terry, R.D.
    Ultrastructural Studies of the Neuropil & Neurofibrillary Tangles
    in Alzheimer's Disease & Post-Traumatic Dementia. J. Neuropath.
    & Exper. Neurol. 35:367, 1976.

Yen, S., Dahl, D., Schachner, M. and Shelanski, M.L. Biochemistry of
    the Filaments of Brain. Proc. Nat. Acad. Sci. USA, 73:529-533,
    1976.

ALUMINUM AND THE GENETIC APPARATUS IN ALZHEIMER DISEASE

Donald R. Crapper and Umberto De Boni

Departments of Physiology and Medicine
University of Toronto
Toronto, Ontario, Canada

Alzheimer disease, unlike certain other central nervous system degenerative processes, is associated with definite histopathological changes. Recent work from several laboratories suggests that it is possible to produce tissue changes in experimental animals resembling those found in Alzheimer disease. The important observation that the infective agent isolated from scrapie tissue induces neuritic plaques in mouse brain, offers a new model for the study of this puzzling manifestation of Alzheimer disease (Bruce and Fraser, 1975; Wisniewski et al., 1975). These observations further support the suspicion, long held by many investigators, that a viral like factor may be involved in the pathogenesis of this disease.

The exact replication of Alzheimer neurofibrillary degeneration has not yet been achieved in experimental animals. It is now generally agreed, however, that the ultrastructural components of the Alzheimer neurofibrillary tangle are paired 100 $\overset{o}{A}$ diameter filaments twisted into a helical configuration (Kidd, 1964; Wisniewski et al., 1976). The chemical composition of the paired helical filaments based on mobility on gel electrophoresis and on polypeptide mapping indicates a close resemblance to normal neurofilamentous protein (Iqbal et al., 1974; Iqbal et al., 1975). However, the nature and distribution of the binding sites which result in the helical configuration of the paired filaments is unknown. The ultrastructure of normal neurofilaments indicates numerous side arm extensions and the twisted helical filaments, while lacking side arms, have poorly defined bridges between the strands. It is conceivable that relatively minor errors in subunit sequence in the synthesis of neurofilaments could lead to and arrangement of side arm binding sites such that a helical array of paired filaments might result.

A remarkable feature of the Alzheimer tangle is the failure of neurons to exhibit morphological evidence of a response which might control the amount of accumulated paired filamentous helical material. This could indicate that affected neurons fail to recognize the material of the tangle as a result of either a disorder in the systems regulating production or breakdown of filaments. It would seem reasonable to speculate that the chemical similarity in the helical protein to the subunits of normal occuring neurofilaments may be sufficiently great that appropriate proteolytic processes fail to respond and remove the excess material. If this assumption were correct, the above line of reasoning would place emphasis on mechanisms of filament production.

Several chemical agents including aluminum, cadmium and certain mitotic blocking agents induce 100 A^O diameter filaments in the soma and dendrites of neurons (Klatzo et al., 1965; Tischner and Schroder, 1972; Wisniewski et al., 1967, 1970). Among these agents, both aluminum and cadmium are found in the human body as normal occurring trace elements. Reports from this laboratory (Crapper et al., 1973, 1973a) indicate that aluminum concentrations which approach those found lethal to experimental animals occur in some brain regions in Alzheimer disease. The increase in aluminum occurs in regions associated with neurofibrillary degeneration and not in brain regions which exhibit only neuritic plaques or perivascular amyloid change (Crapper et al., 1976a).

The origin of the cytoplasmic filamentous material in neurons following exposure to aluminum is unknown. However, rabbit anterior horn cells affected with neurofibrillary degeneration double their organic mass within 10 days after aluminum exposure (Embree et al., 1967). This strongly suggests that the rate of protein synthesis is increased by aluminum as indicated by an active incorporation of labelled amino acids into the neurofibrillary tangle. However, the amount of RNA per cell was not increased. The possibility that aluminum intoxication may be associated with increased synthesis of one particular species of neuronal protein was further supported by the work of Exss and Summer (1973). In addition to a marked increase in {^{3}H}- leucine uptake into protein, indicating increased protein synthesis, the affected neurons accumulated large amounts of an apparently normal protein. Acrylamide disc gel electrophoresis showed no significant differences in mobility of proteins derived from neurons of experimental and control animals: however, a single protein band was reported as more prominent in aluminum treated animals than the same band in control animals. It was concluded that neurons from aluminum treated animals synthesized abnormally large amounts of a protein which was also present in control animals. Similarly, mouse neuroblastoma cells in tissue culture also exhibited a marked increase in protein synthesis following aluminum exposure (Miller and Levine, 1974). Pardoxically, however, despite the high

rate of protein synthesis, the neuroblastoma cells exhibited 20%
less ribosomal RNA per cell than cells of control cultures and the
activity of an enzyme, acetylcholinesterase, was depressed. All of
the above observations are compatible with the hypothesis that
aluminum stimulates the production of a class of proteins capable
of forming 100 A^0 diameter linear filaments closely resembling normal
fibrinous proteins and simultaneously depresses the synthesis of
certain other proteins. The mechanism by which the presence of
aluminum results in these opposite effects is unknown. The increase
in protein synthesis resulting from exposure to aluminum at normal
or depressed levels of ribosomal RNA further supports the hypothesis
of a selective rather than a general increase in protein anabolism.

The size of the nucleolus is generally accepted as an index
of the overall rate of protein synthesis in nerve cells (Hyden, 1960;
Watson, 1968; Brattgard et al., 1957; Bevelander and Ramaley, 1974).
Nucleolar size was used in our laboratory to test whether the increase in protein synthesis associated with aluminum intoxication
was associated with a general increase in anabolic activity. This
study was carried out in a system of cultured goldfish brain cells,
described elsewhere (De Boni et al., 1976), a system not responding
with a filamentous hyperplasia following aluminum exposure.

The cultures were fixed while attached to coverslips by immersion
in 3.5% phosphate buffered gluteraldchyde, washed and stained in a
0.1% aqueous solution of Toluidine blue, adjusted with NH_4OH to pH
9.5. Nucleolar diameters were measured in neuronal and glial nuclei
with the aid of a calibrated ocular graticule under oil immersion.
Nucleolar volumes were calculated as spheres for round nucleoli or
as prolate ellipsoids for nucleoli of oval appearance. In glial
cells containing more than one nucleolus the individual nucleolar
volumes were summed to obtain total nucleolar volumes per cell. All
measurements and calculations, with the exception of the statistical
analysis, were carried out double blind.

Exposure to aluminum of the cultures for duration of 10 min. to
20 days at concentrations ranging between 100 to 500 µM/1t, was
carried out by replacing the growth medium with medium containing
appropriate amounts of aluminum, either as the chloride or the phosphate salt. The pH of the final solution was monitored and the
buffers maintained normal pH values despite addition of acid aluminum
solutions. Nucleolar diameters were measured in 5 separate experiments in a total of 17 cultures involving 597 neurons and 599
glial cells. The measurements included 197 control neurons and 200
control glial nuclei. The number of nucleoli per neuronal nucleus
was never more than 1, but for glial cells ranged from 1 to 5. Total
measurements thus included 597 neuronal nucleoli (197 controls) and
1369 glial cell nucleoli (459 controls). To fulfill homogeneity of
variance criteria, logarithm transform data were employed in the

statistical analysis of nucleolar diameters. The numerical results
are summarized in Table 1 and in the histogram distribution of
nucleolar volumes (Fig. 1). In addition, a scattergram (Fig. 2)
shows the ratio of mean nucleolar diameter of control cells to mean
nucleolar diameter of aluminum exposed cells to be larger than
unity in 19 (95%) of 20 groups analyzed, of which 13 (69%) differ
significantly (p < 0.05). The number of nucleoli per glial cell
decreased significantly at the higher aluminum concentrations only.
Following the exposure to 500 µmoles/1t of aluminum phosphate for 2
weeks (Expt. 1) the mean number of nucleoli per cell decreased from
2.3 ± 0.61 nucleoli per cell, representing a decrease of 26% (Fig.
3). The data clearly indicated that aluminum applied to neurons and
glial cells in culture, depressed nucleolar size and number at
concentrations similar to those found in brain of man with Alzheimer
disease. This concentration also produces neurofibrillary degeneration in susceptible laboratory animals (Crapper and Dalton, 1973a).
These results are compatible with the hypothesis that the increased
protein synthesis observed in neurons undergoing experimental neurofibrillary degeneration (Embree et al., 1967; Exss and Summer, 1973;
Miller and Levine, 1974) is the result of increased production of a
class of filamentous protein and does not reflect a general increase
in anabolism.

Significant decreases in the size of nucleoli have been measured
in neurons exhibiting neurofibrillary degeneration in brain of man
with Alzheimer disease (Dayan and Ball, 1973).

To elucidate the mechanism of aluminum neurotoxicity, our
laboratory undertook a histochemical study of aluminum binding.
Aluminum accumulation was studied in experimental cell systems and
in brain tissue samples from patients with Alzheimer disease following staining of tissues with morin (3,5,7,2', 4'- pentahydroxyflavone,
BDH) by the method of De Boni et al., (1974). This dye fluoresces
bright breen in the presence of trace amounts of aluminum when morin-
stained tissues are examined in a fluorescence microscope with band
pass set at 500 to 650 mµ. For satisfactory application, tissues
must be fixed in aluminum free formalin (<0.01 µg/ml), and aluminum
contamination prevented at all stages of tissue preparation.

The results clearly indicated that aluminum accumulated upon
nuclei of brain cells of animals injected intracranially with aluminum
salts and the intranuclear fluorescent material in neurons and glial
cells exhibited the morphology of chromatin. Selective binding of
aluminum upon constituents other than nuclear chromatin was not
observed. Specifically, arrays of ribosomal aggregates, the Nissl
bodies, cytoplasm or lysosomes, did not concentrate aluminum. To
test the selectivity of aluminum binding to chromatin, human lymphocytes were cultured in medium containing aluminum. Following staining
with morin, the highest intensity of fluorescence arose from the

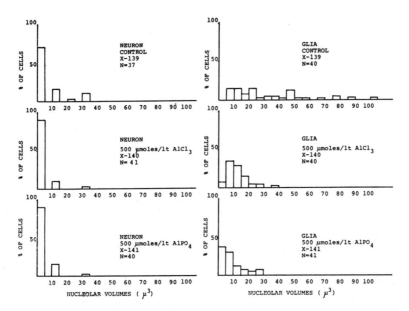

Fig. 1. Histogram distribution of nucleolar volumes of neurons and glial cells exposed to aluminum chloride and aluminum phosphate _in vitro_.
Fig. 1-1, exposure: 14 days.
Concentrations employed are indicated with individual histograms.

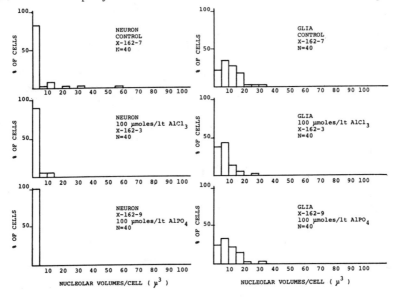

Fig. 1-2, exposure: 7 days.
Concentrations employed are indicated with individual histograms.

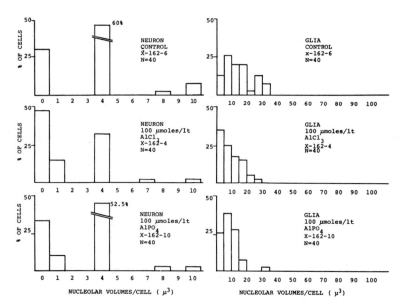

Fig. 1-3, exposure: 14 days.
Concentrations employed are indicated with individual histograms.

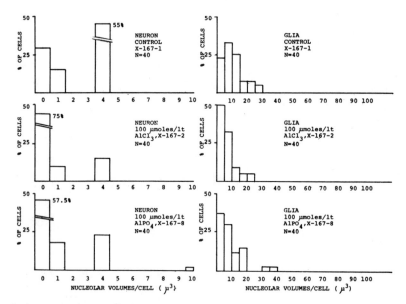

Fig. 1-4, exposure: 7 days.
Concentrations employed are indicated with individual histograms.

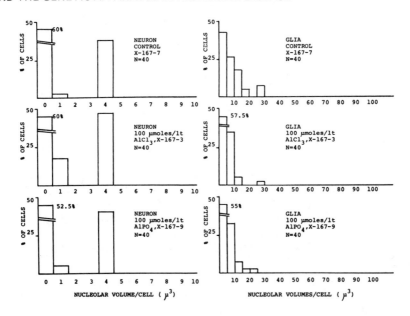

Fig. 1-5, exposure: 14 days.
Concentrations employed are indicated with individual histograms.

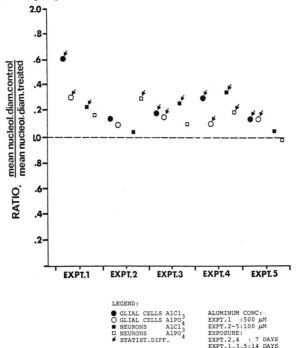

Fig. 2. Scattergram of ratios of nucleolar diameters. Significantly different ratios are identified by arrows. See text for additional detail.

Table 1. Nucleolar diameters following exposure to aluminum of cultured neurons and glial cells. Statistically significant values are identified by line.

EXPT. #	Al μM	EXPO. (DAYS)	CELL TYPE	CONTROL	MEAN NUCLEOLAR DIAMETER			
					AlCl$_3$	DIFF. %	AlPO$_4$	DIFF. %
1	500	14	NEURON	2.2972±0.8118	1.8690±0.6722	-19	1.9624±0.5816	-15
			GLIA	2.6648±0.9429	1.9481±0.5517	-27	2.0571±0.5681	-23
2	100	7	NEURON	2.0374±0.7015	1.9624±0.3985	-4	1.5749±0.4743	-23
			GLIA	1.9175±0.6319	1.6860±0.6280	-12	1.7500±0.6146	-9
3	100	14	NEURON	1.8374±0.5357	1.4624±0.5357	-20	1.6624±0.5236	-10
			GLIA	2.1463±0.6309	1.8043±0.6460	-16	1.8478±0.5583	-14
4	100	7	NEURON	1.6250±0.4493	1.1951±0.3687	-26	1.3624±0.4933	-16
			GLIA	1.9325±0.6270	1.4947±0.5642	-23	1.7445±0.6567	-10
5	100	14	NEURON	1.3874±0.4868	1.3125±0.4189	-5	1.4358±0.4890	+3
			GLIA	1.7447±0.5848	1.5140±0.5068	-13	1.5208±0.4915	-13
MEAN DECREASE:		7	NEURON			-15%		-20%
			GLIA			-17%		-9 %
		14	NEURON			-15%		-7 %
			GLIA			-19%		-17%

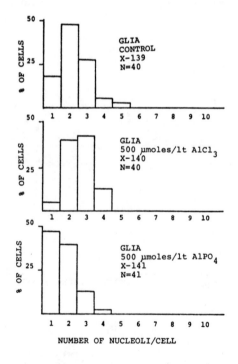

Fig. 3. Histogram distribution of number of nucleoli per glial cell, in cultures exposed to aluminum chloride and aluminum phosphate for 14 days. See text for details.

condensed chromatin of intact cells, and, in fractured cells, was
exclusively associated with the chromosomes. An identical accumulation
of aluminum was found on interphase nuclei and mitotic figures of
meristematic plant tissues germinating in solutions containing
aluminum. Furthermore, this preparation revealed the absence of
fluorescence in the region of the anaphase midbody, a zone known
to contain large aggregates of microtubules. This finding supports
the hypothesis that aluminum does not act by dissociating microtubules into filaments. In addition, nucleoli did not concentrate
aluminum. In plant cells exposed to aluminum the nucleolus appeared
as a well defined non-fluorescent dark body, surrounded by fluorescent
chromatin. In brain cells, the nucleolus was frequently fluorescent,
however, when sectioned, revealed a non-fluorescent dark core.

Samples of human brains stained with morin exhibited an identical
pattern of fluorescence. Five human controls without neurofibrillary
degeneration revealed an occasional nucleus which exhibited defined,
fluorescent chromatin. In material from four Alzheimer cases with
profound dementia and widespread histopathological changes the number
of nuclei with obviously fluorescent chromatin in both neurons and
glial cells was very much larger (Crapper, 1974). Some regions
contained few nuclei with fluorescent chromatin, whereas other areas
were extensively involved. The morin histochemical stain thus
indicated that the distribution of green fluorescent material in
Alzheimer disease is identical to that found in aluminum treated
animals undergoing a progressive encephalopathy. Therefore, the
elevated concentration of aluminum detected by atomic absorption
spectroscopy in some regions from brains of patients with Alzheimer
disease must be considered to be in a potentially neurotoxic compartment.

In the absence of histochemical evidence that significant amounts
of aluminum accumulated on structures other than chromatin of neurons
and glia, a quantitative analysis of aluminum binding to chromatin
was carried out (Crapper et al., 1977). Nuclei from cerebral cortical
grey matter were isolated in heavy sucrose using methods modified
from Yasmineh and Yunis (1970) with special precautions to prevent
aluminum contamination from the reagents or the environment. After
every separation nuclei were stained with toluidine blue and examined
by light microscopy to assure complete removal of cytoplasmic remnants.
This was confirmed by electronmicroscopy of nuclear pellets. Nuclei
were broken by sonication and the resulting suspension of chromatin
separated into three fractions; a heavy fraction of heterochromatin
which was isolated by centrifugation at 4000 g (R_{av}) for 20 minutes,
an intermediate fraction isolated into a pellet by centrifugation at
100,000 g for 1 hour and the supernatant which contained euchromatin.
Aluminum was measured by the method of atomic absorption (Krishnan
et al., 1976), DNA by the method of Levy et al., (1973) and protein
by the Lowry method.

To compare the aluminum content found in Alzheimer disease to that which is lethal to a laboratory animal, chromatin binding of aluminum was also studied in an aluminum encephalopathy in cats.

Human brains were usually bisected in the sagittal plane; one half was fixed in formalin and subsequently submitted to a detailed histological examination. The other half was stored frozen in aluminum free containers until assayed. To establish the aluminum content of normal human chromatin tissue was collected at necropsy from four patients, aged 2, 35, 41 and 52 years. Each had died without focal neurological signs and no neurofibrillary degeneration or neuritic plaques were present in the tissue. For Alzheimer disease, the diagnosis was not based upon age but upon a history of progressive dementia and the necropsy findings of brain atrophy, neurofibrillary degeneration, neuritic plaques, hippocampal pyramidal cell granulovacuolar degeneration and the absence of atherosclerotic vascular lesions. Material from 3 Alzheimer cases aged 52, 81 and 87 was examined.

In five cats an aluminum encephalopathy was induced by injecting 7-10 μmoles of aluminum, as a solution of the chloride salt, into the cerebrospinal fluid of the cisterna-cerebellomedularis (Crapper and Dalton, 1973 a.b.). Animals were sacrificed when motor signs of the encephalopathy were present, usually between 10-15 days post-injection.

The aluminum content of nuclei, heterochromatin, intermediate chromatin and euchromatin of brain cells are shown in Table 2 for control cat and control human, aluminum treated cat and Alzheimer disease. The values are expressed in micrograms of aluminum per gram of DNA. The aluminum content of whole nuclei and each of the chromatin fractions for control cats and humans are closely similar. This is in agreement with previous measures of normal cerebral cortical aluminum content in which the average cerebral cortical grey whole tissue content was 1.4 ± 0.5 SD μg/g dry weight of cortex (n=55) for cats and 1.9 ± 0.7 SD μg/g dry weight (n=208) for humans (Crapper et al., 1976 a). In the cat aluminum encephalopathy with widespread neurofibrillary degeneration, the amount of aluminum found in isolated nuclei and each of the three chromatin fractions was increased by a factor of 3 to 5 times that found in control cat brain. In human brains with Alzheimer disease which exhibited widespread neurofibrillary degeneration , a marked increase in aluminum content was found in all fractions, showing between 3.1 to 3.7 the amount of aluminum than controls. These data indicate that aluminum concentrations almost identical to those associated with a neurofibrillary encephalopathy in an aluminum susceptible species such as the cat occur in human brains with Alzheimer disease. Furthermore, the intracranial dose of aluminum employed in the experimental encephalopathy (7-10 μ moles) is 100% lethal in 21 to 28 days and does not necessarily represent the minimal lethal dose.

Table 2

Al/DNA

μg/gm (S.D.)

	Cat	Human	Al Cat	Alzheimer
Nuclei	705 (248)	771 (231)	2582 (1763)	2611 (1462)
Heterochromatin	1551 (858)	2056 (678)	8394 (4311)	6385 (3425)
Intermediate	299 (136)	286 (95)	886 (335)	980 (879)
Euchromatin	145 (84)	153 (99)	472 (133)	479 (473)
n	8	9	5	7

The above data do not establish, however, that aluminum is toxic to human neurons. Species variation in toxic response to aluminum exist. In two strains of rat (King et al., 1975) aluminum concentrations of 4 to 10 times that employed in cats induced neither a progressive encephalopathy nor neurofibrillary degeneration. In two species of adolescent monkey, rhesus macaque and saimiri sciureus, high doses of aluminum are required to induce an encephalopathy and the encephalopathy does not follow a progressive course similar to that in the cat (Crapper and Dalton, unpublished). Furthermore, widespread neurofibrillary degeneration was not found in these primate species, although limited neurofibrillary degeneration was encountered in regions injected with aluminum 12 months previously. Nevertheless, in susceptible species such as cat, rabbit and guinea pig, the similarity in clinical course, the intracytoplasmic accumulation of filamentous material and the remarkable similarity in the topography of neurons susceptible to neurofibrillary degeneration (Crapper, 1974) taken together with the above observations are sufficiently strong circumstantial evidence to consider aluminum a possible cyto-toxic factor in Alzheimer disease.

Physical-chemical considerations predict that aluminum is likely to bind to the acid protein-DNA complex of chromatin, rather than the histone fraction. Indeed, aluminum treated isolated nuclei subsequently exposed to a process which removes histones (0.14M NaCl washes followed by 0.25 N HCl washes) does not alter morin fluorescence, supporting the possibility that aluminum binding is not altered by histone removal. To quantitatively evaluate chromatin aluminum binding after removal of histones by this method, atomic absorption measures of aluminum binding in human brain cell nuclei were performed and the results are shown in Table 3. In general, little change in aluminum binding was noted following removal of the histones. Thus most of the aluminum is associated with the acid protein-DNA complex.

Table 3

Aluminum Following Deproteinization

	Protein/DNA (mgm/gm)	Al/DNA (µg/gm)
Control Nuclei	2069 (354)	489 (183)
Deproteinized Control Nuclei	936 (183)	431 (201)

Numbers in brackets are standard deviations.
n = 4

The above histochemical evidence of aluminum accumulation upon nuclear chromatin, now supported by direct chemical measurements of aluminum binding, is consistant with the assumption that the increased production of neurofilamentous material induced by aluminum results from an alteration in the transcription of genetic information. Indeed, histochemical methods failed to show an aluminum accumulation in the experimental encephalopathy upon neural membranes, the Golgi or Nissl apparati, ribosomes, liposomes, mitochondria, or the neurofibrillary tangles themselves. However, until the results of a chemical study of the action and binding of aluminum upon RNA in the nucleolus and thus on ribosomal protein synthesis and upon translation processes in the cytoplasm have been completed, effects upon cell components other than chromatin cannot be excluded. Nevertheless, the strongest argument against a direct effect of aluminum upon membranes, transmitter functions or energy metabolism comes from a study of the aluminum encephalopathy in experimental animals. In the early stages of the aluminum encephalopathy surface and depth recorded EEG activity and visual evoked potentials are unchanged. Furthermore, complex motor and higher cerebral functions including performance of learning memory tasks, temporal and spatial discrimination and motivation remain normal for several days after aluminum injection (Crapper and Dalton, 1973 a,b; Crapper, 1976).

In vitro membrane effects have not been observed when aluminum is added to a physiological concentration of other ions. Effects upon cardiac muscle action potentials, aplysia giant neuron action potentials and the frequency and amplitude of frog sartorius miniature end plate potentials have not been observed in our laboratory until concentrations of 10 to 500 times those of the dementia model were reached, or until pH changes induced by the aluminum solutions affected the preparations. Mitochondrial respiration in vitro was not altered (De Boni, unpublished). Measurements, by our associate

Table 4

Metabolite μm/g	Control (n=3)	Saline (n=6)	Aluminum (n=5)
ATP	3.02 ± 0.02	2.96 ± 0.02	2.90 ± 0.06
ADP	0.273± 0.008	0.274± 0.006	0.269± 0.007
AMP	0.016± 0.002	0.019± 0.001	0.016± 0.001
ECP	0.95 ± 0.00	0.95 ± 0.00	0.95 ± 0.00
Phosphocreatine	5.15 ± 0.16	5.15 ± 0.04	5.20 ± 0.14
Glucose	4.03 ± 0.27	3.76 ± 0.006	4.42 ± 0.25
Glucose-6-P	0.116± 0.004	0.105± 0.006	0.101± 0.006
Pyruvate	0.125± 0.009	0.112± 0.007	0.124± 0.002
Lactate	1.60 ± 0.17	1.37 ± 0.05	1.48 ± 0.06
Lactate/Pyruvate	12.8 ± 0.8	12.4 ± 0.6	12.0 ± 0.5
Citrate	0.412± 0.012	0.404± 0.009	0.419± 0.012
α-Ketoglutarate	0.116± 0.014	0.108± 0.009	0.119± 0.007
Malate	0.404± 0.020	0.368± 0.012	0.367± 0.013
Glutamate	15.21 ± 0.55	14.61 ± 0.29	14.28 ± 0.35

Contents of energy metabolites and selected glycolytic – Krebs cycle intermediates in cerebral cortex of control, saline and aluminum injected rats. Values are means ± S.E.M. in um/g wet weight. ECP = {ATP} + 0.5 {ADP} / {ATP} + {ADP} + {AMP}. n = number of animals.

Dr. V. H. MacMillan, of the concentration of products of the oxidative enzymes in cerebral tissue from Wistar rats injected with
aluminum chloride (Table 4) indicated that oxidative metabolism
continued unimpaired in the presence of two to three times the
concentrations of aluminum necessary to induce the encephalopathy
in cats (King et al., 1975). The specific components of oxidative
metabolism measured included phosphocreatine, ATP, ADP, AMP,
pyruvate, lactate, citrate, alphaketoglutarate and malate and did
not differ significantly in 5 aluminum treated rats, 6 saline controls
and 3 sham operated controls.

     Carriers for aluminum and routes of access of this element to
the central nervous system are unknown although access from the
systemic circulation through the blood brain barrier is probable.
This assumption is supported by the findings of elevated brain
aluminum concentrations found in patients with dialysis dementia
(Alfrey et al., 1976). Furthermore, we have recently reported
that elevated systemic aluminum levels result in increased brain
aluminum concentrations and neurofibrillary degeneration in rabbits
(De Boni et al., 1976 a).

     Rabbits were injected daily into the subcutaneous space with
aqueous, neutral solutions of either aluminum lactate or tartrate.
Doses of elemental aluminum exceeding 5.0 mg/kg/day of tartrate or
9.5 mg/kg/day of the lactate induced, after 10 to 28 days, the typical
signs of an aluminum encephalopathy. Histological examination of
brain tissue from these animals showed widespread neurofibrillary
degeneration. The Bielchowski silver stain revealed involvement of
pyramidal cells in cerebral cortex, hippocampus and Purkinje cells
of the cerebellum. Electronmicroscopy confirmed the light microscopical findings of neurofibrillary degeneration and showed the argentophilic structures to be composed of 100 A^O diameter filaments,
occuring in postsynaptic structures. The morin histochemical stain
indicated that aluminum was widely distributed throughout the brain.
Chromatin of all types of brain cells was fluorescent. In addition,
nuclei of capillary endothelial cells showed intense fluorescence,
although nuclei of cells of the choroid plexi did not fluoresce,
indicating that aluminum crossed the blood-brain barrier rather than
the blood cerebro-spinal fluid barrier. Brain aluminum content
measured by atomic absorption spectroscopy was elevated 5 to 10 times
above control levels in all regions sampled; however, concentrations
in cerebral spinal fluid were normal, again supporting the assumption
that aluminum entered the brain via the vascular route. Furthermore,
following subcutaneous administration, aluminum accumulated upon
nuclear chromatin, the locus identical to that found after direct
brain injection of aluminum in experimental animals (De Boni et al.,
1974). These results are in agreement with the report by Liss et al.,
(1975) in which permeability of the blood brain barrier to oral
administered aluminum was demonstrated in newborn rabbits. Aluminum

chloride was fed to pregnant rabbits and resulted in increased concentrations in milk, deposition of aluminum in brain of suckling rabbits and neurofibrillary degeneration.

Specific plasma carriers for aluminum have not been described, however, a spectrum of molecules with different stability constants for aluminum may be postulated. At high systemic loads, aluminum may saturate these carriers and may gain access to the central nervous system by shifting to plasma vectors which normally cross the blood-brain barrier.

In summary, the observations indicate that the neurofibrillary tangle of Alzheimer disease may be composed of a fibrinous protein of near normal composition, although present in excessive amounts in some neurons. It is unclear whether the subunits of this protein are related to normal neurofilaments.

In brain of experimental animals aluminum stimulates the synthesis of a fibrinous protein although the exact relation of this protein to other cell constituents is unknown. Experimentally, aluminum binds to the acidic nuclear protein-DNA complex and in man, aluminum is found on the identical intracellular locus. Furthermore, there is a marked increase in the amount of aluminum on chromatin of patients with Alzheimer disease. The close association of aluminum occurring at concentrations of up to one aluminum atom for every three base pairs on DNA in Alzheimer disease (Crapper et al., 1976) suggests that a mode of action of aluminum neurotoxicity might be the result of changes in the conformation of transcriptionally active components within the cell nucleus. However, at this time, aluminum effects upon translation processes have not been excluded. The known actions of aluminum on brain cells of susceptible mammalian species cannot explain all the histopathological manifestations of Alzheimer disease. Nevertheless, the increased concentration of this element associated with information carrying molecules in brain cells of patients presenting with Alzheimer disease certainly forces a detailed evaluation of the mechanisms of action of this element in selected biological systems.

Acknowledgements: This work was supported by the Ontario Mental Health Foundation.

REFERENCES

Alfrey, A.C., LeGendre, G.R. and Kaehny, W.D. The dialysis encephalopathy syndrome. Possible aluminum intoxication. New Eng. J. Med. 294:184-188, 1976.

Bevelander, G. and Ramaley, J.A. In: Essentials of Histology,
    Seventh Edition, Mosby, St. Louis, 1974.

Brattgard, S.O., Edstroem, J.E. and Hyden, H. The Chemical Changes
    in regenerating Neurons. J. Neurochem. 1:316-325, 1957.

Bruce, M.E. and Fraser, H. Amyloid plaques in the brains of mice
    infected with scrapie: morphological variation and staining
    properties. Neuropathol. and Appl. Neurobiol. 1:189-202, 1975.

Crapper, D.R., Quittkat, S., Krishnan, S.S. and DeBoni, U. Chromatin
    binding of aluminum in Alzheimer disease. Manuscript submitted
    elsewhere, 1977.

Crapper, D.R., Krishnan, S.S. and Quittkat, S. Aluminum, neurofib-
    rillary degeneration and Alzheimer disease. Brain 99:67-79, 1976a.

Crapper, D.R. Functional consequences of neurofibrillary degeneration.
    In: Neurobiology of Aging (Aging, Vol. 3), (Eds. Gershon, S. and
    Terry, R.D.), Raven Press, N.Y., 1976.

Crapper, D.R. Dementia: Recent observations on Alzheimer's disease
    and experimental aluminum encephalopathy. In: Frontiers in
    Neurol. and Neuro. Sci. Research, (Eds. P. Seeman and G.M. Brown),
    University of Toronto Press, Toronto, pp. 97-111, 1974.

Crapper, D.R., Krishnan, S.S. and Dalton, A.J. Brain aluminum dis-
    tribution in Alzheimer's disease and experimental neurofibrillary
    degeneration. Science 180:511-513, 1973.

Crapper, D.R. and Dalton, A.J. Alterations in short term retention,
    conditioned avoidance response acquisition and motivation follow-
    ing aluminum induced neurofibrillary degeneration. Physiol.
    Behav. 10:925-933, 1973a.

Crapper, D.R. and Dalton, A.J. Aluminum induced neurofibrillary
    degeneration, brain electrical activity and alterations in
    acquisition and retention. Physiol. Behav. 10:935-945, 1973b.

Dayan, A.D. and Ball, M.H. Histometric observations on the metabolism
    of tangle bearing neurons. J. Neurol. Sci. 19:433-436, 1973.

DeBoni, U., Seger, M., Scott, J.W. and Crapper, D.R. Neuron culture
    from adult goldfish. J. Neurobiol. 7:495-512, 1976.

DeBoni, U., Otvos, A., Scott, J.W. and Crapper, D.R. Neurofibrillary
    degeneration induced by systemic aluminum. Acta neuropath. (Berl),
    35:285-294, 1976a.

DeBoni, U., Scott, J.W. and Crapper, D.R. Intracellular Aluminum
    Binding; A Histochemical Study. Histochem. 40:31-37, 1974.

Embree, L.J., Hamberger, A. and Sjostrand, J. Qualitative cytochem-
    ical studies and histochemistry in experimental neurofibrillary
    degeneration. J. Neuropath. Exp. Neurol. 26:427-436, 1967.

Exss, E. and Summer, G.K. Basic proteins in neurons containing
    fibrillary deposits. Brain Research 49:151-164, 1973.

Hyden, H. In: The Cell., (Eds. J. Brachet and A.E. Minsky),
    Academic Press, New York, 4:216-324, 1960.

Iqbal, K., Wisniewski, H.M., Grundke-Iqbal, I., Korthals, J.K. and
    Terry, R.D. Neurofibrillary tangles of Alzheimer's presenile-
    senile dementia. J. Histochem. Cytochem. 23:563-569, 1975.

Iqbal, K., Wisniewski, H.M., Shelansky, M.L., Brostoff, S., Liwnicz,
    B.H. and Terry, R.D. Protein changes in senile dementia. Brain
    Research 77:337-343, 1974.

Kidd, M. Alzheimer's disease - An electron microscopy study. Brain.
    87:307-318, 1964.

King, G.A., DeBoni, U. and Crapper, D.R. Effect of aluminum upon
    conditioned avoidance response acquisition in the absence of
    neurofibrillary degeneration. Pharmacol. Biochem. and Behav.
    3:1003-1009, 1975.

Klatzo, I., Wisniewski, H. and Streicher, E. Experimental production
    of neurofibrillary degeneration. J. Neuropath. Exp. Neurol. 24:
    184-199, 1965.

Krishnan, S.S., Quittkat, S. and Crapper, D.R. Atomic absorption
    analysis for traces of aluminum and vanadium in biological tissue.
    A critical evaluation of the graphite furnace atomizer. Can. J.
    Spectroscopy 21:25-30, 1976.

Levy, R., Levy, S., Rosenberg, A. et al. Selective stimulation of
    non-histone chromatin protein synthesis in lymphoid cells by
    phytohemagglutinin. Biochem. 12:224-228, 1973.

Liss, L., Ebner, K., Couri, D. and Cho, N. Alzheimer disease. A
    possible animal model. Abstract: IV Panamerican Congress of
    Neurology, Mexico, 1975.

Miller, C.A. and Levine, E.M. Effect of aluminum gels on cultured
    neuroblastoma cells. J. Neurochem. 22:751-758, 1974.

Tischner, K.H. and Schroder, J.M. The effects of cadmium chloride on organotype cultures of rat sensory ganglia. A light and electronmicroscopy study. J. Neurol. Sci. 16:383–399, 1972.

Watson, W.E. Observations on the nucleolar and total cell-body nucleic acid of injured nerve cells. Physiol. (London) 196:655–676, 1968.

Wisniewski, H.M., Terry, R.D. and Hirano, A. Neurofibrillary Pathology. J. Neuropath. Expt. Neurol. 29:163–176, 1970.

Wisniewski, H.M., Narkiewicz, O. and Wisniewska. Topography and dynamics of neurofibrillary degeneration in aluminum encephalopathy. Acta Neuropath. 9:127–133, 1967.

Wisniewski, H.M., Bruce, M.E. and Fraser, H. Infectious etiology of neuritic (senile) plaques in mice. Science 190:1108–1110, 1975.

Wisniewski, H.M., Narang, H.K. and Terry, R.D. Neurofibrillary tangles of paired helical filaments. J. Neurol. Sci. 27:173–181, 1976.

Yashmineh, W.G. and Yunis, J.J. Localization of mouse satellite DNA in constitutive heterochromatin. Exp. Cell Res. 59:69–75, 1970.

THE FIBROUS PROTEINS OF BRAIN: A Primer for Gerontologists

Dennis J. Selkoe and Michael L. Shelanski

Department of Neuropathology, Harvard Medical School
and Department of Neuroscience, Children's Hospital
Medical Center, Boston, MA. 02115

INTRODUCTION

The morphological hallmarks of the Alzheimer type of presenile dementia and of a major portion of the senile dementias are neurofibrillary tangles and senile plaques. The latter structures are composed of degenerating neuritic processes within a core of congophilic material, presumably amyloid (Terry and Wisniewski, 1970). Neurofibrillary tangles were originally appreciated as fine, argentophilic fibrils in the light microscope. While the neuron normally contains some such fibrils, they are greatly increased in numbers and in thickness in Alzheimer's disease and senile dementia. Electronmicroscopic studies (Kidd, 1963; Terry, 1963) showed quite clearly that these fibrils were composed of linear structures which twisted every 80 nm and had a diameter at these nodes of 9nm and a maximum diameter between the nodes of almost 20 nm. The bulk of morphological evidence points to this pattern being due to a helical twisting of filaments around each other. These structures have been seen only in the human, only in brain and in the brain only within neurons. Nonetheless, the morphology of these twisted filaments combined with the general attention now being received by the normally occurring fibrillary elements of the brain has led to a curiosity about what relationship, if any, exists between the pathological structures and the normal microtubules, neurofilaments and microfilaments of the nervous system. Some aspects of this question will be addressed by Dr. Iqbal later in this symposium.

The task we have chosen is to present to our audience today a primary lesson in the biology and chemistry of the filaments and tubules of brain. These structures have become known, for the most

247

part, since most of us here have finished our studies and the bulk
of the research on them has been published in the basic rather than
the clinical literature. Being aware of the burden facing gerontologists in digesting vast areas of biological, immunological, clinical
and sociological studies germane to their field, we will limit our-
selves to the central themes and questions in this field, making
little effort to delve into the gray areas and numerous unresolved
controversies. It is hoped that this "primer" will aid you in
obtaining a deeper understanding of biochemical research on senile
dementia as it evolves and foster the healthy skepticism which spurs
scientific progress.

Morphological Observations: Light Microscopy

The recent interest in the fibrillar organelles of neurons and
other cells has grown out of electronmicroscopy and the discipline
of cell biology. However, light microscopists, especially those of
the latter nineteenth and early twentieth centuries obtained data
which foreshadowed much of the current work. Remak reported the
existence of neurofibrils in 1847 and the introduction of silver stain
methods, especially the Bielschowsky technique, showed fine neurofibrils as a normal constituent of nerve cells. Later, many neuro-
cytologists felt that neurons were held together in a continuum by
their neurofibrils, though this view lost ground rapidly following
the work of Cajal and the neuron doctrine.

Other anatomical workers were aware that motile flagella have
between 9 and 11 thin fibrils making up their structure, a fact that
was rediscovered only in the past two decades when electron microscopic studies revealed the ciliary and flagellar axoneme to be made
up of nine longitudinal pairs of microtubules forming a circle, plus
two central, unpaired, microtubules (Warner, 1972). In another area,
phase microscopic and birefringence studies of the mitotic spindle
of eukaryotic cells showed that the chromosomes were attached to
a network of fine fibers, the spindle fibres, and that the antimitotic drug colchicine caused a loss of spindle birefringence
(Nicklas, 1971).

What was lacking from these early studies was an ability to
resolve the fibrillar structures directly. Great reliance was placed
on optical tricks and complex staining reactions. Much was made of
the differences in the reactions of filaments to various stains,
but since the actual chemical mechanisms of most coloration methods
were poorly understood, they did little to resolve biological questions. The stage was thus set for an ultrastructural approach and
the application of the techniques of cell biology and biochemistry
to the study of these structures.

Electronmicroscopy

The early years of biological electronmicroscopy were marked by trial and error in methods of preservation and presentation of the specimen. No clear standards existed and many artifactual elements were introduced. However, by the early 1960's most of these problems had been overcome and a more or less standard approach to biological electronmicroscopy evolved. In broad outline, this involves fixation of the tissue in glutaraldehyde, post-fixation in osmium tetroxide, dehydration in graded alcohols and embedding in plastics such as epoxy or methacrylate. The embedded sample is then cut on a precision microtome with either a glass or diamond knife. The optical resolution possible on sectioned biological material is routinely better than 2.5 nm with these techniques and we are therefore able to distinguish many elements which were invisible or only poorly resolved with the light microscope. This added resolving power led very quickly to the discovery that normal cells had at least three types of filamentous structures in them. These were the microtubule (referred to as neurotubule when found in brain), the 10 nm intermediate filament and the 6 nm thin filament. In the sections below, we will concisely describe the major properties of each of these systems and then in the final section we shall relate these facts to what little is known about neuronal filaments in aging and dementia.

Microtubules

Among the fibrous organelles, these structures have received the greatest attention to date and their biochemistry is better understood than that of the other two filaments. Microtubules are long cylindrical organelles of 24 nm diameter with an apparently patent lumen and a 6 nm wall made up of globular subunits arranged as 13 longitudinal protofilaments (Olmsted and Borisy, 1973). They can be up to several microns in length. They are ubiquitous in known eukaryotic cells but found in particularly high concentration in neurons. In the latter cells, they are seen both in the peri-karyon and in the processes. In addition, microtubules make up the spindle fibers of the mitotic apparatus and, as mentioned earlier, are the major structural elements of cilia and flagella. In these motile processes, small "side arms" can be seen on one of each of the tubule pairs and these "arms" are composed of an ATPase called dynein (Gibbons and Rowe, 1965) which is critical for flagellar motion. It is presumed that ciliary and flagellar motility is due to a translation of the tubule pairs with respect to one another by a mechanism which involves movement of the dynein arms (Summers and Gibbons, 1973). The defect in ciliary motility in the Cartegener syndrome is very likely due to an abnormality of the arms, with either an absence or deficiency of the dynein.

Biochemically, microtubules are actually long polymers of a
protein subunit which has been given the name tubulin. Tubulin is
a dimeric molecule with a molecular weight of 110,000 daltons and
a sedimentation coefficient of 6S (Shelanski and Taylor, 1967).
The tubulin dimer is in turn composed of two non-identical monomers
with approximate molecular weights of 55,000 (α-tubulin) and 53,000
(β-tubulin) (Bryan, 1974). Isolated tubulin invariably is found to
have guanine nucleotides bound to it (Weisenberg et al., 1968).
This binding of quanosine 5'diphosphate (GDP) and triphosphate (GTP)
appears to have great importance in the polymerization of tubulin
subunits into microtubules. Following extensive studies in a number
of laboratories, the in vitro polymerization of tubulin was achieved
by Weisenberg in 1972 by keeping the concentration of calcium ions
in the assembly millieu at a low level and supplying exogenous
nucleotide. It is now apparent that the formation of microtubules
from tubulin dimers is remarkably sensitive to a variety of physico-
chemical variables, including pH, ionic strength and temperature.
For example, the warming of a cold solution of tubulin subunits to
room temperature or above in the presence of GTP will allow their
polymerization into ultrastructurally "normal" appearing microtubules.
Cooling the sample to 4°C will result in an equally rapid disassembly into tubulin dimers.

The precise mechanism of such microtubule assembly has been the
subject of much debate. Kinetic studies of the polymerization
reaction have concluded that the assembly of subunits into microtubules involves two distinct steps: initiation of the polymeric
chain and propagation thereof. The finding of a critical concentration (C_c) of tubulin subunits (Gaskin et al., 1974), below which
no polymerization will occur, has been documented by both light-
scattering techniques and viscosity experiments. The occurrence of
a C_c has been interpreted to be the result of a slow or thermo-
dynamically unfavored initiation process in which addition of the
first few tubulin molecules is more difficult than further addition
of subunits. Electronmicroscopic studies have also provided evidence
that microtubule assembly in brain extracts may proceed by a self-
nucleation mechanism. Such studies have documented the presence of
disc or ring-shaped structures composed of microtubule protein that
appear to serve as nucleation centers for tubulin assembly (Borisy
and Olmsted, 1972). The importance of nucleotide binding and
hydrolysis during tubulin assembly has also been recognized, but the
details of this processes are still a matter of controversy.

An important factor in the biochemical study of microtubules
has been their affinity for a number of widely used pharmacological
agents. Foremost among these is colchicine, which binds to tubulin
at a ratio of one mole of tubulin per mole of tubulin dimer. It was
the specific affinity of colchicine for microtubule subunits which
allowed the original isolation and subsequent characterization of

this protein, hence its discriptive name "colchicine-binding protein". Another antimitotic agent, vinblastine, also induces the breakdown of microtubules into subunits by binding to the tubulin molecule at a different site than colchicine does (Marantz and Shelanski, 1970; Owellen et al., 1972). Additional binding sites in tubulin for podophyllotoxin and other mitotic spindle inhibitors, and for cations like calcium have either been demonstrated or postulated (Olmsted and Borisy, 1973). Such sites may have import for both the proper assembly and the function of microtubules.

Although the precise intracellular functioning of the microtubules remains unclear, these organelles have been implicated in the following processes: cellular motility; transport; axoplasmic flow; secretion; chromosome movements in cell division; and determination and maintainance of cell shape (Olmsted and Borisy, 1973).

Neurofilaments

Intracellular filaments of intermediate diameter, ranging from 8 to 11 nm in width have long been recognized by the electron-microscopist but have received considerably less attention from the biochemist, who has concentrated his efforts on the thin filaments and the microtubules. Morphologically, intermediate filaments are defined as long cytoplasmic rods of approximately 10 nm diameter with no apparent lumen and often small projections from their sides ("arms"). When filaments of this type are found in neurons they are called neurofilaments; when seen in astroglia, they have been called glial filaments. Neuropathologists and neuroanatomists have contended that these two filaments are of different morphology and have pointed out their differential histochemical staining. Workers in other fields have referred to similar structures as tonofilaments or 10 nm filaments. Very recently, evidence has accumulated that intermediate filaments may, like the thin filaments and microtubules, be the same or similar from species to species. It is still far from certain that intermediate filaments (IF) are as highly conserved in evolution as are microtubules, nor is it clear that within a single mammalian species all the intermediate filaments are biochemically identical. However, the weight of recent evidence from our laboratory and others points strongly to a marked similarity if not identity of neuronal and glial filaments.

Early ultrastructural studies of brain demonstrated large numbers of intraneuronal 10 nm filaments usually distributed randomly throughout the cytoplasm, as well as tightly packed bundles of filaments of similar diameter in astrocytes. The presence of highly similar but presumably non-identical filaments in those two cell types (Wuerker, 1970) posed serious problems for the biochemist

who wished to isolate and characterize these organelles. It was
necessary to develop a method that would give filaments exclusively
from one source or the other. An intriguing solution to this problem has been the use of the NF-rich myelinated axons of cerebral
white matter as a starting material. Purification of such axons
has been accomplished by homogenization followed by flotation of
the axons, whose myelin acts as a "life-vest" in aqueous media,
away from cell bodies and organelles (DeVries and Norton, 1972).
The axons can then be denuded of myelin and purified by gradient
centrifugation.

Biochemical studies of this presumably neuronal filamentous
material have shown that the neurofilament is markedly different
than the microtubule. To begin with, neurofilament is highly
insoluble in aqueous media of various ionic strengths compared to
the readily disassembled microtubules. Solubilization can be
achieved in urea, guanidine or detergents such as SDS (Shelanski
et al., 1971). If dissolved filaments are then run on protein
separating gels, the major subunit constituent has a molecular
weight of approximately 53,000 (Shelanski et al., 1971; Davison
and Winslow, 1974).

The presumptive subunit of filament in glial cells has also
been isolated recently. In contradistinction to neurofilament (NF)
the glial filament protein is quite soluble in part, and appears
to exist in both soluble and particulate forms, the former of which
makes up at least 50% of the glial fibrillary protein. Originally,
the glial protein was isolated from highly gliotic areas in the
plaques of multiple sclerosis patients (Eng et al., 1971). Antisera
prepared against this protein give apparently specific glial
staining by indirect immunofluorescence methods (Bignami et al.,
1973), and the protein has therefore been termed the glial fibrillary
acidic protein (GFA). Its molecular weight in polyacrylamide gel
electrophoresis is approximately 54,000 (Dahl, 1976).

A major effort of this laboratory in recent months has been a
comparison of the presumptive NF and GFA proteins (Yen et al., 1975).
Bovine and neuronal filament proteins have been found to electro-
phorese with similar mobilities on urea SDS gels. Bovine GFA
migrates with the tubulin bands and the neurofilament protein migrates
slightly ahead of them. Comparative tryptic peptide maps of the two
proteins are highly similar but not identical (Yet et al., 1975).
Immunological comparison of the GFA and NF proteins by reacting
them against their respective antisera prepared in rabbit or guinea
pig reveals a reaction of identity on Ouchterlony immunodiffusion
plates (Yet et al., 1975). These antisera are now being used in
immunohistological studies using immunofluorescence and immunoperoxidase techniques to differentially localize neurofilaments
and glial filaments in normal and pathological states.

In summary, available biochemical and immunologic data on the intermediate filaments from brain suggest a high degree of similarity although not identity between these protein organelles in neurons and glia, as well as their distinction from neuronal microtubules and microfilaments.

Recent experiments in our laboratory on cultured aortic endothelial cells from the guinea pig lend support to the idea that the intermediate filaments are similar in diverse organs. These cells have a perinuclear ring of 100 $\overset{o}{A}$ filaments which reorganizes into a perinuclear cap in response to treatment with colcemid (Blose and Chacko, 1976). The antibody prepared against the axonal neurofilament will stain this ring and this staining is not lost during or after the reorganization suggesting that the antibody binding is not only specific to the filaments but also unaffected by colcemid (Blose et al., In press).

Similar immunofluorescent studies on the bundles of filaments induced in cultured chick cardiac muscle cells by colchicine or colcemid (Croop and Holtzer, 1975) and which are similar to the filaments seen in vincristine intoxication (Shelanski and Wisniewski, 1969) show strong staining of the bundles which is not blocked by the addition of either actin or tubulin, but is very strongly absorbed by the addition of neurofilaments or of their subunit protein. Thus these results would suggest that the intermediate filament protein of brain and nerve is a highly conserved protein, similar to other such systems in its evolutionary stability.

Microfilaments

The third class of neuronal fibrillar organelles, microfilaments, has only recently received much attention. These are the thinnest of the fibrous structures under consideration, averaging 5-6 nm in diameter. They are found in highest concentration in the growing tip, or growth cone, of the axon in the embryonic neuroblast or in cultured nerve cells (Yet et al., 1975; Tennyson, 1970; Yamada et al., 1971). Because of their prominence in the growth cone, a motile role for the microfilaments was proposed. It has now been shown biochemically that these thin filaments are in fact composed of actin (Puszkin, 1968; Fine and Blitz, 1974). As would be expected, the microfilaments can combine with heavy meromyosin or with subfragment 1 of the myosin molecule (Ishikawa et al., 1969). No role for these filaments in cellular aging or any disease state has yet been proposed and we will not consider them further here.

The Neurofilament in Disease

In the past several years, an increasing number of neurological disorders have been shown to be characterized by striking accumulations of normal or abnormal neuronal fibrous proteins. In virtually all of these conditions, the fibrillary structures which accumulate most closely resemble the neurofilament. Indeed, no neurologic disorder has yet been associated with a specific alteration of microtubules or microfilaments. Clinically, the most important diseases in this category are the late-life dementias, which are marked by the accumulation of abnormal filament-containing structures generally referred to as "twisted tubules". These disorders will be considered in detail in the following section. In this section, we wish to call attention to the numerous human and experimental states which are marked by axonal and perikaryal accumulation of masses of apparently normal neurofilaments.

Various recent ultrastructural studies have shown us that an increase in 9-10 nm filaments can be seen in spontaneously occurring and hereditary disease states, in response to axonal injury, and in a variety of exogenous intoxications. The most common examples of neurofilamentous proliferation in human disease are sporadic motor neuron disease (Schochet et al., 1969) and infantile neuroaxonal dystrophy (Martin and Martin, 1972). Hypertrophy of the inferior olive in man has been associated histopathologically with an increase in NF. In experimental axonal injury, marked neurofilamentous accumulation has been observed in the red nucleus after sectioning the tecto-spinal tract (Barron et al., 1975). These reactions to injury do not occur at once but rather develop over a period of days to weeks.

The toxins which lead to an increase in neurofilaments are a heterogeneous group, of which only the mitotic spindle inhibitor are felt to show an obvious site of action. Colchicine, vinblastine and podophyllotoxin, all of which were mentioned earlier as capable of binding to and precipitating microtubules in vitro, can cause striking perikaryal masses of NF in anterior horn cells if injected intracisternally (Wisniewski et al., 1968). Similar neurofilamentous proliferation can be induced by the lathyrogenic agent and its analog, B-B'-iminodiproprionitrile (IDPN) (Chou and Hartmann, 1965).

In man, a growing list of industrial and commercial toxins has been associated with profound peripheral neuropathies that are marked pathologically by axonal bundles of apparently normal NF. Examples are acrylamide intoxication (Prineas, 1969) and "glue-sniffing" neuropathy, the latter caused by inhalation of the aliphatic solvent n-hexane (Asbury et al., 1974). Most recently, 86 workers in a fabric printing plant in Ohio came down with a sensorimotor neuropathy found to be due to a purchasing agent's substitution of methyl n-butyl ketone (MBK) for methyl isobutyl ketone (MIBK) in the plant's standard organic solvent mixture (Mendell et al., 1974). In both MBK and n-hexane neuropathies, distal peripheral nerves have shown ballooned focally swollen axons stuffed with 10 nm filaments (Spencer et al., 1975). An additional dimension to the interest in these disorders has been provided by the discovery of Asbury et al. (1972) of a genetically determined progressive neuropathy of childhood marked by a neurofilamentous proliferation indistinguishable from that of n-hexane and MBK neuropathies.

The mechanism whereby any of these agents might induce the aggregation of neuronal filaments remains entirely obscure. In the case of colchine and the other antimitotics, for example, the proliferation occurs to a significant extent even in the presence of almost complete inhibition of protein synthesis by cycloheximide. Furthermore, the removal of the drugs results in a gradual disappearance of the filaments and the reappearance of the microtubules in the neuron (Wisniewski et al., 1968). These findings, as well as observations on the relationship of tubules and filaments during neural development (Peters and Vaughn, 1967), have led to the suggestion that the filaments and tubules might actually represent polymorphic assembly forms of the same tubulin subunits. However, other filament-inducing agents such as n-hexane and MBK do not show any direct effect on microtubules in cells and we have found that these chemicals and their derivitives do not affect the in vitro ability of tubulin to assemble into microtubules (Selkoe et al., in preparation). These results suggest that the induction of filamentous proliferation by these toxins is independent of their effect on microtubules.

Among the neurotoxins which can cause neurofibrillary pathology, aluminum has aroused the greatest interest, both in experimental and clinical circles (Editorial, 1976; Selkoe, 1976). Remarkably, the neurotoxicity of aluminum was first established in 1897, when, for reasons known only to himself, a German worker, Dolken, injected aluminum tartrate into rabbits and found that they came down with a neuronal degeneration in different parts of the brain (Dolken, 1897). During the 1930's and 1940's, aluminum paste began to be injected intracortically to produce experimental epileptogenic foci (Kopeloff et al., 1942). In 1965, Klatzo et al. first studied the ultrastructure of aluminum lesions in cortex and discovered that they contained intraneuronal bundles of 10 nm neurofilaments which showed argophyillic staining and bore a striking light microscopic resemblance to neurofibrillary tangles. A major ultrastructural difference was the fact that the aluminum-induced filaments did not contain the periodic twists that are the hallmark of the so-called twisted tubule (Terry and Pena, 1965).

When aluminum salts are injected into brain or subarachnoid space, the animals maintain an asymptomatic interval of 10-15 days,

after which a rapidly progressive encephalomyelopathy ensues, marked
by seizures and quadriparesis and leading to death from status
epilepticus or inanition in a few days. Crapper et al. (1973)
studied the early course of the intoxication, when the animals were
overtly asymptomatic, and found: (1) their performance on a task
requiring retention of new information (short-term memory) progressively declined, and (2) the level of performance was linearly correlated
with cortical aluminum levels.

Moving from experimental to human pathology, Crapper et al.
(1973) assayed aluminum in the biopsied and autopsied cortex of
4 patients with verified Alzheimer's Disease and found levels 3-4
times that of control cortex in some areas. The highest levels
were noted in mesial frontal and temporal cortex. A later study by
the same group extended these observations to 12 demented patients,
including 2 with Down's Syndrome and Alzheimer's Disease, and again
found significantly elevated aluminum levels in an average of 28%
of the cortical samples from each of the 12 brains (Crapper et al.,
1976). The distribution of cortical aluminum levels closely matched
the topographic distribution of NFT's while it did not seem to
correlate with the presence of senile plaques. The source of the
aluminum and its possible etiologic relevance to the dementia remain
entirely obscure. Although these results are clearly preliminary,
they are given additional credence by the report this year (Alfrey
et al., 1976) of elevated cortical aluminum levels in 12 patients
with chronic renal failure who developed the syndrome of dialysis
dementia. These patients had been taking high doses of aluminum-
containing antacids daily for longer than 3 years.

Our laboratory is presently engaged in efforts to characterize
the aluminum-induced filament biochemically and compare it to the
abnormal fibrillary structures of Alzheimer's Disease.

"Twisted Filaments" in Aging and Dementia

We shall conclude this primer on the biology of the tubules
and filaments of brain by discussing the aspect of the subject which
is of greatest interest to gerontologists. We speak, of course,
about the bizarre intraneuronal organelles which were originally
called twisted tubules but are now increasingly referred to as
"paired helical filaments" or simply "twisted filaments". As mentioned
earlier, these structures appear only in humans and only in the
brain. The fibrillary changes occasionally demonstrated in extremely
old dogs and monkeys are of quite different morphology (Wisniewski
et al., 1973).

The twisted filaments are the most widespread and specific
ultrastructural finding in Alzheimer's Disease, a term which is now

accepted to include both presenile and senile varieties. These
abnormal cytoplasmic organelles have a smaller maximum diameter
(19 nm) than normal microtubules and appear to have regular con-
strictions or "twists" where their girth decreases to just 9 nm.
There has been debate in the past as to whether this structure was
actually a twisting tube or a pair of hellically wound filaments.
Morphological data (Kidd, 1963) now strongly favor the latter
hypothesis, revealing two filaments, each 7-8 nm in diameter, arranged
in a helix with a periodicity of 80 nm. On a light microscopic level,
they comprise the neurofibrillary tangle which is found in the
perikaryon of neurons in certain predilection areas, particularly
the hippocampal formation and the mesial-frontal cortex. The
abnormal filaments are also found in the neuropil where they exist
inside the tangled neuronal processes which make up the senile
plaque.

In addition to Alzheimer's Disease, twisted filaments have been
found in Guam Parkinson - Dementia complex (Hirano, 1970) and
postcephalitic Parkinsonism. Of particular interest is their widespread presence in the brains of older patients with Down's Syndrome.
It has been apparent for many years (Jervis, 1948) that Down's patients
often develop a neurofibrillary degeneration after the age of 40,
and recent electron microscopic studies have demonstrated its
morphological identity with Alzheimer's Disease (Ellis et al., 1974).
Crapper and his colleagues have shown that the clinical development
of superimposed "presenile" dementia can be appreciated in these
retarded adults if carefully looked for (Crapper et al., 1975).
These findings have lead to the hypothesis (Elam and Blumenthal,
1971) that neurofibrillary degeneration may be a manifestation of
accelerated cellular aging, as seen in other organs of the progeric-
like mongols.

The potential relevance of these unusual organelles to the
process of normal neuronal aging is emphasized by the work of Matsuyama
et al. (1966). These authors found a remarkably high incidence of
neurofibrillary tangles in the temporal cortex of supposedly non-
demented older individuals. In their series, 4% of patients between
ages 50 and 59 showed greater than 50 such affected neurons per
section. This percentage rose to 23% in the seventh decade, 53% in
the eighth, and 72% in the ninth. Neuritic (senile) plaques were
also present in many patients, although not as commonly as were the
tangles. In the case of demented individuals, quantitative studies
(Tomlinson et al., 1970) have recently demonstrated a correlation between the number and distribution of both these lesions and the degree
of psychometric deficiency. These various findings underscore the
appropriateness of studying the biochemistry of these organelles as
an approach to understanding normal and pathological neuronal aging.

Very little is presently known about the molecular biology of the abnormal neurons in these conditions. An attempt to study the proteins of the neurofibrillary tangle in Alzheimer's Disease by isolating a brain fraction enriched in twisted filaments revealed that the major protein of this fraction had the same molecular weight as the normal neurofilament (Iqbal et al., 1974). Further studies by Iqbal and his associates showed that peptide maps of the enriched filament fraction were similar to those of the neurofilament (Iqbal et al., 1976). Although the authors originally felt that this data supported the notion that the abnormal structure is made up of paired normal neurofilaments, this work must now be re-examined in light of the recent results on biochemical similarity, if not identity, of the NF and the glial fibrillary acidic protein (GFA), the presumed subunit of glial filaments (Yen et al., 1975). Since the enriched protein in the TF cell fractions had the same molecular weight as the NF, it is probably the same as the GFA as well. Because the neuronal fractions used were taken from severely gliotic areas and because the TF were not purified to morphological homogeneity, it is possible that the protein the authors identified as the presumptive TF subunit is actually a GFA contaminant. Further progress in clarifying the relationship of abnormal and normal neurofilaments awaits purer filament preparations and the application of immunohistological techniques.

CONCLUSION

In these brief pages, we have attempted to present a glossary of the fibrous elements of brain, both anatomically and biochemically, and to point to their prospective roles in a variety of disease states but particularly in the human non-vascular dementias. As more knowledge of the chemistry and molecular pathology of the fibrous proteins accumulates this information may aid in understanding the rapid and malignant loss of intellectual function that so frequently accompanies aging, the pathogenesis of which is at present totally unexplained. Work in this area may prove to have relevance to the problem of intellectual deficit at the opposite end of the chronological scale that is, mental retardation. It may also shed light on the fundamental processes of neuronal aging at the macromolecular level.

REFERENCES

Alfrey, A.C., LeGendre, G.R., et al. The dialysis encephalopathy syndrome: possible aluminum intoxication. N. Eng. J. Med. 294: 184, 1976.

Asbury, A.K., Gale, M.K., et al. Giant axonal neuropathy. Acta Neuropathol. 20:237, 1972.

Asbury, A.K., Neilson, S.L., Tefler, R. Glue-sniffing neuropathy.
    J. Neuropath. Exp. Neurol. 33:191, 1974.

Barron, K.D., Dentinger, M.P., Nelson, L.R. and Mincy, J.E. Ultra-
    structure of axonal reaction in red nucleus of cat. J. Neuro-
    pathol. Exp. Neurol. 34:222, 1975.

Bignami, A., Eng, L.F., Dahl, D. and Uyeda, C.T. Localization of the
    glial fibrillary acidic protein in astrocytes by immunofluorescence.
    Brain Res. 43:429, 1973.

Blose, S.H. and Chacko, S. Rings of Intermediate (100 Å) Filaments
    in the Perinuclear Region of Vascular Endothelial Cells. J.
    Cell Biol. 70:459-466, 1976.

Blose, S.H., Shelanski, M.L. and Chacko, S. Localization of Antibody
    prepared against brain filaments to intermediate filaments in
    guinea pig vascular endothelial cells. Proc. Nat. Acad. Sci.,
    in press.

Borisy, G.G. and Olmsted, J.B. Nucleated assembly of microtubules in
    procine brain extracts. Science 177:1196, 1972.

Bryan, J. Biochemical properties of microtubules. Fed. Proc. Fed.
    Amer. Exp. Biol. 33:152, 1974.

Chou, S.M. and Hartmann, H.A. Electronmicroscopy of focal neuroaxonal
    lesions produced by iminodipropionitrile (IDPN) in rats. Acta
    Neuropathol. 4:590, 1965.

Crapper, D.R., Krishman, S.S., et al. Brain aluminum distribution in
    Alzheimer's Disease and experimental neurofibrillary degeneration.
    Science 180:511, 1973.

Crapper, D.R., Krishnan, S.S. and Quittkat, S. Aluminum, neuro-
    fibrillary degeneration and Alzheimer's Disease. Brain 99:67,
    1976.

Crapper, D.R., Skopitz, M., Scott, J.W. and Hachinski, V. Alzheimer
    degeneration in Down's syndrome: electrophysiological alterations
    and histopathology. Arch. Neur. 32:618-623, 1975.

Croop, J. and Holtzer, H. Response to myogenic and fibrogenic cells
    to cytochalasin B and to colcemide. I. Light microscopic observa-
    tion. J. Cell Biol. 65:271-285, 1975.

Dahl, D. Glial fibrillary acid protein from bovine and rat brain.
    Degradation in tissue and homogenates. Biochim. Biophys. Acta
    420:142, 1976.

Davison, P.F. and Winslow, B. The protein subunit of calf brain neurofilament. J. Neurobiol. 5:119, 1974.

DeVries, G.H. and Norton, W.T. Axons: Isolation from mammalian central nervous system. Science 175:1370, 1972.

Dollken, V. Uber die wirkung des aluminiums mit Berucksichtingung der aluminium verursachten Lasionen im CNS. Archiv. Exp. Path. Pharm. 40:98, 1897.

Editorial. Aluminum and Alzheimer. Lancet, June 12, 1976.

Elam, L.H. and Blumenthal, H.T. Aging in the mentally retarded. In: Interdisciplinary Topics in Gerontology, (Ed. H.T. Blumenthal), S. Karger, New York, Vol. 7, p. 87, 1971.

Ellis, W.G., McCulloch, J.R. and Corley, C.L. Presenile dementia in Down's syndrome. Neurology 24:101, 1974.

Eng, L.F., Vanderhaegen, J.J., Bignami, A. and Gerstl, B. An acidic protein isolated from fibrous astrocytes. Brain Res. 28:351, 1971.

Fine, A. and Blitz, A.L. Muscle-like contractile proteins and tubulin in synaptosomes. Proc. Nat. Acad. Sci. 71:4472, 1974.

Fine, R.E. and Bray, D. Actin in growing nerve cells. Nature (London) 234:115, 1971.

Gaskin, F., Cantor, C.R. and Shelanski, M.L. Turbidimetric studies of the in vitro assembly and dissembly of porcine neurotubules. J. Mol. Biol. 89:737, 1974.

Gibbons, I.R. and Rowe, A.J. Dynein: a protein with ATPase activity from cilia. Science 149:424, 1965.

Hirano, A. Guam-Parkinsonism Dementia. In: Ciba Foundation Symposium: Alzheimer disease and related conditions, (Eds. G.E.W. Wolstenholme and M. O'Connor), Churchill, London, p. 185, 1970.

Iqbal, K., Grundke-Iqbal, I., Wisniewski, H., Korthals, J.K. and Terry, R.D. Chemistry of the neurofibrous proteins in aging. In: Neurobiology of Aging, (Eds. R. D. Terry and S. Gershon), Raven Press, New York, 1976.

Iqbal, K., Wisniewski, H.M., Shelanski, M.L., Bostoff, S., Liwnicz, B.H. and Terry, R.D. Protein changes in senile dementia. Brain Res. 77:337, 1974.

Ishikawa, H., Bischoff, R. and Holtzer, H.   Formation of arrowhead
    complexes with heavy meromyosin in a variety of cell types.
    J. Cell Biol. 43:312, 1969.

Jervis, G.A.   Early senile dementia in mongoloid idiocy.   Am. J.
    Psych. 105:102, 1948.

Kidd, M.   Paired helical filaments in electron microscopy of Alzheimer's
    disease.   Nature 197:192, 1963.

Klatzo, I., Wisniewski, H. and Streicher, E.   Experimental production
    of neurofibrillary degeneration. I. Light microscopic observations.
    J. Neuropath. Exp. Neurol. 24:187, 1965.

Kopeloff, L.M., Barrera, S.E. and Kopeloff, N.   Recurrent convulsive
    seizures in animals produced by immunologie and chemical means.
    Am. J. Psych. 98:881, 1942.

Marantz, R. and Shelanski, M.L.   Structure of microtubular crystals
    induced by vinblastine in vitro.   J. Cell Biol. 44:234, 1970.

Martin, J.J. and Martin, L.   Infantile neuroaxonal dystrophy: Ultra-
    structural study of the peripheral nerves and of the motor end
    plates.   Eur. Neurol. 8:329, 1972.

Matsuyama, H., Namiki, H. and Watanabe, I.   Senile changes in the brain
    in the Japanese: Incidence of neurofibrillary change and senile
    plaques.   In: Proceedings of the 5th International Congress of
    Neuropathology, (Eds. F. Luthy and A. Bischoff), Amsterdam,
    Excerpta Medica, pp. 979-980, 1966.

Mendell, J.R., Saida et al.   Toxic polyneuropathy produced by methyl
    n-butyl ketone.   Science 185:787, 1974.

Nicklas, R.B.   Mitosis.   Advan. Cell. Biol. 2:225-98, 1971.

Olmsted, J.B. and Borisy, G.G.   Microtubules.   Ann. Rev. Biochem.
    42:507, 1973.

Owellen, R.J., Owens, A.H., Jr., Donigien, D.W.   The binding of
    vincristine, vinblastine and colchicine to tubulin.   Biochem.
    Biophys. Res. Commun. 47:685, 1972.

Peters, A. and Vaughn, J.E.   Microtubules and filaments in the axons
    and astrocytes of early post-natal rat optic nerves.   J. Cell.
    Biol. 32:113, 1967.

Prineas, J.   The pathogenesis of dying-back polyneuropathies. II:
    An ultrastructural study of experimental acrylamide intoxication
    in the cat. J. Neuropath. Exp. Neurol. 28:598, 1969.

Puszkin, S., Berl, S., Puszkin, E. and Clark, D.D. Actomyosin-like
    protein isolated from mammalian brain. Science 161:170, 1968.

Schochet, S.S., Jr., Hartman, J.M., Ladewig, P.P. and Earle, K.M.
    Intraneuronal conglomerages in sporadic motor neuron disease.
    Arch. Neurol. 20:548, 1969.

Selkoe, D.J. Aluminum intoxication. N. Eng. J. Med. (letter) 294:
    119, 1976.

Shelanski, M.L., Albert, S., DeVries, G.H. and Norton, W.T. Isolation
    of filaments from brain. Science 174:1242, 1971.

Shelanski, M.L. and Taylor, E.W. Isolation of a protein subunit from
    microtubules. J. Cell. Biol. 34:549, 1967.

Shelanski, M.L. and Wisniewski, H. Neurofibrillary Degeneration
    induced by vincristine therapy. Arch. Neurol. 20:199-206, 1969.

Spencer, P.S., Schoumberg, H.H., Raleigh, R. and Terhaar, C.J. Nervous
    system degeneration produced by the industrial solvent methyl
    n-butyl ketone. Arch. Neurol. 32:219, 1975.

Summers, K.E. and Gibbons, I.R. Effects of trypsin digestion of
    flagellan structures and their relationship to motility. J.
    Cell. Biol. 58:618, 1973.

Tennyson, V.M. The fine structure of the axon growth cone of the
    dorsal root neuroblast of the rabbit embryo. J. Cell. Biol.
    44:62, 1970.

Terry, R.D. The fine structure of neurofibrillary tangles in Alzheimer's
    disease. J. Neuropathol. Exp. Neurol. 22:629, 1963.

Terry, R.D. and Pena, C. Experimental production of neurofibrillary
    degeneration. 2. Electron microscopy, phosphate histochemistry and
    electron probe analysis. J. Neuropath. Exp. Neurol. 24:200, 1965.

Terry, R.D. and Wisniewski, H. The ultrastructure of the neuro-
    fibrillary tangle and senile plaque. In: Ciba Foundation
    Symposium: Alzheimer's disease and related conditions, (Eds.
    G.E.W. Wolstenholme and M. O'Connor), Churchill, London, p. 145,
    1970.

Tomlinson, B.E., Blessed, G. and Roth, M. Observations on the brains
    of demented old people. J. Neurol. Sci. 11:205, 1970.

Warner, F.D. Macromolecular Organization of Eukaryotic Cilia and
    Flagella. Advan. Cell. Mol. Biol. 2:193–235, 1972.

Weisenberg, R.C. Microtubule formation in vitro in solutions contain-
    ing low calcium concentrations. Science 117:1104, 1972.

Weisenberg, R.C., Borisy, G.G. and Taylor, E.W. The colchicine-
    binding protein of mammalian brain and its relation to micro-
    tubules. Biochemistry 7:4466, 1968.

Wisniewski, H.M., Ghetti, B. and Terry, A.D. Neuritic (senile)
    plaques and filamentous changes in aged rhesus monkey. J.
    Neuropath. Exp. Neurol. 32:566, 1973.

Wisniewski, H., Shelanski, M.L. and Terry, R.D. Effects of mitotic
    spindle inhibitor on neurotubules and neurofilaments in anterior
    horn cells. J. Cell. Biol. 38:224, 1968.

Wuerker, R. Neurofilaments and glial filaments. Tissue and Cell.
    2:1, 1970.

Yamada, K.M., Spooner, B.S., Wessels, N.K. Ultrastructure and function
    of growth cones and axons of cultured nerve cells. J. Cell. Biol.
    49:614, 1971.

Yen, S.H., Dahl, D., Schachner, M. and Shelanski, M.L. Biochemistry
    of filaments of brain. Proc. Nat. Acad. Sci. 73:529, 1975.

CEREBRAL CIRCULATORY AND ELECTROENCEPHALOGRAPHIC CHANGES IN AGING

AND DEMENTIA

Walter D. Obrist

Department of Neurosurgery
University of Pennsylvania
Philadelphia, PA

A full understanding of senescent behavioral changes requires
information from in vivo physiologic studies, including both the
electroencephalogram (EEG) and cerebral blood flow (CBF). The
purpose of the present paper is to review some of the recent
findings on cerebral physiology in the dementias of old age. Earlier
EEG and CBF findings have been extensively reviewed elsewhere
(Obrist 1972; Obrist 1975) and will only be summarized here.

The electroencephalogram and cerebral blood flow undergo changes
associated with age, but the magnitude of these changes is primarily
a function of health status. Thus, both variables deviate minimally
from young adult standards in healthy individuals over age 60. On
the other hand, elderly subjects with various physical and mental
disorders, particularly those with diseases of the cardiovascular
system and/or signs of organic dementia, undergo more pronounced
alterations of their EEG and CBF. The EEG changes consist of a
slowing of the dominate alpha rhythm from 10 to 9 or 8 cps, and an
increase in the prevalence of slower theta (4-7 cps) and delta
(1-3 cps) waves. These findings correlate well with the severity
of intellectual deterioration. Although the slowing is usually
diffuse, there is a predilection for the temporal lobe to become
more involved.

CBF changes in vascular disease and dementia consist of a
generalized reduction in blood flow associated with increased
cerebral vascular resistance. Because there is a concomitant decrease in cerebral metabolic rate for oxygen, the question arises
whether the blood flow reductions are responsible for the alterations
in metabolism, or whether the lower blood flow is simply an

265

autoregulatory response to the lesser metabolic demands of the tissue. Although CBF reductions may produce metabolic changes in the early acute stages of vascular disease, decreased metabolic demand is more likely to be the primary variable in cases with extensive neuronal degeneration.

In contrast to earlier studies that measured global CBF by the Kety-Schmidt technique, the newer radioisotope methods make it possible to estimate blood flow in specific brain regions. While confirming a generalized blood flow reduction in senile dementia and its correlation with the degree of mental impairment, Obrist et al. (1970) obtained significantly greater CBF decreases in the temporal and prefrontal areas where EEG abnormalities were maximal. This focal decrease has also been observed by Ingvar and Gustafson (1970) and by Simard and co-workers (1971). It is consistent with the greater atrophy found in the temporal lobe of such patients (Tomlinson, Blessed and Roth 1970).

Recent pathological studies on the brains of elderly people provide a basis for classifying the etiology of dementia, which has direct relevence for the interpretation of CBF findings. Tomlinson, Blessed and Roth (1970) have distinguished two types of dementia in old age: (1) primary parenchymal degeneration, designated "senile", and (2) multiple cerebral infarction, designated "arteriosclerotic". Whereas the former is associated with typical Alzheimer changes (senile plaques and neurofibrillary tangles), the latter consists of multiple areas of cerebral softening secondary to ischemic vascular disease. Fifty-eight percent of the 50 elderly patients studied by Tomlinson and co-workers revealed extensive senile plaque formation and/or neurofibrillary tangles. In contrast, only 32 percent showed widespread cerebral softening with a volume exceeding 50 milliliters; a third of these patients also had severe Alzheimer changes. Less marked, but nevertheless significant, instances of one or both types of pathology were found in an additional 12 percent of the cases.

In an extension of the same study, Roth (1971) obtained significant correlations between the magnitude of pathological changes and a quantitative "dementia score". Thus, the severity of the dementia gave a product-moment correlation of 0.77 with the number of senile plaques per low-powered field, and 0.69 with the total amount (in ml) of cerebral softening. Differentiation of the two types of pathology was possible on purely clinical grounds, using the absence or presence of cerebrovascular disease as the principal criterion. Whereas a significant degree of cerebral softening was found in only 7 percent of 29 patients diagnosed senile, it occurred in 73 percent of 22 patients diagnosed arteriosclerotic. Furthermore, cerebral softening (as opposed to number of plaques) accounted for a much greater amount of the variance in dementia score among the latter patients. More sophisticated neuropsychological methods for differentiating the two types of dementia have recently been described (Perez et al. 1975).

The above quoted pathological studies have had considerable impact on the neurological diagnosis of dementia. Contrary to the traditional assumption that "cerebral arteriosclerosis" is the cause of dementia in old age, it is now recognized that cerebral infarction plays a dominant role in only one-third of the cases, with perhaps a few more in which it is a contributing factor. This contrasts with the almost 60 percent of cases where Alzheimer-type pathological changes are a major determinant. The distinction between the two types of dementia has been clearly documented by Fisher (1968) and, more recently, by Hachinski, Lassen and Marshall (1974). These authors emphasize that arteriosclerotic narrowing of blood vessels, per se, is not sufficient to cause dementia, which regularly occurs only in the presence of multiple, widespread small or large infarctions. In order to avoid confusion with the older concept of cerebral arteriosclerosis, Hachinski and co-workers have redesignated the vascular type, "multi-infarct dementia", a term widely used in the literature today. Although lower than previously believed, the incidence of multi-infarct dementia is of sufficient magnitude to justify continued investigation of cerebral ischemia in elderly patients with mental deterioration.

The possibility that cerebral blood flow might distinguish between the two types of dementia was first suggested by O'Brien and Mallett (1970). Using the xenon-133 inhalation technique, they found a significantly greater reduction in CBF among demented patients with clinical evidence of cerebrovascular disease than in patients with dementia of non-vascular origin; in fact, the latter tended to have normal flows. They interpreted the decreased blood flow in the vascular cases as a sign of cerebral ischemia. It was argued that the differentiation is valid only in the early stages of dementia, before massive cell loss produces CBF reductions in both etiologic types.

These findings have recently been confirmed by Hachinski and co-workers (1975), using the xenon-133 intracarotid injection technique and a compartmental analysis that distinguishes between grey and white matter. Dementia was classified clinically as multi-infarct or primary degenerative on the basis of the presence or absence of cerebral ischemia. Both types of dementia showed a reduction in the relative size of the grey matter compartment. However, a significant blood flow reduction was obtained only in the multi-infarct group. This suggested that blood flow was adequate to meet the brain's lesser metabolic needs in the primary degenerative group, but inadequate for those with multi-infarct dementia. Of special interest is the significant correlation between the degree of dementia and CBF in the multi-infarct group, a relationship that was absent in patients of the primary degenerative type.

Differences in CBF between the two types of dementia are paralleled by variations in cerebral metabolic pattern. In a mixed series of 115 patients diagnosed as primary degenerative and multi-infarct dementia, Hoyer and Weinhardt (1976) observed a bimodal distribution of cerebral glucose uptake, comparable to the one obtained for blood flow. Because cerebral metabolic rate for oxygen was more uniformly depressed, the glucose-to-oxygen ratio (G/O) paralleled differences in glucose uptake; i.e., a biomodal distribution was obtained. When the patients were divided into two groups on the basis of their G/O ratio, it was found that those with a high G/O had relatively lower CBFs. Hoyer and Weinhardt interpreted this as evidence for two distinct cerebral metabolic patterns in elderly demented patients. Since an elevated G/O ratio indicates a shift to anaerobic metabolism, which is characteristic of cerebral ischemia, it was speculated that the high G/O group represented cases of multi-infarct dementia. The possibility of differentiating the two pathological types of dementia on the basis of in vivo cerebral metabolic patterns is an intriguing one that clearly deserves further study.

Vascular reactivity to changes in arterial carbon dioxide tension ($PaCO_2$) is another potential means of distinguishing the two types of dementia. The normal response to elevated $PaCO_2$ produced by 5-7 percent CO_2 inhalation is a 30-50 percent increase in CBF due to cerebral vasodilatation. On the other hand, hyperventilation, which reduces $PaCO_2$, results in a corresponding decrease in CBF due to cerebral vasoconstriction. In 1953, Schieve and Wilson reported differences in the CBF response to inhaled CO_2 between patients with clearcut strokes and those with dementia who had no evidence of vascular disease. Whereas the latter group revealed a normal CBF increase, the patients with stroke had significantly smaller responses. Unfortunately, the problem of CO_2 reactivity in dementia has received little further attention, particularly as it relates to differential diagnosis.

Although Simard and co-workers (1971) claim normal CO_2 reactivity in vascular dementia, their evidence is based on a single case subjected to hyperventilation. Dekoninck, Collard and Jacquy (1975) obtained normal CBF responses to both hyperventilation and CO_2 inhalation among relatively healthy old people, and a reduction in reactivity among patients with cerebrovascular disease. A highly variable response was found in patients with dementia, but unfortunately they were not classified according to the presumed etiology. Hachinski and colleagues (1975) carried out systematic observations on hyperventilation in dementia, and found a tendency (not significant) for smaller CBF decreases in patients of the multi-infarct type than in those with primary neuronal degeneration. CO_2 inhalation was not attempted. From this, it would appear that the vasoconstrictor response to hyperventilation does not clearly differentiate the two types of dementia. Whether there is a difference in the vasodilator response to CO_2 inhalation has not, until this time, been satisfactorily tested.

Still another potential means of studying dementia is the hemodynamic response to psychological stimuli. According to Ingvar, Risberg and Schwartz (1975), CBF is normally augmented in cortical association areas during activation by mental tests. Comparable increases in blood flow were not obtained, however, in demented patients with either Alzheimer's disease or normal pressure hydrocephalus. The functional response of regional CBF to psychologoical stimulation is a new area of investigation, which conceivably could contribute to a better understanding of dementia.

In this brief review, emphasis has been placed on the distinction between two types of dementia in old age which, on pathological grounds, are believed to have different etiologies. Not only do these two types of dementia present a different clinical course, but recent evidence suggests that they differ in their cerebral hemodynamic and metabolic patterns. Whether the electrical activity of the brain also differs, remains to be established. Further investigation of these possibilities would seem indicated, particularly since such a differentiation may have therapeutic implications.

REFERENCES

Dekoninck, W. J., Collard, M. and Jacquy, J. Comparative study of cerebral vasoactivity in vascular sclerosis of the brain in elderly men. Stroke, 6:673-677, 1975.

Fisher, C. M. Dementia in cerebral vascular disease. In: Cerebral Vascular Diseases: Sixth Conference. (Eds. J. F. Toole, R. G. Siekert and J. P. Whisnant), Grune & Stratton, New York, pp. 232-236, 1968.

Hachinski, V. C., Iliff, L. D., Zilhka, E., DuBoulay, G. H., McAllister, V. L., Marshall, J., Russell, R. W. R. and Symon, L. Cerebral blood flow in dementia. Arch. Neurol., 32:632-637, 1975.

Hachinski, V. C., Lassen, N. A. and Marshall, J. Multi-infarct dementia: A cause of mental deterioration in the elderly. Lancet, 2:207-210, 1974.

Hoyer, S. and Weinhardt, F. Absence of correlation of age to reduction of cerebral blood flow and metabolism in patients with dementia of the multiple infarct and Alzheimer types. In: Cerebral Vascular Disease: Seventh International Conference. (Eds. J. S. Meyer, H. Lechner and M. Reivich), Georg Thieme, Stuttgart, pp. 84-88, 1976.

Ingvar, D. H. and Gustafson, L.   Regional cerebral blood flow in
    organic dementia with early onset.   Acta Neurol. Scand., 43:42-73,
    1970.

Ingvar, D. H., Risberg, J. and Schwartz, M. S.   Evidence of subnormal
    function of association cortex in presenile dementia.   Neurology,
    25:964-974, 1975.

O'Brien, M. D. and Mallett, B. L.   Cerebral cortex perfusion rates
    in dementia.   J. Neurol. Neurosurg. Psychiat., 33:497-500, 1970.

Obrist, W. D.   Cerebral physiology of the aged: Influence of
    circulatory disorders.   In: Aging and the Brain.   (Ed. C. M.
    Gaitz), Plenum Press, New York, pp. 117-133, 1972.

Obrist, W. D.   Cerebral physiology of the aged: Relation to psycho-
    logical function.   In: Behavior and Brain Electrical Activity.
    (Eds. N. Burch and H. L. Altshuler), Plenum Press, New York,
    pp. 421-430, 1975.

Obrist, W. D., Chivian, E., Cronqvist, S. and Ingvar, D. H.   Regional
    cerebral blood flow in senile and presenile dementia.   Neurology,
    20:315-322, 1970.

Perez, F. I., Rivera, V. M., Meyer, J. S., Gay, J. R. A., Taylor,
    R. L. and Mathew, N. T.   Analysis of intellectual and cognitive
    performance in patients with multi-infarct dementia, vertebro-
    basilar insufficiency with dementia, and Alzheimer's disease.
    J. Neurol. Neurosurg. Psychiat., 38:533-540, 1975.

Roth, M.   Classification and aetiology in mental disorders of old
    age: Some recent developments.   In: Recent Developments in
    Psychogeriatrics.   (Eds. D. W. K. Kay and A. Walk), Headley
    Bros., Ashford, U. K., pp. 1-18, 1971.

Schieve, J. F. and Wilson, W. P.   The influence of age, anesthesia
    and cerebral arteriosclerosis on cerebral vascular activity to
    CO_2.   Amer. J. Med., 15:171-174, 1953.

Simard, D., Olesen, J., Paulson, O. B., Lassen, N. A. and Skinhoj
    Regional cerebral blood flow and its regulation in dementia.
    Brain, 94:273-288, 1971.

Tomlinson, B. E., Blessed, G. and Roth, M.   Observations on the brains
    of demented old people.   J. Neurol. Sci., 11:205-242, 1970.

SENILE DEMENTIA AND DRUG THERAPY

Roland Branconnier and Jonathan O. Cole

Boston State Hospital
591 Morton Street
Boston, MA. 02124

As far as we can tell from the available literature, there
are no specific drug therapies of major clinical benefit in
senile dementia (Prien, 1973). Since the pathology of the condition
has not been elucidated to the point of any specific remediable
biochemical defect, specific therapy of the insulin – diabetes
mellitus type has not been possible.

The best therapeutic results in patients who appear to suffer
from senile dementia are achieved by treating some condition which
is really masquerading as the dementia (Foley, 1972). Physical
conditions – heart failure, pneumonia, metabolic derangements,
space occupying lesions, normal pressure hydrocephalus can all
present as dementia and sometimes the defect in brain function
will clear remarkably when the underlying condition is treated.
Depressed elderly often show memory and cognitive difficulty or
"pseudo-dementia" which clears when the depression is treated by
drugs or electroconvulsive therapy (Grauer and Kral, 1960). Drugs
e.g. alcohol, anticholinergics or L-Dopa can sometimes cause toxic
confusional states in the elderly which clears up when the offending
drug is removed.

Magnesium pemoline (Cylert) was developed as a "specific"
memory drug which increased cell RNA in the brain. This finding
however was shown to be in error (Eisdorfer, 1968). Further
investigation demonstrated that the drug was a CNS stimulant, the
exact mode of action of which is undetermined. The compound is now
marketed for use in children with minimal brain dysfunction and/or
hyperkinetic behavior.

Roumanian procaine (Gerovital H3) has had a reputation, at

271

least in Roumania, for improving memory in senile patients. At
present it seems most likely that this effect, if it exists, is a
result of the drug's mild antidepressant action (Jarvik and Milne,
1975).

There remains for serious study in senile dementia mainly
cerebral vasodilators. The justification for using these drugs in
senile dementia is of course, weak. There is no real evidence that
senile dementia is caused by narrowing of cerebral arteries or
arterioles. It has recently been estimated that only 10% of elderly
patients with memory difficulty, confusion, or disorientation are
suffering from cerebral arteriosclerosis. The vast majority of these
patients have a neurofibrillary degeneration as the primary neuropathology (Obrist, 1972). Even if dementia in the elderly is caused
by arteriosclerosis, it seems unlikely that a vasodilator will be
able to dilate a sclerosed artery.

There is evidence that cerebral blood flow (CBF) is reduced
in senile dementia, but it is generally assumed that this is a
result of cell death, not a cause. The recent paper by Hagberg and
Ingvar (1976) adds to the data in this area by demonstrating that
regional reductions in CBF strongly correlates with the degree and
type of neuropsychological impairment. Nevertheless, the only
animal screening method available in recent years for selecting
drugs for use in senile conditions relates to the identification
of vasodilating drugs.

None of these drugs have dramatic ameliorating effects on the
neuropsychologic symptoms in the elderly. Hydergine, the best
studied of these drugs has repeatedly been shown to be more effective
than placebo in elderly patients. However, its effects become most
evident after three months of therapy. Drug – placebo differences
are less clear at earlier samplings (Roubicek, 1972). To confuse
matters further, the exact criterion measures showing Hydergine –
placebo differences vary markedly from study to study. Mood, ward
adjustment, sociability or memory tests may all show small effects
but the total body of data fails to suggest any clear major key
effect for the drug. Emmenegger, et al. (1968) suggest that Hydergine
may act not as a vasodilator, but may improve the metabolic capacity
of the brain under conditions of anoxic or hypovolemic stress,
acting via the cyclic AMP system and on the cationic pump. This
postulation perhaps may be extended to other vasodilators claimed
to be effective in senile dementia. In that case, "useful treatments" for senile dementia initially tried because they are vasodilators, actually are effective because of their other, presumably
unrelated, pharmacological properties.

Vasodilators in clinical use in the U.S. include, in addition
to Hydergine, Papaverine, Cyclandelate, Isoxsuprine and Nylindrin.

For papaverine, Cyclandelate and Isoxsuprine there are only a limited number of studies in various older patient groups.

Our interest in this area grew out of an opportunity to utilize quantitative computerized EEG analysis to examine drug effects. A pilot cross over study of a long-acting Papaverine preparation (Pavabid) in a single dose of 300 mgs. v.s. placebo in elderly volunteers showed a trend (p<.10) for Papaverine to increase alpha and decrease theta activity in the EEG, changes in a "good" direction (Cole et al., 1975).

We have since developed a recruiting system for mildly to moderately impaired elderly individuals perhaps best described as "symptomatic volunteers". They or their relatives respond to newspaper ads, and after testing to see if they meet study criteria, they volunteer to take drug or placebo for 2-3 months. They are paid a modest amount to reliably ensure their participation in periodic neuropsychological testing. In addition they receive routine physical examinations, electrocardiograms and blood and urine tests of a routine clinical sort e.g. complete blood count, SMA-12. This subject group shows heterogenous pathology on such tests and EEGs. About 80% of all volunteers are clearly impaired in one or more psychological test e.g. Wechsler Memory Scale (WMS), Bender Gestalt (BG) or tests of recent memory like the Peterson and Peterson Test (P&P).

We have now completed 3 prolonged administration studies in elderly symptomatic volunteers comparing: 1. Papaverine (Pavabid), 2. Isoxsuprine (Vasodilan) and 3. Naftidrofuryl (Praxilene) with placebo. The specific criteria measures have been changed from study to study.

Papaverine

Papaverine is an ancient drug, an alkaloid found in opium. It lacks any analgesic morphine-like activity. It has been shown to produce an increase in cerebral blood flow in man when given intravenously in a single dose (Jayne et al., 1952). It has a dopamine-blocking effect at dopaminergic synapses (Ernst, 1962).

Our study involved elderly subjects. They were not specifically prescreened for evidence of neuropsychological defect or EEG abnormality but almost all showed some impairment as rated by psychiatric Clinical Global Impression (CGI). Patients took either 300 mgs. of Papaverine b.i.d. in a long-acting preparation (Pavabid) or placebo for three months.

In this first study we had the psychiatrist rate the degree of

clinical improvement while the patient completed, with or without
our assistance, a mood scale (The Profile of Mood States or POMS)
as a measure of their subjective status. The P&P test of recent
(3-18 second) memory which includes a component of pro-active
inhibition, The Continuous Performance Test (CPT) and the Self
Paced Digit Symbol Test (SPDT) were used to assess cognitive function.
EEGs were collected on magnetic tape and analyzed by computer. The
quantities of delta, theta, alpha and two ranges of beta activity
were calculated.

Analysis of covariance revealed that on the three second version
of this P&P test there was greater impairment with Papaverine compared
to the placebo at three months. Pre-post t-tests carried out
separately for the two treatment groups showed improvement with
Papaverine but not with placebo on the depression and confusion
subscales of the POMS. There was also a significant decrease in
delta-theta activity and an increase in alpha activity in the
quantitative EEG in the Papaverine condition only.

Vasodilan

Forty physically healthy elderly volunteers with either clinical
evidence of organic brain syndrome or an abnormal baseline EEG
(slow-1 or fast-1 according to the Gibbs classification) were randomly
assigned to Isoxsuprine or placebo groups. The drug was given in a
dose of 20 mgs. four times a day. Medications were taken double
blind for three months.

When analysis of covariance was performed on the P&P test,
both medication groups showed improvement in the intermediate (9
second) phase of the test. Additionally, Vasodilan alone showed
a decrease in theta and an increase in alpha on the quantitative EEG.
The POMS, the CGI, the SCL-90, a list of symptoms seen in neurotic
outpatients, the Paced Digit Symbol Test (PDS), the Reaction Time
(RT), the WMS, and the quantified BG test all failed to show
Significant drug or time effects.

Praxilene

This vasodilator is widely used in France for the treatment of
senile states. It increases cerebral ATP by activating succinic
dehydrogenase i.e. by changing enzyme conformation, increasing the
velocity of the reaction and thereby activating the Krebs cycle
(Fontaine et al., 1968). Two controlled studies have shown it to
be superior to placebo in elderly patients with "cerebral incompetence"
or senile dementia (Judge and Urquihart, 1972; Bouvier et al.,
1974).

For our study, 60 symptomatic volunteers were selected who showed impairment on at least two of four neuropsychological tests, the BG, Visual Reaction Time, the WMS or the PDS. They were randomly assigned to placebo or Naftidrofuryl (N), 100 mgs. t.i.d., groups for 90 days. Covariance analyses were again non-significant in terms of clear drug-placebo differences. A composite impairment index derived by adding scores on all tests used, analyzed by a non-parametric Friedman two-way Anova showed a significant difference in degree of improvement in favor of N.

The three second (shortest) portion of the P&P test showed a significant improvement on N but not on placebo, while placebo patients worsened on the 18 second (longest) portion of the test. Reaction time improved significantly on N only. The BG improved both on placebo and drug, presumably a practice effect. The Perceptual Trace, a visual memory task, improved only on N. No difference or significant changes occurred on the CGI, POMS, WMS, Gottschaldt Hidden Figures, tests of spatial orientation, analogies, or the PDS. EEG data from this study has not yet been analyzed.

DISCUSSION

The results obtained from our three vasodilator studies are enticing but not conclusive. We have not seen any marked clinical improvement attributable to the drugs. However, statistically demonstrable changes do occur. Our most sensitive measures, to date, have been the quantitative EEG and the P&P test. These are relevant to the problems of patients with early signs of dementia i.e. poor memory, transient confusion. Attempts to increase the sensitivity of covariance analysis by a prior stratification of our patient population have not been successful in clarifying drug effects. We are left with the impression that these drugs have modest but measurable effects on brain function.

In the absence of more clearly effective drug therapies for senile dementia, we can't tell whether our mildly impaired elderly patients are relatively unresponsive to these drugs or whether the drugs are relatively weak in senile dementia. A previous study of Pavabid carried out in moderately to severely impaired patients on the geriatric wards at Boston State Hospital failed to show any drug-placebo differences. This led us to examine a community-resident elderly group who were both cooperative and testable. Our next step should logically be the study of Hydergine as the most potent of this group of subtly effective drugs.

PSYCHOMETRIC TESTS COMMON TO ALL STUDIES

TESTS	PBO	PAVA	PBO	VASO	PBO	PRAX
CLINICAL GLOBAL IMPRESSION						
Global Improvement	ns	ns	ns	ns	ns	ns
Efficacy Index	ns	ns	ns	ns	ns	ns
PETERSON & PETERSON						
3 second	.025(I)	.10(I)	ns	ns	ns	.01(I)
9 second	.01 (I)	ns	.05(I)	.05(I)	ns	ns
18 second	ns	ns	ns	ns	.05(W)	ns
PROFILE OF MOOD STATES						
Depression	ns	.05(I)	ns	ns	ns	ns
Anger	ns	ns	ns	ns	ns	ns
Vigor	ns	ns	ns	ns	ns	ns
Fatigue	ns	ns	ns	ns	ns	ns
Confusion	ns	.025(I)	ns	ns	ns	ns
Tension	ns	ns	ns	ns	ns	ns
EEG						
delta	ns	.05(I)	ns	ns	data being processed	
theta	ns	ns	ns	.05(I)		
alpha	ns	.05(I)	ns	.05(I)		
beta 1	ns	ns	ns	ns		
beta 2	ns	ns	ns	ns		

ADDITIONAL PSYCHOMETRIC TESTS USED IN VARIOUS STUDIES

TESTS	PBO	PAVA	PBO	VASO	PBO	PRAX
CONTINUOUS PERFORMANCE TEST						
omissions	ns	ns			*	
SELF PACED DIGIT SYMBOL TEST						
corrects	ns	ns			*	
PACED DIGIT SYMBOL TEST						
corrects	*	*	ns	ns	.10(I)	.10(I)
omissions	*	*	ns	ns	ns	ns
SYMPTOM CHECK LIST						
somatization	*		ns	ns	*	*
obsessive - compulsive	*		ns	ns	*	*
interpersonal sensitivity	*		ns	ns	*	*
depression	*		ns	ns	*	*
anxiety	*		ns	ns	*	*
anger	*		ns	ns	*	*
phobic anxiety	*		ns	ns	*	*
paranoid ideation	*		ns	ns	*	*
psychotism	*		ns	ns	*	*
positive symptom total	*		ns	ns	*	*
positive symptom distress index	*		ns	ns	*	*
REACTION TIME	*		ns	ns	ns	.01(I)

TESTS	PBO	PAVA	PBO	VASO	PBO	PRAX
SELF RATING SYMPTOM SCALE						
neurotic feelings	*				ns	ns
somatization	*				ns	ns
cognitive performance	*				ns	ns
depression	*				ns	ns
fear–anxiety	*				ns	ns
WECHSLER MEMORY QUOTIENT	*		ns	ns	ns	ns
BENDER GESTALT TOTAL	*		ns	ns	.01(I)	.10(I)
TACTILE EXTINCTION	*			*	ns	ns
STEREOGNOSIS	*			*	ns	ns
YERKES	*			*	ns	ns
HANDS	*			*	ns	ns
PARALLELOGRAMS	*			*	.10(W)	ns
LOGICAL GRAMMATIC RELATIONSHIPS–SIMPLE	*			*	ns	ns
LOGICAL GRAMMATIC RELATIONSHIPS–COMPLEX	*			*	ns	ns
LOGICAL GRAMMATIC RELATIONSHIPS– ECHOPRAXIC SUPPRESSION	*			*	ns	ns

TESTS	PBO	PAVA	PBO	VASO	PBO	PRAX
ANALOGIES		*		*	ns	ns
GOTTSCHALDT FIGURES		*		*	ns	ns
PERCEPTUAL TRACE		*		*	ns	.01(I)
IMPAIRMENT INDEX		*		*	ns	.01(I)

PBO = placebo
PAVA = Pavabid
VASO = Vasodilan
PRAX = Praxilene
*   = not performed
ns   = not significant
I   = improved
W   = worsened

FRIEDMAN TWO-WAY ANOVA USING CHANGE SCORES

TESTS	PRAX (Xr^2)	p	PBO (Xr^2)	p
Reaction Time	11.90	.01(I)	.75	ns
Digit Symbol Substitution Test	4.86	.10(I)	4.86	.10(I)
Peterson & Peterson				
3 second	9.29	.01(I)	1.27	ns
9 second	2.12	ns	1.18	ns
18 second	.16	ns	6.45	.05(W)
Wechsler Memory Scale – Memory Quotient	3.81	ns	1.53	ns
Bender Gestalt	5.12	.10(I)	13.74	.01(I)
Profile of Mood States				
depression	.33	ns	2.16	ns
anger	4.40	ns	2.12	ns
tension	2.12	ns	1.18	ns
fatigue	3.03	ns	.73	ns
vigor	2.25	ns	1.27	ns
confusion	.23	ns	.23	ns
Yerkes	1.51	ns	3.03	ns
Hands	.75	ns	2.49	ns
Parallelograms	.99	ns	5.29	.01(W)

TESTS	PRAX (Xr^2)	p	PBO (Xr^2)	p
Analogies	2.12	ns	.75	ns
Gottschaldt Figures	1.97	ns	4.31	ns
Perceptual Trace	10.08	.01(I)	1.86	ns
Impairment Index	11.71	.01(I)	1.27	ns
	n=23		n=23	

PRAX = Praxilene
PBO = Placebo
I = improved
W = worsened

REFERENCES

Bouvier, J.B., Passeron, O. and Chapin, M.P. Psychometric study of praxilene. J. Int. Med. Res., 2:59–65, 1974.

Cole, J. O., Branconnier, R.J. and Martin, G.F. Electroencephalogram and behavioral changes associated with papaverine administration in healthy geriatric subjects. J. Am. Geriatric Soc., 23:295–300, 1975.

Eisdorfer, C., Conner, J.F. and Wilkie, F.L. Effects of magnesium pemoline on cognition and behavior. J. Gerontol., 23:283–288, 1968.

Emmenegger, H. and Meier-Ruge, W. The action of hydergine and the brain, A histochemical, circulatory and neurophysiological study. Pharmacology, 1:65–78, 1968.

Ernst, A. M. Experiments with an o-methylated product of dopamine on cats. Acta Physiol. Pharmacol. Neerl., 11:48–53, 1962.

Foley, J. M. Differential diagnosis of the organic mental disorders in the elderly patients. In: Aging and the Brain, (edited by Charles M. Gaitz), pp. 153–161, Plenum Press, New York, 1972.

Fontaine, L., Brand, M., Charbert, J., Szavasi, E. and Bayssat, M. Cerebral pharmacology of a new vasodilatory drug, Naftidrofuryl. Bull. Chem. Ther., 6:463–469, 1968.

Grauer, H. and Kral, V.A. The use of imipramine (tofranil) in psychiatric patients of a geriatric outpatient clinic. Con. Medical Association J., 83:1423–1426, 1960.

Hagberg, B. and Ingvar, D. H. Cognitive reduction in presenile dementia related to regional abnormalities of the cerebral blood flow. Br. J. Psychiatry, 128:209–222, 1976.

Jarvik, L. F. and Milne, J. F. Gerovital-H3: A review of the literature. In: Aging Vol. 2, Genesis and treatment of psychologic disorders in the elderly, (edited by Gershon, S. and Raskin, A.), pp. 203–227, Raven Press, New York, 1975.

Jayne, H. W., Scheinberg, P., Rich, M. and Belle, M. S. The effects of intravenous papaverine hydrochloride on the cerebral circulation. J. Clin. Invest., 31:111–114, 1952.

Judge, T. G. and Urquihart, A. Naftidrofuryl – A double blind crossover study in the elderly. Curr. Med. Res. Opinion, 1:166–172, 1972.

Obrist, W. D. Cerebral physiology of the aged. Influence of
    circulatory disorders. In: Aging and the Brain, (edited by
    Charles M. Gaitz), pp. 117-133, Plenum Press, New York, 1972.

Prien, R. F. Chemotherapy in chronic organic brain syndrome. A
    review of the literature. Psychopharmacology Bulletin, 9:5-20,
    1973.

Roubicek, J., Geiger, C. H. and Abt, K. An ergot alkaloid preparation
    (hydergine) in geriatric therapy. J. Am. Geriatric Soc., 20:
    222-229, 1972.

SENILE AND PRE-SENILE DEMENTIA:

A CLINICAL OVERVIEW

Ira Sherwin and Benjamin Seltzer

Veterans Administration Hospital
Department of Neurology, Harvard Medical School
Bedford, MA
Boston, MA

INTRODUCTION

Age related brain dysfunction, in particular senile dementia explored at this symposium, is one of the country's most serious health problems. This is true not only in terms of the human suffering experienced by patients and their families but also in terms of its enormous social and economic impact.

Senile dementia is very common. Of the patients in state and county mental hospitals over the age of sixty-five, more than half have the diagnosis of senile dementia (Riley and Foner, 1968). Similarly more than 50% of the large number of elderly persons living in nursing homes carry the same diagnosis (Goldfarb, 1962). Undoubtedly there are many more persons with the same problem who remain at home. Thus the statistics on the institutionalized elderly may reflect only the "tip of the iceberg." As the mean age of the American population rises and ever improving medical care allows still more individuals to reach advanced age, senile dementia and related disorders will inevitably become one of the most serious health care problems we face.

Physicians as a group tend to find these patients uninteresting and unattractive. Since senile dementia is generally held to be a hopeless disorder, these patients receive superficial examinations and then are consigned to medical neglect.

Moreover the common use of the term "chronic brain syndrome" in referring to these patients obfuscates the problem and impedes possible progress. This diagnostic catch-all term is also used to refer to a variety of **other** organic mental disorders, and subsumes entities as diverse as Korsakoff's syndrome, post-traumatic encephalopathy, and Huntington's chorea. We recently completed a survey of eighty patients given the diagnosis of Chronic Brain Syndrome (unpublished data). Table I shows the specific diagnostic makeup of this group.

To group all of these patients together into one diagnostic category clearly masks the important differences that exist amongst them. A therapeutic trial conducted on such a vaguely defined and heterogeneous group of patients can only give indeterminate and confusing results. In the same way, any attempt to validate a new diagnostic test in such a diverse collection of disorders may be expected to fail just because of the meaningful differences that in fact exist amongst them. Furthermore, if the results of research efforts are to be compared in a significant way, then, it is essential that there be congruence between the patient groups studied.

TABLE I.

SPECIFIC DISORDERS IN EIGHTY* PATIENTS DIAGNOSED "CHRONIC BRAIN SYNDROME"

Senile dementia	22
"Alcoholic dementia"	15
Korsakoff's syndrome	11
Schizophrenia	10
Post-traumatic encephalopathy	6
Senile dementia supervening upon schizophrenia	3
Aphasia	3
Presenile dementia	2
Post-anoxic encephalopathy	2
Post-infectious encephalopathy	2
Multi-infarct dementia	1
Multiple sclerosis	1
Parkinson's disease	1
Schizophreniform psychosis with temporal lobe epilepsy	1
Affective psychosis	1
Mental retardation	1
Personality disorder	1

*Total is greater than eighty since some patients had two diagnoses.

It should be stressed that these data do not purport to be statistics describing the prevalance and relative frequency of occurrence of these specific disorders. They are presented rather to show that using only conventional diagnostic methods it is possible to fractionate such a markedly heterogenous group. It seems likely that more precise delineation of these clinical syndromes may, in turn, provide further insight into the significance of related biomedical research findings, some of which have been presented at this symposium.

Dementia may be defined as a multi-faceted deterioration of intellect, personality, and behavior resulting from definable disease of the brain. It must be distinguished from mental retardation, in which an individual may never have fully acquired all of these attainments, and from disorders such as the aphasias and Korsakoff's syndrome which result from some highly focal insult to the brain. Dementia may be stable or progressive. Stable dementias are usually the sequel of some clearly defined insult to the brain, for example post-anoxic encephalopathy. Senile dementia and the other entities discussed in this symposium belong to the category of "progressive dementias."

We divide the progressive dementias into two major groups. Primary dementias are those in which the abnormality of the mental state is the major feature of the disease and the etiology is unknown. Secondary dementias are those in which the mental deterioration occurs as part of some other, definable pathological process.

Although numerically much less common than the primary dementias, these latter conditions acquire a special significance because they represent, at the present time, the only potentially treatable forms of dementia. A selected list of the secondary dementias is given in Table II. This table is not intended to present an exhaustive list; rather it is a guide to diagnostic considerations which should be taken before making the diagnosis of a primary dementia.

TABLE II.

SECONDARY DEMENTIAS

1. Chronic CNS infection
    a. General paresis
    b. Tuberculous meningitis
    c. Fungal meningitis
    d. Presumed viral, e.g. Jakob-Creutzfeldt
        disease

2. Trauma: Chronic subdural hematomas

3. Toxic and metabolic
    a. Pernicious anemia; folate deficiency
    b. Hypothyroidism
    c. Bromides and certain industrial toxins

4. Neoplasms
    a. Subfrontal Meningiomas
    b. Slow growing, CSF-obstructing
        intraventricular tumors

5. Specific Neurological Disorders
    a. Multiple Sclerosis
    b. Huntington's Disease
    c. Parkinson's Disease

6. Normal-Pressure Hydrocephalus

7. Vascular Disease

Dementia due to vascular disease is a type of secondary dementia which deserves special mention. Until recently, dementia occurring in the senium was uncritically attributed to atherosclerosis. The diagnosis "cerebral arteriosclerosis" was often used a a synonym for senile dementia. On careful post-mortem examination, however, workers such as Fisher (1968) find the amount of atherosclerosis involving the cerebral vessels bears little, if any, relationship to the degree of clinical dementia. In fact, Tomlinson et al (1970) have shown that these brains are affected by precisely the same pathological changes as those classically described in Alzheimer's presenile dementia. For these reasons many neurologists have come to agree with the position articulated by Katzman and Karasu (1975), that presenile dementia and senile dementia are basically the same disease albeit with onset at different ages.

The clinical similarities between these disorders parallel the pathological similarities. Intellectual deficits in the spheres of memory, language, and constructional ability are hallmarks of both disorders. Personality and behavioral changes are also prominent. In the early stages, these patients are often quiet, apathetic, and withdrawn. They lack spontaneity but remain neat and socially appropriate. These features probably reflect the predominance of early pathological changes in the parietal and temporal lobes. Later, as the frontal lobes are affected, patients become indifferent to social decorum, and, in the final stages, they may be boisterous, hyperactive, and assaultive. It sometimes appears that patients with senile dementia do not deteriorate as markedly as patients with Alzheimer's disease, and unlike the rather sterotyped clinical picture in pre-senile dementia, there may be more variability in the course of senile dementia.

Pick's disease, a rare disorder, and the third member of the triad of primary dementias, may be clinically difficult to distinguish from Alzheimer's disease. Some authors claim that early involvement of the frontal lobes makes a clinical distinction possible (Sjogren, et al, 1952).

An important consideration in the evaluation of patients with dementia is the differential diagnosis with depression. Some patients in the early stages of dementia do experience true subjective depression. On the other hand, the apathetic, withdrawn appearance of a demented patient may closely mimic a depression. The elderly, who are, of course, the primary candidates for dementia, also have a high incidence of depression. Furthermore, some depressed patients are so profoundly dejected that they do badly on the clinical tests usually employed to diagnose dementia. This "pseudodementia" (Kiloh, 1961) may then be mistaken as evidence of degenerative brain disease. To mistake depression for dementia is a very serious diagnostic error. Even in the elderly, depression has a far better prognosis than dementia (Roth, 1955). Careful consideration of the history and future course are usually sufficient to settle the diagnosis on clinical grounds alone. If the situation is uncertain, however, it is preferable to treat the patient as though he were depressed. In this way, a treatable case of depression will not be missed, and a demented patient may receive some temporary, symptomatic relief.

Pathology

Because of the similarities mentioned above, senile dementia and Alzheimer's disease are usually considered together in descriptions of brain pathology and speculations on etiology. On gross examination, the brains of patients suffering from both conditions reveal marked cortical atrophy and, to a lesser degree, ventricular dilatation (Corsellis, 1976a). The gross degenerative changes are particularly prominent in the cortical association areas of the parietal, temporal, and frontal lobes. Primary motor and sensory areas, such as the pre- and post-central gyri and the occipital lobe, tend to be relatively preserved. Microscopic examination reveals neuronal loss and the presence of three unique pathological changes. One of these, the intraneuronal skein of fibers known as the "neurofibrillary tangle," has been studied in great detail by Wisniewski and co-workers (1970). They have found these argentophilic structures to be composed of bundles of paired helical filaments (PHF). The filaments in these helical pairs differ in size and chemical composition from the unpaired filaments normally found in healthy neurones (see Chapter by Iqbal). The quantity of PHF per unit volume of brain appears to correlate with the degree of mental deterioration observed in life (Wisniewski et al, 1976).

The second characteristic neuropathological feature is the senile plaque, consisting of an amyloid core surrounded by degenerating neurites. A third and less dramatic finding, often limited to the hippocampus, is a form of neuronal degenerative change referred to as granulovacuolar degeneration. Although plaques, tangles and granulovacuolar degeneration remain the hallmarks of both senile and presenile dementia, these morphological changes may also be seen, but in lesser numbers, in the brains of elderly individuals without apparent dementia. It must be stressed however that the correlation of the intensity of these changes with the degree of intellectual deterioration (Blessed et al, 1968), is less than perfect.

Morphological changes in the aging brain have also been analyzed at a quite different level. The chapters by Scheibel and Scheibel and Feldman detail how Golgi-stained material from aging brains has demonstrated a selective loss of the dendritic spines of neurones and a shortening of the dendrites. The basal dendrites of the fifth neocortical layer appear to be particularly vulnerable, a finding which might relate to the changes

in association cortex described above (see also Strehler's
Chapter). Brody, in his chapter, and Corsellis (1976b) have
demonstrated an age-related loss of neurones. Interestingly, Corsellis suggests that the loss is greater in the
left than in the right hemisphere (personal communication).

A characteristic feature of the morphological changes
that occur in the brain during maturation and, ultimately,
aging, seems to be that the last structures to appear
developmentally are the first to be affected in the senium.
This "last in, first out" relationship, has given rise to
the notion of a reverse maturation hypothesis. Thus,
the association areas, the last to develop in maturation
seem to bear the brunt of the pathological changes of
aging.

Certain age-related EEG findings (Walter and Dovey,
1947) and epidemiological data concerning epileptic children (Taylor, 1971), both of which reflect changing maturational states, also suggest that the left hemisphere may
lag behind the right during development. These findings,
taken together with those of Corsellis, not only support
this reverse maturational hypothesis but suggest a peculiar vulnerability for the left side of the brain. They
also strongly suggest the importance of genetic factors
in the pathophysiology of presenile and senile dementia.

ETIOLOGY

Several risk factors, predisposing to Alzheimer's
disease and senile dementia, have been suggested. A
genetic factor, mentioned above, is also suggested by the
high incidence of Alzheimer's disease in certain families
and by its marked association with Down's syndrome (Pratt,
1970). Tissue cultures of skin fibroblasts from patients
with Down's syndrome show "premature aging" (Martin et al,
1970). Interestingly, the same study showed a difference
in the rate of cell aging depending upon whether the skin
biopsy was taken from the right or the left side of the
body. In this connection it is noteworthy that the skin
lesions in certain neurocutaneous syndromes, such as
Sturge-Weber disease, always appear ipsilateral to the
pathology in the brain. Taken together, these findings
support the genetic hypothesis of neuronal aging. Moreover,
they increase the plausibility of the left hemisphere
vulnerability argument, which we propose.

At present, how any of these characteristic pathological changes come about is far from clear. Recently,
Wisniewski et al (1975) reported the induction of neuritic

plaques in the brains of mice injected with the causative
agent of scrapie, isolated from sheep or goats. These
studies strongly suggest the possibility of an infectious (viral) and/or immunological causative factor.
A possible immunological basis for Alzheimer's disease
and senile dementia is also in keeping with the loss of
immunological competence that characterizes the aging
process (Makinodan et al, 1971). This notion gains
further support from the findings of Nandy (1973) which
demonstrate an age- related increase in circulating antibrain antibodies in mice. It is noteworthy, that
this finding has been confirmed in man by Ingram et al
(1974). Such an immunological mechanism might, in turn,
depend upon an alteration in the blood brain barrier
(BBB). With the barrier intact, the CNS has been considered an "immunological sanctuary". If, however, the
BBB should be breached, either as a result of some specific aging effect or as a result of brain damage, e.g.
trauma, infarction, etc., such privilege would be abro-
gated. In the former case, a pre-existing circulating
antibody which can react with brain tissue might enter
the brain to produce the changes discussed. In the
second case, brain proteins might escape into the general circulation and provoke antibody formation. These
specific antibrain antibodies, in turn, could recross
the defective BBB and produce the changes previously
outlined. The problem of the BBB and aging is explored
in more detail in the Chapters by Rappaport and Nandy.

   Another animal model (see Chapter by Crapper) suggests a possible role for aluminum and/or cadmium in
producing neurofibrillary degeneration. Wisniewski and
his co-workers (1970) have shown that aluminum salts are
capable of inducing neurofibrillary tangles, consisting
of 100 Å diameter filaments, similar although not identical, to those occurring in the brains of patients dying
from Alzheimer's disease. In their study of brains taken
from such patients Crapper et al (1973) have found high
concentrations of aluminum in those regions showing neurofibrillary degeneration, but not in regions containing
only neuritic plaques. Although provocative and sugges-
tive, all of the possible etiological agents discussed
above require much additional study before a specific
relationship to senile or presenile dementia can be
established. Until then extrapolations from animal
models to man must be interpreted with great caution.

Hemispheric Lateralization

There is a tendency amongst clinicians to consider presenile and senile dementia as diffuse brain disorders. From the foregoing, it should be obvious that such a view is without foundation. As we have seen, the left side of the brain may be selectively vulnerable to neuronal loss, at least in the early stages of aging. Similarly, there may be regional selective vulnerability, e.g. parieto-temporal involvement in Alzheimer's disease. Moreover, in a given region (lobe), the association cortex is selectively vulnerable as compared to primary cortex. We, have also seen that there is a selective vulnerability with respect to the different cortical layers and the neural elements lying within these layers. This principal of selective vulnerability, and the extent to which it is applicable, has important implications for all aspects of research in this field and, in particular, for studies involving the evaluation of diagnostic tests and therapeutic approaches.

To date, neuropsychological tests appear to provide the most sensitive markers of subtle regional brain abnormalities. A variety of neuropsychological tests sensitive to localizable age-related brain dysfunction have been cross correlated with focal changes in the EEG (Obrist et al 1963) and regional reductions in cerebral blood flow (Lassen et al, 1957). It is probable that such reductions in cerebral blood flow (CBF) are the result of neuronal loss rather than the cause of it. Lassen et al (1957) compared the two cerebral hemispheres in normal aged individuals and in patients with "organic dementia". No significant lateralizing difference was found when the normal elderly were studied. In the elderly demented patients, however, blood flow in the left cerebral hemisphere was significantly decreased compared to the right. Using the same blood flow data, Obrist, Lassen and their co-workers (1963) correlated unilateral CBF with EEG slow wave activity (see also Obrist's Chapter). They found the correlations to be consistently higher in the left hemisphere. Feinberg et al (1960) have found certain psychometric test scores in demented patients to be consistently better correlated with left hemispheric oxygen uptake values than with right sided values. Taken together, and viewed in the context of previously mentioned left-right differences, we interpret these data as demonstrating selective age-related deterioration of the left half of the brain. Thus, the aphorism "You're only as old as you feel" might be more aptly restated, "You're only as old as your left hemisphere thinks you feel."

Therapy

To date, the results of therapy in both presenile and senile dementia have been uniformly disappointing. Hyperbaric oxygen, and various drugs, including vasodilators, vitamins and numerous psychotropic agents, have been tried unsuccessfully (for a review see Prien, 1973). Drugs which are possible candidates for clinical trials are discussed in the chapters by Cole and Samorajski. One agent, used primarily in Europe, which appears promising is the plant hormone centrophenoxine. Nandy (1968) has shown that this agent can reduce the amount of age pigment (lipofuscin) accumulated in the neurons of senescent mice. His studies indicate this action may improve learning scores in treated animals (1977).

Until such time when the fundamental mechanisms underlying these disorders are clarified therapeutic intervention is likely to remain a matter of trial and error. For the present, accurate diagnosis and the use of those more or less specific therapies appropriate to the secondary and pseudodementias holds the greatest promise.

REFERENCES

Blessed, G., Tomlinson, B.E., and Roth, M. The association between quantitative measures of dementia and of senile change in the cerebral grey matter of elderly subjects. Brit. J. Psychiat. 114:797-811, 1968.

Corsellis, J.A.N. Ageing and the dementia. In: W. Blackwood, JAN Corsellis (Eds.) Greenfield's Neuropathology, 3rd ed. pp. 796-848, 1976a.

Corsellis, J.A.N. Some observations on the Purkinje cell population and on brain volume in human aging. In: R.D. Terry and S. Gershon (Eds.) Neurobiology Of Aging. Raven Press, N.Y. pp. 205-209, 1976.

Crapper, D.R., Kirshnan, S.S. and Qwlttkat, S. Aluminum neurofibrillary degeneration and Alzheimer's disease. Brain 99:67-69, 1976.

Feinberg, I., Lane, M.H. and Lassen, N.A. Bilateral studies of cerebral oxygen uptake measured on the right and left sides. Nature. 188:962-964, 1960.

Fisher, C.M. Dementia in cerebrovascular disease. In, R.G. Siekert & J.P. Whisnant (Eds.), Cerebral Vascular Disease, Sixth Conference. Grune & Stratton, N.Y. pp. 232-236, 1968.

Goldfarb, A.I. Prevalance of psychiatric disorders in metropolitan old age and nursing homes. J. Amer. Geriat. Soc. 10:77-80, 1962.

Ingram, C.R., Phegan, R.J. and Blumenthal, H.T. Significance of an age-linked neuron-binding gamma globulin fraction of human sera. J. Geront.,29: 20-27, 1974.

Katzman, R. and Karasu, T.B. Differential diagnosis of dementia. In: W.S. Fields (Ed.), Neurological & Sensory Disorders in the Elderly. Stratton, New York, pp. 103-134, 1975.

Kiloh, L.G. Pseudodementia. Acta Psychiat. Scand. 37: 336-351, 1961.

Lassen, N.A., Munck, O., and Tottey, E.R. Mental func-
    tion and cerebral oxygen consumption in organic
    dementia. Arch. Neurol. Psychiat. 77:126-133,
    1957.

Makinodan, R., Perkins, E.H. and Chen, M.G. Immunologic
    activity of the aged. In: B. Strehler (Ed).
    Advances in Gerontological Research, Vol. 2.
    Academic Press, New York, 1971.

Martin, G.M., Curtis, A., Sprague, B.S. and Epstein,
    C.J. Replicative life-span of cultivated human
    cells. Effects of donor's age, tissue, and geno-
    type. Lab Invest. 23:86-90, 1970.

Nandy, K. Further studies on the effects of Centropheno-
    xine on the lipofuscin in neurones of senile guinea
    pigs. J. Geront. 23:82-92, 1968.

Nandy, K. Brain-reactive antibodies in serum of aged
    mice. In: D.H. Ford (Ed.) Neurological-Aspects of
    Maturation and Aging. Elsvier, Amsterdam. pp.
    437-454, 1973.

Nandy, K. and Lal, H. Neuronal lipofuscin and learning
    difficulties in aging mammals. In: Proceedings 10th
    Collegium International Neuro-psychopharmaco-Logicum
    Congress. Pergamon, (in press), 1977.

Obrist, W.D., Sokoloff, L., Lassen, N.A., Lane, M.D.,
    Butler, R.N. and Feinberg, I. Relation of EEG to
    cerebral blood flow and metabolism in old age.
    Electroencephalogr. Clin. Neurophysiol. 15:610-619,
    1963.

Pratt, R.T.C. The Genetics of Alzheimer's Disease. In:
    GEW Wolstenholme and M. O'Connor (Eds.) Alzheimer's
    Disease and Related Conditions. London, Churchill,
    pp.137-143, 1970.

Prien, R.F. Chemotherapy in chronic organic brain syn-
    drome. A review of literature. Psychopharmacology
    Bulletin 9:5-20, 1973.

Riley, M.W. and Foner, A. Aging and Society Russell
    Sage Foundation, New York, 1968.

Roth, M. The natural history of mental disorder in old
     age. J. Ment. Sci., 101:281-301, 1955.

Sjogren, T., Sjogren, H., and Lindgren, A.G.H. Morbus
     Alzheimer & Morbus Pick: a genetic, clinical, and
     pathological study. Acta. Psychiatr. Scand. 82:1-152,
     1952.

Taylor, D.C. Ontogenesis of chronic epileptic psychoses:
     A reanalysis., Psychol. Med. 1:247-253, 1971.

Tomlinson, B.E., Blessed, G. and Roth, M. Observations
     on the brains of demented old people. J. Neurol.
     Sci., 11:205-242, 1970.

Walter, G.W. and Dovey, V.J. Clinical and EEG studies
     of temporal lobe function. Proc. Roy. Soc. Med.
     42: 891-904, 1947.

Wisniewski, H.M., Bruce, M.E. and Fraser, H. Infectious
     etiology of neuritic (senile) plaques in mice.
     Science 190:1108-1110, 1975.

Wisniewski, H.M., Narang, H.K., Corsellis, J.A.N. and
     Terry, R.D. Ultrastructural studies of the neuropil
     and neurofibrillary tangles in Alzheimer's disease
     and post-traumatic dementia. J. Neuropath., Exper.
     Neurol. 35:367, 1976.

Wisniewski, H.M., Terry, R.D., and Hirano, A. Neuro-
     fibrillary pathology, J. Neuropath., Exper. Neurol.
     29:163-176, 1970.

CONTRIBUTORS

Donald Armstrong, Ph.D.
   Assistant Professor, Department of Neurology, University of
   Colorado School of Medicine, Denver, Colorado

Mark P. Bear
   Geriatric Research, Educational and Clinical Center, Veterans
   Administration Hospital, Bedford, Massachusetts

Roland J. Branconnier
   Research Director, Geriatric Psychopharmacology, Boston State
   Hospital, Boston, Massachusetts

Harold Brody, M.D., Ph.D.
   Professor and Chairman, Department of Anatomical Sciences,
   State University of New York, Buffalo, New York

Virgil R. Carlson, Ph.D.
   Laboratory of Psychology, National Institute of Mental Health,
   National Institutes of Health, Bethesda, Maryland

Jonathan Cole, M.D.
   Chief, Psychopharmacology Program, Alcohol and Drug Abuse Research
   Center, McLean Hospital, Belmont, Massachusetts; Director of
   Clinical Research, Boston State Hospital, Boston, Massachusetts

Donald R. Crapper, M.D.
   Professor of Physiology, University of Toronto, Toronto, Ontario,
   Canada

Umberto De Boni, Ph.D.
   Ontario Mental Health Foundation Research Fellow, Department of
   Physiology, Medical Sciences Building, University of Toronto,
   Toronto, Ontario, Canada

Irwin Feinberg, M.D.
   Chief, Psychiatry Service, Veterans Administration Hospital,
   and Professor, Department of Psychiatry, University of California,
   San Francisco, California

Martin L. Feldman, Ph.D.
     Assistant Professor of Anatomy, Boston University Medical
     Center, Boston, Massachusetts

Paul A. L. Haber, M. D.
     Assistant Chief Medical Director for Professional Services,
     Department of Medicine and Surgery, Veterans Administration,
     Washington, D. C.; Assistant Clinical Professor of Medicine,
     George Washington University School of Medicine, Washington,
     D. C.

Satoshi Hibi, M.A.
     Psychiatry Service, Veterans Administration Hospital, San
     Francisco, California

Inge Grundke-Iqbal, Ph.D.
     Assistant Professor of Pathology, Albert Einstein College of
     Medicine, The Bronx, New York

Khalid Iqbal, Ph.D.
     Assistant Professor of Pathology, Albert Einstein College of
     Medicine, The Bronx, New York

Nils Koppang, V.M.D.
     Professor of Pathology, Norwegian Veterinary Institute, Oslo,
     Norway

Jans Muller, M.D.
     Professor of Pathology (Neuropathology), Indiana University
     School of Medicine, Indianapolis, Indiana

Kalidas Nandy, M.D., Ph.D.
     Associate Director, Geriatric Research, Educational and Clinical
     Center, Veterans Administration Hospital, Bedford, Massachusetts;
     Research Professor of Anatomy, Boston University School of
     Medicine, Boston, Massachusetts

Walter Obrist, M.D.
     Research Professor of Neurosurgery and Neurology, University of
     Pennsylvania, Philadelphia, Pennsylvania

Stanley I. Rapoport, M.D.
     National Institute of Mental Health, Laboratory of Neurophysiology,
     National Institutes of Health, Bethesda, Maryland

Suzanne G. Rehnberg
     Geriatric Research, Educational and Clinical Center, Veterans
     Administration Hospital, Bedford, Massachusetts

Carolyn Rolsten, M.S.
  Research Associate, Texas Research Institute of Mental Sciences,
  Houston, Texas

Thaddeus Sammorajski, Ph.D.
  Chief, Biological Section, Texas Research Institute of Mental
  Sciences, Houston, Texas

Arnold B. Scheibel, M.D.
  Professor of Psychiatry and Anatomy, University of California
  at Los Angeles, School of Medicine, Los Angeles, California

Madge E. Scheibel, M.D.
  Professor of Psychiatry and Anatomy, University of California
  at Los Angeles, School of Medicine, Los Angeles, California

F. Howard Schneider, Ph.D.
  Research Pharmacologist, Geriatric Research, Educational and
  Clinical Center, Veterans Administration Hospital, Bedford,
  Massachusetts; Associate Professor of Pharmacology, University
  of Massachusetts Medical Center, Worcester, Massachusetts

Dennis J. Selkoe, M.D.
  Instructor of Neurology, Harvard Medical School, and Research
  Associate in Neuroscience, Childrens' Hospital Medical Center,
  Boston, Massachusetts

Benjamin Seltzer, M.D.
  Clinical Investigator, Geriatric Research, Educational and
  Clinical Center, Veterans Administration Hospital, Bedford,
  Massachusetts; Instructor of Neurology, Harvard Medical School,
  Boston, Massachusetts

Michael L. Shelanski, M.D., Ph.D.
  Associate Professor of Neuropathology, Harvard Medical School,
  and Senior Research Associate, Childrens' Hospital Medical
  Center, Boston, Massachusetts

Ira Sherwin, M.D.
  Associate Chief of Staff for Research and Development, Veterans
  Administration Hospital, Bedford, Massachusetts; Assistant
  Professor of Neurology, Harvard Medical School, Boston,
  Massachusetts

Aristotle N. Siakotos, Ph.D.
  Associate Professor of Pathology, Indiana University Medical
  Center, Indianapolis, Indiana

F. Marott Sinex, Ph.D.
Professor and Chairman, Department of Biochemistry, Boston
University School of Medicine, Boston, Massachusetts

Bernard L. Strehler, Ph.D.
Professor of Biological Sciences, University of Southern
California, Los Angeles, California

Albert Sun, Ph.D.
Research Professor of Biochemistry, Sinclair Comparative
Research Farm, University of Missouri, Columbia, Missouri

Robert D. Terry, M.D.
Professor and Chairman, Department of Pathology, Albert
Einstein College of Medicine, The Bronx, New York

N. Vijayashankar, M.D.
Assistant Professor of Anatomy, State University of New York,
Buffalo, New York

Henryk M. Wisniewski, M.D., Ph.D.
Director, New York State Institute for Basic Research in
Mental Retardation, Staten Island, New York

INDEX